HOW TO NURSE:

Relational Inquiry with Individuals and Families in Changing Health and Health Care Contexts

Gweneth Hartrick Doane, RN, PhD
Professor, School of Nursing
University of Victoria
Victoria, British Columbia

Colleen Varcoe, RN, PhD
Professor, School of Nursing
University of British Columbia
Vancouver, British Columbia

Wolters Kluwer | Lippincott Williams & Wilkins
Health

Philadelphia · Baltimore · New York · London
Buenos Aires · Hong Kong · Sydney · Tokyo

Acquisitions Editor: Patrick Barbera
Product Development Editor: Staci Wolfson
Production Project Manager: Marian Bellus
Senior Marketing Manager: Nicky Dunlap
Designer: Holly McLaughlin
Developmental Editor: Laura Bonazzoli
Art Director: Jennifer Clements
Compositor: Absolute Service, Inc.
Printer: R. R. Donnelley

351 West Camden Street   Two Commerce Square
Baltimore, MD 21201   Philadelphia, PA 19103

Printed in China

9781451190267
Library of Congress Cataloging-in-Publication Data
available upon request

DISCLAIMER
Care has been taken to confirm the accuracy of the information present and to describe generally accepted practices. However, the authors, editors, and publisher are not responsible for errors or omissions or for any consequences from application of the information in this book and make no warranty, expressed or implied, with respect to the currency, completeness, or accuracy of the contents of the publication. Application of this information in a particular situation remains the professional responsibility of the practitioner; the clinical treatments described and recommended may not be considered absolute and universal recommendations.

To purchase additional copies of this book, call our customer service department at (800) 638-3030 or fax orders to (301) 223-2320. International customers should call (301) 223-2300.

Visit Lippincott Williams & Wilkins on the Internet: http://www.lww.com. Lippincott Williams & Wilkins customer service representatives are available from 8:30 am to 6:00 pm, EST.

To all of those nurses and those *becoming* nurses who, on a daily basis, strive to make compassionate, socially just nursing care a reality—may you never lose touch with the relational possibilities that exist in each moment. And if you ever feel alone and adrift when in the hard spots of nursing, please know that we are with you in "optimistic" spirit, compassionately and confidently cheering you on.

Reviewers

Verna Pangman, MEd, MN, RN
Senior Instructor
Faculty of Nursing
University of Manitoba
Winnipeg, Manitoba, Canada

Donna Romyn, PhD, MN, BScN
*Acting Associate Vice President Research/
 Associate Professor*
Research Centre
Athabasca University
Athabasca, Alberta, Canada

Joan Martin Saarinen, MN, BSN
RN Professor of Nursing
Northern College
South Porcupine, Ontario, Canada

Wilma Schroeder, MMFT BN RN
Nursing Faculty
Red River College
Winnipeg, Manitoba, Canada

Karen Silvester, MN, BSN, RN
Nursing Faculty, BSN Program
North Island College
Courtenay , British Columbia, Canada

Holly Symonds-Brown, MSN, BNSc
Faculty Instructor
Bachelor of Science Program
MacEwan University
Edmonton, Alberta, Canada

Elsie Tan, MSN, RN
Senior Instructor
School of Nursing
University of British Columbia
Vancouver, British Columbia, Canada

Landa Terblanche, PhD, RN
Associate Professor
School of Nursing
Trinity Western University
Langley, British Columbia, Canada

Karyn Unrau, MN, RN
Nurse Educator
Aurora College, Yellowknife Campus
Yellowknife, Northwest Territories,
 Canada

Stephen VanSlyke, MN, RN
Senior Teaching Associate
Faculty of Nursing
University of New Brunswick
Fredericton, New Brunswick, Canada

Nicola Waters, PhD(c), MSc, RN
Assistant Professor
School of Nursing
Mount Royal University
Calgary, Alberta, Canada

Acknowledgments

In acknowledgment . . .

While we have always believed that ideas cannot be owned by individuals—that as living phenomena, ideas, and understandings arise and are "known" in and through relational spaces—writing a book makes us realize to what extent our ideas have been shaped and influenced by others. Thus, we wish to acknowledge the countless others who have contributed to the ideas we offer in this book. While it is impossible to individually name all of them, we would like to offer a heartfelt thanks.

To our colleagues Dr. Janet Storch, Dr. Paddy Rodney, and Dr. Rosalie Starzomski, who initially brought us together in a research ethics team and who recognized the common ground of our shared passions. We continue to draw on our learning from that work together.

To all of the people with whom we have worked on the many research teams spanning a range of topic areas—relational practice, violence, public health nursing, primary health care, family health, women's health, palliative and end-of-life care, nursing education, professional development, and so forth. Those experiences and the wisdom gained from the patients, staff in the various health care settings, all our co-investigators, and research staff are threaded throughout the pages of this book.

To the students and the nurses with whom we have worked who have both inspired and challenged us and who, through their honest willingness to be uncertain, continue to teach us about relational inquiry.

To all of the people who graciously allowed us to include their stories or art as illustrations—students, colleagues, friends, relatives (named or not named in this book according to your preference)—your experiences and words not only enriched our understanding but also helped us bring the ideas to life.

To our teaching colleagues with whom we have shared the joys and challenges of working the edges of knowledge and reimagined possibilities for nursing education.

To Ms. Kelly Gray, a doctoral candidate at the University of British Columbia School of Nursing, for her excellent assistance with supporting literature and to Ms. Karen Mahoney for her expertise in nephrology nursing and for her careful review of Dana and Helene's case study.

To Jessica Peart, Corey Atwell, Sarah Wolfson, Ananda Clotier, Kayla Brolie, and Katie Mayer, who at the time were undergraduate nursing students, for their detailed and thoughtful reviews of early chapters.

To our supporters at Lippincott Williams & Wilkins: Christina Burns, for your enthusiastic belief in our ideas and your support in making this book a reality; Staci Wolfson, for your patience as we worked out the flow and reordered everything "just one more time"; and to Laura Bonazzoli, for seeing what we were doing even during the muddled times and cheering us on by stringently editing our work. Finally, we would like to acknowledge our multiple teachers who we are not able to reference in an academic way. In particular, indigenous scholars and colleagues have greatly influenced and enriched our understanding of relationality, for which we are grateful. All my relations.

To the funding agents who have offered generous support for the multiple studies we have drawn upon to inform this book, including the Associated Medical Services, the Social Sciences and Humanities Research Council (SSHRC), the Canadian Institutes of Health Research (CIHR), the Institute of Aboriginal People's Health, the Institute of Gender and Health, the Michael Smith Foundation for Health Research, and the Institute of Population and Public Health.

About the Authors

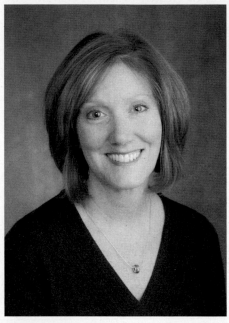

Gweneth Hartrick Doane, RN, PhD
Professor, School of Nursing
University of Victoria
Victoria, British Columbia

Gweneth brings an interdisciplinary practice background as a nurse and psychologist. Her clinical work in nursing has included neonatal and adult intensive care, emergency, psychiatry, and community. Her scholarly work and research has focused on relational inquiry in nursing practice, family nursing, ethics, knowledge translation in clinical nursing settings, and, most recently, a palliative approach in acute and long-term care settings. She has published papers in each of those areas, has taught and developed curricula across a wide range of face-to-face and online courses, and has extensive administrative and faculty development experience. Gweneth has won several teaching awards, including the highest award for university teaching in Canada, the 3M Teaching Fellowship, and The Canadian Schools of Nursing Teaching Excellence Award.

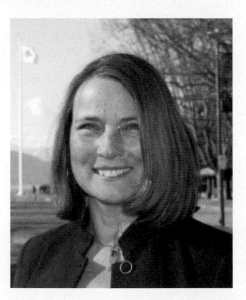

Colleen Varcoe, RN, PhD
Professor, School of Nursing
University of British Columbia
Vancouver, British Columbia

Colleen had the great privilege and experience of being a hospital-trained nurse before completing an undergraduate degree in nursing and graduate degrees in education and nursing. Her clinical practice has been in critical care and emergency nursing with more recent shifts to women's health and primary health care. Her research focuses on all forms of violence and inequity, including interpersonal violence and structural forms of violence such as racism and poverty. Colleen has worked with other nurse educators to enhance teaching toward cultural safety. She has won awards for both her research and teaching.

Preface

PREFACE TO TEACHERS

Thank you for picking up this book—we want to invite you to join us in making this book useful to nursing students at a wide range of places in their learning. For that reason, we thought it might be helpful if we highlighted and/or explained a few things about this book—what inspired it and how we have approached the presentation of the ideas and strategies offered within this book.

The Background Context

Preparing nurses to meet the demands of contemporary health care contexts poses an enormous challenge for nurse educators today. As Diekelmann, Ironside, and Gunn (2005) contend, covering and delivering the overwhelming amount of available content while ensuring that students have the opportunity to integrate that content into practice has become virtually impossible. At the same time, Duchscher and Myrick (2008) have described how the interrelated forces and normative patterns that exist in most North American health care settings often serve to transform creative, vibrant nurses into disillusioned, exhausted practitioners. "New graduates who work in the hospital setting consistently express frustration and a sense of demoralization as a direct result of the dissonance they experience between their perception of nursing and what they find nursing to 'really' be" (Duchscher & Myrick, 2008, p. 196). These authors describe the emotional distress that builds over time when nurses are unable to provide the kind of care they have been educated to provide. This distress includes frustration and resentment directed at themselves for failing to provide the quality of care they believed they should be providing, at their managers who the nurses' perceived as putting them in such compromising positions, and at educators who did not prepare them for the nursing "realities" they faced.

As educators/researchers, we have witnessed this disillusionment first-hand. We have watched deeply committed nurses feel disempowered and bereft in their practice as they try to provide high-quality care to patients/families. We ourselves have also felt despair—questioning the implications of this current nursing reality for nursing education and what we are and are not doing in response. We have brought the question *How can we better prepare nurses to navigate the complexities of contemporary health care settings and confidently, competently enact and meet their nursing obligations?* to our conversations with each other, our educator colleagues, colleagues from our various research teams (including point-of-care practitioners and nursing practice leaders), and, importantly, to our conversations with students. Those conversations and experiences have informed and inspired this book.

We believe that the complexities of contemporary nursing have moved us beyond the point of being able to offer any certainties or prescriptions for practice. Thus, while in this book we outline knowledge and strategies and a process that we believe has the potential to support nurses in their practice (what we call relational inquiry), *how to nurse* needs to be a question brought to each new situation. In outlining relational inquiry, we offer a process that provides *a way* of orienting, focusing, checking in with nursing values and commitments, enlisting knowledge, discerning action, and moving forward, especially in the face of uncertainty. Importantly, we are *not* proposing that relational inquiry be taken up as a defined method for nursing practice but rather as a strategic way for nurses to effectively navigate within the complexities of contemporary health care and determine "best practice" in particular situations. *Relational inquiry is a way of proceeding*—a way in which nurses might be, move, and relate within their work to address their nursing concerns (Hartrick Doane, in press).

The Focus of This Book

The discussion in this book begins and is oriented toward the question of *how* to nurse within the complexities and realities of contemporary nursing practice. Having taught undergraduate students entering the profession, post-RN diploma students studying at the baccalaureate degree level, and graduate students in master's and doctoral programs, we have come to believe that a relational inquiry process in both nursing practice and nursing education can be helpful in directly responding to the complex nature of nursing in contemporary health care. Illustrating how relational inquiry can provide structures and processes to inform the translation of nursing values, knowledge, skills, ideals, and imperatives into effective action, we take a pragmatic approach to knowledge and knowledge development. *We suggest that the way to foster knowledgeable and competent nursing practice is to develop a more conscious, intentional, and responsive way of living knowledge.* To that end, we draw upon a broad range of knowledge (empirical, ethical, sociopolitical, and aesthetic), employing and explicitly showing the relationship between those differing forms and ways of knowing. We illustrate how nursing theories from the human science tradition, critical and experiential theories, contemporary ethical theories, biomedical knowledge, and research evidence work in concert to inform nursing action. *Our goal is to help readers engage in a thoughtful process of inquiry to more intentionally and consciously develop their knowledge and nursing practice, develop their confidence and ability to act in alignment with their nursing values, and to navigate the complexities of contemporary health care settings as they care for patients and families.* Throughout our discussion, we assume that both expert knowledge and local differences are of fundamental importance in nursing practice. Students need to develop a strong nursing standpoint and, at the same time, the confidence and ability to focus their attention and their knowledge very specifically—to discern their nursing obligations and act on those obligations in specific nursing situations and know *how* to draw upon different forms of knowledge to inform their actions.

Who Might Use This Book?

We envision this text as an undergraduate, graduate, and continuing education–level nursing text. The conversational style and concrete examples are intended to make complex ideas accessible for undergraduate students and practicing nurses and at the same time invite in-depth explorations by graduate-level students. It is important to be clear that we believe there is no theory or concept that is too difficult for a first-year nursing student to grasp. In our experience, students of all levels have the capacity to engage with complex material if it is presented in a meaningful way and if teachers provide the needed support to help students make meaning of the concepts. Toward that end, we have attempted to present the ideas in such a way that allows readers of all levels to make meaning of them and to be able to link them to their everyday nursing experiences. Pedagogical strategies we have used to help us do so include introducing the concepts and then building and further elaborating those concepts gradually throughout this book. This strategy has implications for the way that you, as a teacher, use this book. Because concepts are built upon throughout the book, this book makes most sense when read from the beginning. That is, a chapter later in the book assumes students have the knowledge from earlier chapters and will build upon those earlier ideas, examples, and learning activities. Thus, we suggest using this book by assigning each chapter in sequence.

Within What Courses Might You Use This Book?

We see this book as a "fundamentals" text—one that can be used across courses and throughout a curriculum. The ideas are ones that, when looked at from different vantage points, can reveal and inspire new and ongoing learning. We ourselves find that the ideas are continually teaching us and showing new connections and implications for our understandings and actions as nurses/educators/researchers. In addition, many students, nurses, and nurse educators have affirmed that revisiting ideas from different vantage points and across time enables them to make meaning of the ideas and strategies in more in-depth ways. It also enables them to make connections *between* different content areas they may have studied—for example, to see the connections between nursing ethics, cultural safety, biomedical treatment, and nursing theory within a particular context of care.

I. Clinical Courses:

This book can serve as a valuable resource for clinical courses. Clinical courses and practicums, which make up a large portion of nursing curricula, are often undertaken atheoretically. That is, while clinical experiences are intended to support a praxis process and an opportunity for students to translate classroom learning into clinical practice, students and educators tell us (and we ourselves have observed) that this does not always happen. As Dall'Alba and Barnacle (2007) have pointed out, the relevance of classroom knowledge is implied and assumed rather than explicitly addressed or linked. Thus, the task of integrating knowledge into practice often falls to the students who may be more or less able to see those connections. We have written this book for the explicit purpose of creating a bridge between conceptual/theoretical courses and the "how to" of nursing action in clinical courses (or said another way—to address the supposed theory–practice gap). With clinical translation in mind, the learning activities have intentionally been created for students to use in their practice settings. The strategies and checkpoints we provide offer specific conceptual areas and translation techniques to link conceptual ideas and clinical action. We further outline the use of this book in clinical courses and offer concrete learning activities in the ancillary teaching package that accompanies this book.

II. Classroom Courses that This Book Could Serve as a Textbook for Include:

- Communication and relational practice courses
- Knowledge development courses
- Nursing inquiry and theory courses
- Cross-cultural, transcultural, and culture and health nursing courses
- Family nursing courses
- Professional issues courses

We suggest using this book in its entirety in at least one course and then revisiting sections and/or ideas in subsequent courses to support further translation and integration of the ideas and strategies across conceptual and practice domains.

RECURRING FEATURES

In order to support the understanding and translation of complex concepts, we have included some recurring features in each chapter.

Learning Objectives

Each chapter begins with identified learning objectives. These learning objectives align with each of the main sections of the chapter.

To Illustrate

This feature focuses on illustrating particular ideas and/or some larger and more general arguments. So, for example, we focus upon the media as an example of how ideas are shaped by broader contexts. We also include a number of real stories from patients and families, former students, practicing nurses, clinical nurse specialists, and ourselves to bring the ideas in the text to life. Often, we return to the story in the chapter in which it is presented and in subsequent chapters.

Try It Out

"Try it Out" features are learning activities that feature a range of ways of engaging with the content in the chapter. Typically, we have three or four per chapter. These learning activities can be incorporated into activities in classrooms, clinical settings, online, or other teaching–learning settings.

Text Boxes

Many of the chapters include text boxes to summarize and highlight some of the key relational inquiry ideas and/or strategies.

Figures and Visual Images

We have included figures that depict the relationship between ideas as well as visual images (e.g., photos) that symbolize or depict the ideas about which we are writing. These images are focused on stimulating critical thinking through visual means as well as through written text.

This Week in Practice

Each chapter has a learning activity at the end of the chapter that integrates the ideas presented in the chapter and draws upon readers' past or current practice experiences. These activities provide opportunities for the students to practice translating the chapter ideas into their clinical practice.

An Example

This feature presents a story that illustrates a point being made in the text. Often, we return to the story in the chapter in which it is presented and in subsequent chapters.

Relational Inquiry Toolbox

Each chapter describes tools (in the form of knowledge, strategies, inquiry frameworks, and checkpoints) students can enlist in everyday nursing practice. At the end of Chapters 2–11 we identify tools to add to the toolbox.

USING THIS BOOK AS A TEACHER

While we have written this book for the individual reader, we hope that individuals will learn together with colleagues or classmates. To that end, our "Try It Out" activities and suggestions for "This Week in Practice" often incorporate ideas for working together with the hope that teachers will expand these creatively. We expand on these and offer further suggestions in the ancillary materials that go with this book on thePoint. We have also incorporated art into each chapter with the intention that teachers might use the art to create learning activities.

REFERENCES

Dall'Alba, G., & Barnacle, R. (2007). An ontological turn for higher education. *Studies in Higher Education, 32*(6), 679–691.

Diekelmann, N., Ironside, P., & Gunn, J. (2005). Recalling the curriculum revolution: Innovation with research. *Nursing Education Perspectives, 26*(2), 70–77.

Duchscher, J., & Myrick, F. (2008). The prevailing winds of oppression: Understanding the new graduate experience in acute care. *Nursing Forum, 43*(4), 191–206.

Hartrick Doane, G. A. (in press). Cultivating relational consciousness in social justice practice. In P. Kagan, M. Smith, & P. Chinn (Eds.), *Philosophies and practices of emancipatory nursing: Social justice as praxis*. New York: Routledge.

A NOTE OF THANKS

We appreciate that your use of this book will determine its relevance and so we thank you for joining us in this work.

Foreword

RELATIONAL INQUIRY BY GWENETH DOANE AND COLLEEN VARCOE

Let me start with a brief biographical story, pieces of which kept entering my consciousness as I read this wonderful text. My story may be unusual in that I have encountered many circumstances that cause me to have a particular affinity for the concepts in this book. But I am reminded that, despite so many circumstances that tend to detract us from our own mission and purposes, nurses worldwide somehow come to share the fundamental values and ideals expressed in this book. I believe that my story illustrates some of the contextual circumstances that sustain these central values regardless of forces that pull us in other directions.

When I was an undergraduate nursing student at the University of Hawaii in the early 1960s, our curriculum was modeled after that of UCLA, which was based on Dorothy Johnson's Behavioral Systems model. At the time, baccalaureate education was still rare, and master's programs were even rarer. Most of the theoretical frameworks and models we know of today had yet to be created, so having an introduction to nursing based on a theoretical model was a gift that I only came to recognize many years later. At the heart of this curriculum was the concept of "integrating" psychiatric nursing concepts into every course in the curriculum. The intent of this integration was to teach us, to socialize us, to value and create meaningful relationships with those for whom we provided nursing care. Unbeknownst to me, I embarked on a lifelong nursing career that centered around relationships.

By the time I entered a master's program later in the decade, a number of nurses from all areas of the United States had begun to recognize a mutual interest in developing formal expressions of nursing knowledge. The University of Kansas sponsored a series of nursing theory conferences (Norris, 1969), and articles began to appear in nursing journals that set forth theoretical ideas about nursing (Dickoff & James, 1968, 1971; Dickoff, James, & Wiedenbach, 1968; Ellis, 1968, 1969; Folta, 1971; Walker, 1971).

In my master's program, I pursued a child health clinical focus. There were two important contextual circumstances surrounding my master's experience. First, the program was conceptualized deliberately to focus on child health (instead of pediatrics) and offered a strong orientation to the child's family as the focus of care, as well as an emphasis on health in the context of child and family development and promotion and maintenance of health.

Second, even though my master's education coincided with the emergence of the nurse practitioner movement, my own program remained relatively untouched by the medical model that eventually began to dominate advanced practice education. The relationships that surrounded a child as a member of a family were recognized as essential to the child's health and well-being, and application of theory related to child health and family development was the focus of our advanced nursing practice. Our mission was to promote the health and well-being of children in the context of their families. Partly as an outcome of my master's education, I authored a child health textbook that some remember to this day, entitled *Child Health Maintenance: Concepts in Family-Centered Care* (1974).

My doctoral program in Educational Psychology offered the option to focus on development of theory and research methods. At the time, there were only six nursing doctoral programs in the United States, so the best option for me was to pursue doctoral education in a department willing to support a collaboration with the nursing program. As an outcome of that background, in the late 1970s/early 1980s, Maeona Kramer and I embarked on writing a book (Chinn & Kramer, 1983) that focused on theory development, later emerging as a broader text focusing on knowledge development related to the fundamental patterns of knowing described by Barbara Carper (1978).

Carper's work came at a time when many in the academic world of nursing were striving to earn respect in academic circles based on their achievements using empirical scientific methods. But many also recognized the inadequacy of empirical methods alone to address pressing needs of people and families from a nursing standpoint. Carper's explanation of the fundamental patterns of nursing was received with a huge "ah-ha" for many—her description put into language the broad, encompassing aspects of human experience that we knew to be at the heart of nursing.

I began to focus my own scholarly work on the conceptualization and development of aesthetic knowing and the art of nursing. Over and over in my conversations with nurses exploring their notion of the art of nursing, I heard phrases like "It is the relationship" and "It is the connection" (Chinn, 1994, 2001). Through this work, I began to recognize elements of the artistry of nursing, including the artistry involved in grasping the meaning of a situation in its entirety and using skilled action to move the situation from what is to what it can become.

In the seventh edition of our text (Chinn & Kramer, 2007), we introduced our conceptualization of emancipatory knowing. By this time, there had emerged a worldwide host of nurses who recognized the significance of social and political aspects of nursing, health and well-being, and the role that these social dynamics play in creating systems of injustice, inequality, and disparity in people's experiences of health and illness. Even though I had not initially recognized the connection, my work using the concepts of peace and power (Chinn, 2013a, 2013b) as a form of group process had been a sort of "fieldwork" for the conceptualization of emancipatory knowing.

Fast-forward to the present and the publication of this book. When the authors of this book asked me to write the foreword for the book, I was delighted, but I had no idea that reading it would not just be a "read" but instead an experience. Yes, the book resonates with many aspects of my own background and experience, but it represents a major achievement that parallels the importance of Carper's work years ago. The processes of "relational inquiry" presented here are of nursing that I believe many have sensed, some have attempted to teach, and that many nurses still hold as an image of what their practice could be. As students in my classes have consistently stated over the years, nursing is characterized by fundamental complexity, covering a vast realm of human experience. But they struggle to articulate more specifically what this means in terms of explaining and defining nursing.

The concept of relational inquiry and the detailed chapters that build on this concept in this book resonate with what I know of nursing and with what I hear students attempting to express. We already "know" these ideas, but at the same time we do not have a language, a mental image, or a framework that structures our understanding of these complex ideas. This book provides that language and structure that nursing needs.

However, this is not a mundane "read" of conceptual and theoretical ideas. The authors do provide explanations of very sophisticated philosophic and theoretic ideas, but just as you might be tempted to zone out, along comes a fascinating story—a story from the experience of the authors or stories other nurses have told them—to bring the complex ideas to life. In addition to the stories, the authors approach the text as a conversation with us, the readers. They speak directly to us. They ask us questions to ponder. They share their struggles in reaching for the ideals they seek, they reveal who they are, and they invite us to reflect on our own experiences to better know ourselves.

At the same time, this is a practical book for nurses in all areas of practice. There are "Try It Out" features throughout all the chapters—invitations and guidelines to apply ideas in practice, in one's own life. The "This Week in Practice" features guide specific applications of the ideas of the book in real nursing practice situations. There are checkpoints and reference points throughout that provide guidelines and pose questions for readers to ask themselves, leading to a personal experience of the content of the book that includes forming a path to make conscious decisions about practice. Each chapter ends with a "Relational Inquiry Toolbox," a list of actions, ways of thinking, and ways of being as a nurse that shift toward relational inquiry nursing.

Throughout, the authors resist the typical pattern to reject one thing in favor of another. They acknowledge the most persistent problems that nurses everywhere decry (e.g., lack of collaboration, acrimony between and among nurses), but rather than placing blame or attempting to analyze the problems in terms of "right" or "wrong," they apply the relational inquiry approach to examine the interacting social and cultural circumstances that frame the situation on all sides. They offer insights that guide shifts that nurses can make to address these complex issues without judgment of what one is shifting from and offer a way to move into a way of being and practicing that is consistent with the values of relational nursing.

The authors present an exemplar of that which is "relational" in nursing in the context of the wider world of health care and society. They bring together complex issues of social norms and cultural practices that shape nursing, along with a vision of how nursing is vital in shaping health care. I found myself wishing that I could have read this book as a young student but celebrate the appearance of this book at this moment in time. I believe that the world right now desperately needs nursing—and nursing needs the guiding light of this book to do its part in shaping our practice and, in turn, health care.

Peggy L. Chinn, RN, PhD, FAAN
July 31, 2013

REFERENCES

Carper, B. A. (1978). Fundamental patterns of knowing in nursing. *Advances in Nursing Science, 1*(1), 13–23.

Chinn, P. L. (1974). *Child health maintenance: Concepts in family-centered care*. St. Louis: CV Mosby.

Chinn, P. L. (1994). Developing a method for aesthetic knowing in nursing. In P. L. Chinn & J. Watson (Eds.), *Art and aesthetics in nursing* (pp. 19–40). New York: National League for Nursing Press.

Chinn, P. L. (2001). Toward a theory of nursing art. In N. L. Chaska (Ed.), *The nursing profession: Tomorrow and beyond* (pp. 287–297). Thousand Oaks, CA: Sage.

Chinn, P. L. (2013a). *Peace & power*. Retrieved March 19, 2013, from http://peaceandpowerblog.wordpress.com

Chinn, P. L. (2013b). *Peace & power: New directions for building community* (8th ed.). Burlington, MA: Jones and Bartlett Learning.

Chinn, P. L., & Kramer, M. (1983). *Theory & nursing: A systematic approach*. St Louis: Mosby.

Chinn, P. L., & Kramer, M. (2007). *Integrated theory and knowledge development in nursing* (7th ed.). St Louis: Mosby.

Dickoff, J., & James, P. (1968). A theory of theories: A position paper. *Nursing Research, 17*(3), 197–203.

Dickoff, J., & James, P. (1971). Clarity to what end? *Nursing Research, 20*(6), 499–502.

Dickoff, J., James, P., & Wiedenbach, E. (1968). Theory in a practice discipline. Part 1: Practice-oriented theory. *Nursing Research, 17*(5), 415–435.

Ellis, R. (1968). Characteristics of significant theories. *Nursing Research, 17*(3), 217–222.

Ellis, R. (1969). The practitioner as theorist. *American Journal of Nursing, 69*, 1434.

Folta, J. R. (1971). Obsfucation or clarification: A reaction to Walker's concept of nursing theory. *Nursing Research, 20*(6), 196–199.

Norris, C. M. (1969). Proceedings: First Nursing Theory Conference, University of Kansas Medical Center, Department of Nursing Education, March 20–21, 1969: University of Kansas Medical Center.

Walker, L. O. (1971). Toward a clearer understanding of the concept of nursing theory. *Nursing Research, 20*(5), 428–435.

Contents

Contents

Reviewers xx

Acknowledgments xi

About the Authors xiii

Preface ix

Foreword xv

1 How to Nurse: An Introduction to Relational Inquiry in Nursing Practice

LEARNING OBJECTIVES

By engaging with the material in this chapter, you will have an introductory understanding of:

1. The components of relational inquiry

2. The limitations of an individualist approach to nursing practice

3. The connections among patient/family well-being, nurse well-being, and the well-being of the health care system

4. Relational conceptualizations of people, families, and communities

5. A pragmatic approach to knowledge development and its implications for learning how to nurse as a relational inquirer

In this chapter, we introduce relational inquiry as an approach to nursing practice. Distinguishing it from an individualist orientation, we provide a beginning look at how relational inquiry can address and support patient/family well-being, nurse well-being, and the well-being of the health care system.

WHAT IS A RELATIONAL INQUIRY APPROACH TO NURSING PRACTICE?

We come to know nursing in the fullest sense by experiencing it. Although concepts, theories, and methods guide us in our work (and we will certainly get to these), they do not reveal what it is like to be in the complexities and uncertainties of contemporary nursing situations. They do not speak to what goes on inside of us as we strive to "do good" and meet our professional obligations. They do not fully reveal *how* nursing knowledge, competencies, goals, values, ideals, and obligations are brought together and integrated into safe, competent, health-promoting, socially just nursing care. To understand what it means to be a nurse in our complex world— a world that is shaped by relationships, economics, history, politics, values, and normative ideologies—and how our own well-being and the well-being of our patients, families, communities, and health care system are integrally connected, we need to explore that place where they are intricately interwoven—everyday nursing at the point-of-care.

Drawing on multiple examples from acute care, long-term care, community care, and mental health contexts, this book focuses on *how to nurse*. Outlining a relational inquiry approach to nursing practice, we provide structures and processes to support the translation of nursing values, knowledge, skills, ideals, and imperatives into effective action. Paying attention to the common ingredients of any illness, trauma, and/or injury experience, we examine how to nurse individuals and families as they live through birth, pain, anguish, suffering, disability, uncertainty, extraordinary life experiences, and death. Whether providing postoperative care to a man who has just had a thoracotomy, a middle-aged woman who has just been diagnosed with diabetes, a family with a child undergoing cancer treatment, a community facing a tuberculosis outbreak, or any other nursing situation, relational inquiry and the strategies offered in this book provide a way to optimize your knowledge and effectiveness as a nurse.

TO ILLUSTRATE

The *Relational* Experience of Contemporary Nursing Practice

Recently, I (Gweneth) was asked to make a presentation to an audience of nurses who came from a range of clinical areas and positions: direct care positions, administration, education, and research. Guided by the goal of improving nursing care across all sectors (acute, long-term, and community), the conference organizers had asked me to speak about how we might prepare "reflective and relational nurses." I began the presentation with a story that had been told by a nurse working on an acute medical unit when she participated in a recorded interview during a research project focused on improving end-of-life (EOL) care (Hartrick Doane, Stajduhar, Bidgood, Causton, & Cox, 2012; Stajduhar et al., 2008). The nurse's own words offered a vivid description of nursing in contemporary health care settings. She explained how a man had been sent up to their unit from the emergency room (ER) with the diagnosis of a toxic megacolon. *"They were actively treating him until within probably about 10 minutes before they sent him up to us and they decided, no, this isn't going to work so we're just going to send him up to you to die."*

She described how during the transfer, she asked the ER nurse, *"Have you guys put these things in place before you send him up so that I can just kind of make sure that he's comfortable?"* *"No, we don't do that down here; you're going to have to arrange that."* Relating the *"nightmare"* scene as she scrambled to get an IV line in for pain control, follow the isolation protocols, deal with the interdepartmental and interprofessional dynamics

continued on page 3

TO ILLUSTRATE *continued*

The *Relational* Experience of Contemporary Nursing Practice

---

that were happening and "*at least establish some sort of rapport*" with the man and his wife, she described how everything had happened so quickly, how the man had gone from being lucid on admission to dying an hour later. She described how at the end of that hour she was left struggling to find something to say to his wife who "*stood there with her mouth gaping open*" as she tried to take in what had just happened. The nurse told of how, unable to convince the wife to take a taxi home or call someone, "*I walked her to the parking lot and sat with her in her car and stayed out there and talked to her a little bit longer [about] what she was expecting when she got home and who she could call over to her house so that she wouldn't be alone there.*" She also described how for her as a nurse, the experience had not ended there—how later that night she had gone home and cried as she thought about what had transpired and where the care had fallen short. She ended her story by declaring, "*I still think about that woman.*"

When I finished reading the nurse's words to the audience, I invited them to respond. A young nurse raised her hand and in a shaky voice declared, "That could be my story—it is so similar to what I experience just about every day." In response, heads around the room began to nod. It was clear that the story resonated with all of us. Regardless of the clinical area in which we practiced, all of us had walked in that nurse's shoes. We knew what it was like to be in a complex, fast-paced situation scrambling to meet our professional obligations, to "do right" by patients, and to meet the needs of the circumstances at hand. And we had all come to appreciate that what ultimately happened for patients and families was not simply a matter of what *we* did but rather how nursing care rested in and arose through the complex *relational interplay* of people, situations, and contexts.

It is this relational interplay and the *how* of nursing that we focus on in this book. Our goal is to provide the opportunity for you as a reader/student/nurse to carefully examine the contingent and ever-changing nature of contemporary health care situations and enlist a relational inquiry approach to nursing to enhance your knowledge and effectiveness as a nurse.

When we use the word "relational" and speak of a relational inquiry approach to nursing practice, many people think we are merely emphasizing the touchy-feely, emotional side of nursing and particularly "nurse–patient" relationships. However, relational inquiry is far more encompassing than that. Although relationships between people are certainly part of relational inquiry, in this book, the term "relational" refers to the complex interplay of human life, the world, and nursing practice. Specifically, relational inquiry involves highly reasoned, skilled action. Relational inquiry requires (a) a thorough and sound knowledge base; (b) sophisticated inquiry and observational and analytical skills; (c) strong clinical skills including clinical judgment, decision-making skills, and clinical competencies; and

(d) particular ways of being. Thus, relational inquiry is about nursing competence in its fullest sense.

A Relational Inquiry Approach Has Two Essential Components

A relational inquiry approach to nursing practice includes two essential components: a relational consciousness and inquiry as a form of action. These components are interrelated and overlapping. Like ingredients in a cake, each enhances and informs the other to create a whole approach— relational inquiry.

Relational Consciousness

First, relational inquiry involves bringing a relational consciousness to our work as nurses (Hartrick Doane, in press). A relational consciousness is grounded in the assumption that people are relational beings who are situated in and constituted through social, cultural, political, and historical processes and communities (Thayer-Bacon, 2003). A relational consciousness extends your attention beyond the individual level to the *relational interplay* occurring at and between the intrapersonal, interpersonal, and contextual levels. Looking *intrapersonally*, you consider what is going on *within* all the people involved. For example, you think about what might be going on within an individual patient you are caring for, what is going on within you, and what others in the situation (such as family members or colleagues) might be experiencing. Focusing on the *interpersonal*, you notice what is going on *among and between* people—how people are acting in the situation, what they are prioritizing, what they are ignoring, and so forth. *Contextually*, you consider what is going on *around* the people and situation—the structures and forces that are influencing the situation and shaping the intrapersonal and interpersonal responses. To use an analogy, a relational consciousness is like getting up on a balcony during a dance so that you can see everything going on in and around the room. *It positions and guides you to intentionally turn your attention to the details*—to notice the people, their attire, the way they are moving, what kind of experience they seem to be having (are they smiling, frowning), how they are interacting with each other or not, the music that is playing and how that music is shaping the way they are dancing, how the surroundings contribute to what is occurring, and so forth.

In the opening To Illustrate story, a relational consciousness draws attention beyond the nurse and the patient to the multiple elements that were shaping what happened for him, his wife, and the nurse. Intrapersonally, we can hear the nurse feeling distressed and overwhelmed and the wife feeling stunned. Interpersonally, we see a flurry of activity—the nurse scurrying to try and set things in place for the man, the tense interaction between the ER nurse and the medical nurse, and the compassionate actions of the nurse as she walks the wife out to her car. Contextually, the ER transfer policy comes into focus as does the dominance of biomedical imperatives throughout the health care system that lead to, among other things, a dramatic shift in priorities once it was decided that the man was dying. From this example, it becomes apparent that providing high-quality nursing care is not simply a matter of the nurse having up-to-date knowledge and skills. Rather, a relational consciousness highlights the interplay of a number of factors affecting the point-of-care for the man and his wife. This heightened awareness enables more informed decisions and more effective action.

Overall, a relational consciousness

- Sensitizes us to the relational complexities that affect what happens at the point-of-care
- Directs attention toward the "relational transactions" that are occurring within and among people and contexts
- Enables us to be very intentional and consciously choose how to act in response to these complexities and transactions

Specifically, relational consciousness is the *action* of being mindfully aware of the relational complexities that are at play in a situation and intentionally and skillfully working in response to those relational complexities (Hartrick Doane, in press). For example, the nurse in the story

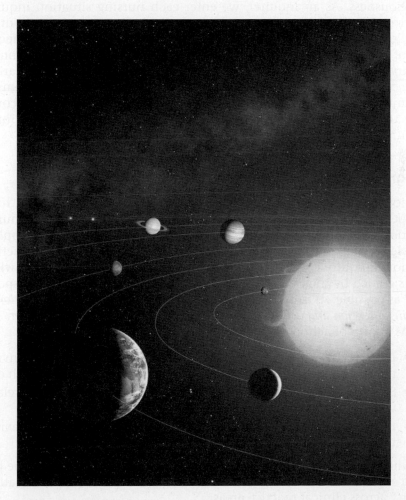

Relational consciousness.

wanted to provide quality nursing care to the man, but she felt over-whelmed by the competing obligations she faced. She was obligated to her organization to work within the ER transfer policy, she was obligated to maintain collegial relationships with the ER staff, she was enabled and limited by the resources that were and were not available (e.g., resources to assist her with setting up the admission and isolation protocols), and so forth. Thus, her nursing decision making and actions were not simply a matter of applying her knowledge of comfort care at EOL and/or infection control procedures. If she was to provide quality care to the man and his wife, she required the knowledge and skillfulness to see the relational complexities, consciously enlist knowledge that could help her discern and make decisions within the competing obligations, and choose actions that would enable her to intentionally navigate within this complex situation.

Inquiry as a Form of Action

Inquiry offers a method for this process of navigation, mediation, and decision making. In essence, inquiry is the "how to" of a relational consciousness. As an inquirer, we enter each nursing situation inquiring into the relational experiences of people (including ourselves), contexts, knowledge, meaningful purposes, excellence of practices, and effective-ness of outcomes (Hartrick Doane & Varcoe, 2008). Like a scientific inquiry, inquiry-based nursing practice involves being in that in-between relational space of knowing/not knowing, being curious, looking for what seems sig-nificant, examining the interrelatedness among the elements, and consid-ering the relevance of those interrelationships in the moment to inform action toward patient, nurse, and system well-being.

Integrating the Two Components

Relational inquiry orients you to consciously examine and relate to the intrapersonal, interpersonal, and contextual forces shaping each nursing situation. At the same time, it leads you to examine how you are applying knowledge, making clinical decisions, and determining the "right" actions. Relational inquiry is a way of relating to people, situations, and knowledge and is guided by the overriding goal of being as responsive and "response-able" as possible. *At its very core, relational inquiry is a practice of attention—of focusing attention and acting in a more conscious and intentional manner.*

As a form of action, relational inquiry leads us to:

- Look for the ways in which people, situations, contexts, environ-ments, and processes are integrally connected and shaping each other
- See how we ourselves are being present, responding, and relating within the situational circumstances
- Inform and form our practice responsively within the complexity of those relational realities

We will expand this description of relational inquiry throughout the book as we explore the knowledge, skills, and capacities that support relational inquiry across clinical practice areas.

WHY A RELATIONAL INQUIRY APPROACH TO NURSING PRACTICE?

The main reason for developing a relational inquiry approach is that it is consistent with the realities of contemporary nursing situations. Currently, an individualist, decontextualized approach dominates nursing in most health care settings. An individualist approach to nursing practice focuses on individual nurses without considering the influences that shape their actions and possibilities. Subsequently, nurses see themselves as individually responsible to ensure good care for their patients. Yet given contextual constraints that shape the options available to them, nurses may feel powerless to affect the quality of care. As with the nurse in the opening story, this disjuncture often leads to a focus on what has *not* been provided (Doane, 2004; Hartrick Doane, 2002). We call it the "half-empty" view and have observed its incredibly demoralizing impact.

For example, in an ethics research study (Varcoe et al., 2004), nurses described situations that had happened several years earlier. They had never shared these stories with anyone before, not even their life partners, because they felt so guilty or ashamed at not being able to change the outcomes for patients and/or families. While telling the stories, their emotions were as intense as if the situations had happened the day before (Doane, 2004; Hartrick Doane, 2002). What was significant is that in hearing the stories, it was evident that many of the nurses had in fact done a lot for the patients or families; many times, they had actually offered exemplary nursing care. However, being so focused on what they had *not* been able to change or do in the situation and feeling responsible, they had failed to see what they *had* done.

This same half-empty view was also evidenced in the nurse's words in the opening story. Given the complexities of the situation, she had been highly responsive, offering high-quality nursing care to the man who had died. She had also provided profoundly meaningful care to his wife following his death (as evidenced by the wife phoning the next day and asking to speak to her specifically). Yet the nurse saw her care as inadequate and herself as "too involved" and "too emotional." She had narrated the experience as a failure to provide good care.

Overall, an individualist approach to nursing is not only incongruent with the relational complexities that are part and parcel of most contemporary nursing situations but also insufficient for understanding and working within those complexities (Hartrick Doane, in press). Similar to Walker's (2003) description of moral oblivion where there is a lack of awareness of the moral demands that are being made, when nurses are oblivious to the intrapersonal, interpersonal, and contextual elements shaping their decisions and actions, they are more likely to be at the mercy of those influences. That is, they are more likely to be practicing in *relational oblivion*. Practicing without awareness of the relational complexities impacts nursing care in a very practical way and ultimately makes meeting nursing obligations all but impossible (Hartrick Doane & Varcoe, 2007).

Within the existing individualist frame, we have observed that over time, the "half-empty" view can come to shape nurses' views of patients.

As contextual forces require nurses to make choices about who to provide more or less care to, nurses can unintentionally align with broader social ideas regarding "who" is more or less deserving of care. For example, in an ethics study (Rodney, Hartrick, Storch, Varcoe, & Starzomski, 2002), we encountered staff in one emergency room who referred to patients whose conditions were not acute and who were awaiting placement in long-term care facilities as "bed blockers." Using this depersonalizing phrase seemed to help nurses accept or even justify the limited care they were able to provide to these patients, who often waited for placement on stretchers in hallways for days at a time, with no privacy while using bedpans, and received minimal care. The nurses felt bad about the care they provided but simultaneously justified it by seeing the "bed blockers" as problem patients who were diverting resources from more acute patients who were more deserving of emergent care.

Simply put, relational inquiry is aimed toward patient well-being, nurse well-being, and system well-being, and it recognizes the way in which those elements are integrally connected. In situations such as the story told earlier, that integral connection becomes glaringly evident. For example, in telling her story, the nurse described being "frustrated and angry" with the ER, stating, *"Maybe the emergency room isn't the best place for somebody to die either, but like you know, (the patient) all of a sudden gets a whole new set of hands and faces."* What the nurse is pointing to is the disjuncture between the system-level ER transfer policy and patient/family well-being. It is obvious to her that experientially, from the perspective of the patient's well-being, a transfer to a new unit with new people does not make sense. How can good EOL care be provided given his imminent death and what is *not* in place on the medical unit? Rationally, she knows that the ER is not necessarily better equipped, yet a transfer to a new unit does not make sense either. The nurse is left with deep and unresolved feelings about the situation, yet she actually dispels the significance of her response and the questions that arise from it, going on to explain, *"So to be honest, I usually chalk it up to the fact that I'm more emotional than most people and that I'm probably getting more involved than I need to be, especially around death."* She concludes that her emotional response indicates a problem in *her* and that she needs to change something in herself.

Whereas through an individualist lens the nurse's frustration and anger might be considered just *her* response, through a relational lens, her response (including her emotions) are seen as arising through the interplay *between* the patient/family, the nurse, the health care situation, and the system. Moreover, her response is seen as having the potential to inform both her nursing action and ultimately the patient/family and system well-being. Specifically, her response is pointing to crucial aspects that need to be addressed if good EOL care is to be offered in her facility. However, coached to see her practice through an individualist lens, the nurse responds negatively toward the ER staff (whose practice is also highly constrained by contextual forces); receives little support from other colleagues who contend that "that is just the way things are"; and is left feeling something is wrong with *her*, that she should dampen her compassion. In addition, the factors that fail to support patient/family well-being, her nurse well-being, and the well-being of the system are left unaddressed.

Ultimately, an individualist approach to nursing practice results in a normative pattern in which good care, and subsequently patient/family well-being, is continually compromised; nurses are left feeling like they have done all they can, but it is still not "good enough"; nurses lose sight of the way in which they are making a difference and promoting well-being; and the discourse between nurses becomes one of "that's just the way it is," and thus system problems go unaddressed. Nurses feel powerless to change the system, yet they are ambivalent and unsettled at participating in it. The nurse in the opening story describes this normative pattern of powerlessness quite eloquently: *"I know a lot of nurses have similar experiences but they're just like, 'Well that's just what happens. Like emerg sends them up; they're imminent death; we help them die, and hopefully we do it as best that we can.' And so that's kind of that, you know . . . It's kind of matter-of-fact."*

Bringing a relational inquiry approach to nursing practice serves to both interrupt this normative pattern and provide an avenue for action. For example, returning to the nurse in the story, if you listen carefully, you can hear something in between the nurse's words that is quite vital—a little niggling question that she has within herself: *"But . . . I don't know, in nursing I feel like sometimes . . . we deal with a lot of emotional relational stuff and sometimes there's an expectation that you need to suck it up and keep going, and by the way, your next admission's coming in an hour."* One can hear her ambiguity. While the individualist orientation has schooled her to discount her emotions as irrelevant and to fault herself for not having found a matter-of-fact way of dealing with death, there is an uncertainty within her and a little voice asking, "Can it really be right to just have to 'suck it up'?"

We believe these questions and unsettled responses that arise in the relational spaces of practice are crucial areas for knowledge and practice development. Moreover, when we bring our attention to things that do not seem quite right and inquire further—intentionally listening to and enlisting the questions that arise—we have the potential to enhance patient well-being, nurse well-being, and system well-being.

TO ILLUSTRATE
Acting beyond the Coffee Room

As part of the ethics research team mentioned earlier, we conducted a series of focus groups across a range of clinical areas to examine the meaning and enactment of ethics in everyday nursing practice (Varcoe et al., 2004). Our research team wanted to learn what ethics actually meant to practicing nurses and thus began by defining ethics in the

continued on page 10

TO ILLUSTRATE *continued*

Acting beyond the Coffee Room

---

broad sense of "doing good." We began each focus group by asking the nurses to tell us a story from their perspectives of a time when they had practiced ethically. Consistently across the focus groups that opening request was followed by silence, and then often one brave nurse would declare, "I can tell you a time when I *didn't* practice ethically." Their experience of ethics—of doing good—paradoxically had been one of *not* doing good.

Interestingly, the stories we heard of "not doing good" were surprisingly similar across contexts. Like the one earlier, they were stories of nurses constantly working *between* their own values and the values of others, *between* competing interests and concerns, and *between* their nursing ideals and health care realities. The nurses described their deep personal struggle as they sought to do what they could to live up to their nursing ideals and how they felt "unethical" as contextual forces constrained their ability to choose and act in ways they deemed to be "good." They also described the deleterious impact on themselves and the patients/families for whom they cared.

On completion of the research, our team conducted a series of presentations throughout the health regions in which the research had taken place. The presentations defined ethics from the perspective of everyday nursing practice and included examples of the ethical issues nurses faced. At the end of one of the presentations, a nurse in the audience exclaimed, "*You mean to say that's ethics? I thought that was just bitching in the coffee room!*" While she said it in a joking way, her comment was profoundly astute. She was pointing to the way in which the deeply felt concerns of nurses are often expressed indirectly and in ways that have no impact— for example, as "bitching in the coffee room." Deeply feeling the gap *between* what constitutes good care and what actually transpires, nurses can eloquently describe (in the coffee room) how their practice is constrained by systemic realities (such as system policies, resources, staffing ratios, etc.). Yet, coached to see themselves as individual, autonomous moral agents, they often express and see their concerns about patient/ family care and/or system limitations as merely *their* reactions. Thus, they "blow off steam" in the coffee room to diffuse their distress about situations they feel powerless to affect, to gain reassurance that their situations are not unique, or to gauge the appropriateness of their responses. Worse yet, they blame other individuals, or as with the nurse in the opening story, they see their emotional turmoil as a personal limitation. Regardless, the outcome is most often the same: they feel they have not met their nursing obligations, and the conditions that need to be changed to support the well-being of patients/families, nurses, and the health care system go unaddressed.

TRY IT OUT 1.1
Review a Situation that Bugged You

Recall a nursing situation from practice that bothered you. It could be yesterday, last week, or, if you have been in practice for a while, years ago. Think of any situation in which you felt bad, uncomfortable, disturbed, or unsettled. Purposefully look through an "individualist lens"; that is, see if you can ascribe as much responsibility as possible to the nurses involved, yourself, any patients or families, any physicians, or managers. Imagine "blaming" particular individuals. Next, look at the situation with relational inquiry in mind. If you look "relationally," how does your view change? What intrapersonal elements do you consider? What interpersonal dynamics stand out? How were all the players interrelating? And how were they all "positioned" in the larger system? What competing obligations were operating in the situation? What priorities were held by different people? And what system priorities influenced the situation? How did the interrelationships between the intrapersonal, interpersonal, and contextual domains shape the situation? How does your understanding expand when you consider the intrapersonal, interpersonal, and contextual factors? What questions arise for you? How might you have responded to affect the situation? As you look "relationally," do your thoughts about responsibility shift? Share your thoughts about the situation with one other person doing the same exercise.

A Relational Inquiry Approach Increases Nurses' Abilities to Affect Well-Being

A relational inquiry approach enables nurses to consciously navigate within these kinds of complexities and enhance their ability to affect the well-being of patients, nurses, and the health care system. As Dickoff and James (1968) contend, "A professional is a doer who shapes reality rather than a doer who merely attends to the cogs of reality according to prescribed patterns" (p. 102). We hope to empower you to become this situation-producing "doer" as you consider your nursing practice at the point-of-care. To be such a doer, you need to be proactive in self-selecting, self-directing, and self-generating knowledge. You also need to inquire and act at all three levels (intrapersonal, interpersonal, and contextual) to support and foster the creating and recreating of realities (Hartrick Doane & Varcoe, 2007).

It is our contention that nurses are obligated to all persons, most immediately on an individual basis to all those within their care, and also collectively to those who require their care. We are greatly concerned about the inattention to the complexities of nursing practice and the iatrogenic impact of an *individualist, decontextualized* approach on patients/families;

on nurses; and on the health care system. We believe that relational inquiry is a far more effective approach to promoting patient/family well-being, nurse well-being, and system well-being. We begin with the premise that these three concerns are inherently related and dependent on one another. That is, as part of the same relational whole, each influences and shapes the others. Thus, specific attention to all three of these elements is necessary for effective nursing action.

Patient/Family Well-Being

If you read any nursing textbook, you will come across the terms "health" and "health promotion." If you pay close attention, however, you will notice that those terms are used in very different ways (Hartrick Doane & Varcoe, 2005a, 2005b; Labonte, 1993). One of the most dominant understandings of health has come from biomedicine that understands health as the "absence of disease or infirmity." Based on this definition of health, nursing practice focuses on *treating or preventing disease* by correcting problems. Another fairly prominent understanding of health is one that rests in *a behavioral model*. Within a behavioral model, health is more than the absence of disease and includes physical and emotional well-being. Subsequently, health-promoting nursing practice based on a behavioral perspective includes secondary and primary prevention, and emphasis is given to *changing behaviors and lifestyle* (such as quitting smoking, increasing fitness) in order to decrease disease risks and maintain well-being.

During the latter part of the 20th century, the World Health Organization (WHO) conducted work that balanced the dominance of a biomedical orientation to health care. The Ottawa Charter for Health Promotion (WHO, 1986) marked a shift from strictly medical and behavioral health determinants to health determinants defined in psychological, social, environmental, and political terms. This groundbreaking document moved health promotion far beyond a disease and/or behavioral perspective to a socio-environmental one, emphasizing that health is deeply rooted in human nature and societal structures (WHO, 1986). A socio-environmental understanding of health incorporates sociologic and environmental aspects as well as the medical and behavioral ones. From this perspective, health is considered to be "a resource for living . . . a positive concept . . . the extent to which an individual or group is able to realize aspirations, to satisfy needs, and to change or cope with the environment" (WHO, 1986, p. 1). Subsequently, empowerment—the capacity to define, analyze, and act upon concerns in one's life and living conditions—joined treatment and prevention as an essential goal of health promotion (Labonte, 1993).

Relational inquiry rests in a socio-environmental understanding of health and health promotion. Nursing practice enacted as a process of relational inquiry is oriented toward enhancing the capacity and power of people to live meaningful lives. Although this may involve treating and preventing disease or modifying lifestyle factors, the primary motivation (e.g., the reason disease is treated or certain lifestyles are promoted) is to enhance people's well-being and the capacity and resources for meaningful life experiences. This socio-environmental view of health and well-being moves beyond thinking of health as an individual choice and responsibility and highlights how *health is a sociorelational experience* that is strongly shaped by contextual factors. We will be exploring this sociorelational perspective of health in detail throughout the book.

Nurse Well-Being

Relational inquiry is also oriented toward nurse well-being. Similar to the experience of the nurse in the earlier story, Duchscher and Myrick (2008) have described how the interrelated forces and normative patterns that exist in most North American health care settings can serve to transform creative, vibrant nurses into disillusioned, exhausted practitioners. "New graduates who work in the hospital setting consistently express frustration and a sense of demoralization as a direct result of the dissonance they experience between their perception of nursing and what they find nursing to 'really' be" (Duchscher & Myrick, 2008, p. 196). These authors describe the emotional distress that builds over time when nurses are unable to provide the kind of care they have been educated to provide. This distress included frustration and resentment directed at themselves for failing to provide the quality of care they believed they should be providing, at their managers who the nurses perceived as putting them in such compromising positions, and at educators who did not prepare them for the nursing "realities" they faced. Consistent with a socio-environmental understanding of health and well-being, relational inquiry intentionally and explicitly enlists these workplace realities to examine ways nurses might more effectively mediate and work within them. Relational inquiry practice includes particular skills and strategies that can aid in the prevention of deleterious effects on you as a nurse and also offers a way of navigating through the often conflicting and competing interests and values inherent in contemporary settings.

System Well-Being

Health care reform over the past few decades has dramatically shaped the systems within which nursing happens. Globally, health care has been oriented increasingly to business models, even in countries where there is some level of public funding and "for-profit" health care is limited. Emphasis is on efficiency, limiting the use of resources and optimizing profit, often without accompanying attention to the longer-term consequences for health of individuals and populations. Relational inquiry draws attention to the ways in which nursing practice and the well-being of patients and populations are shaped by changing health care systems, including the organizations and units within which nurses practice, and by wider social, political, and economic trends. For example, increasing acuity in hospitals combines with changing skill mix and more patients per nurse to make practice situations more challenging for the delivery of good care. Throughout this book, we suggest that each moment of practice has potential for improving the care of both those immediately in front of us and for those who will receive care in the future. Throughout, we simultaneously point to how, from a stance of relational inquiry, nurses can practice more effectively and with greater well-being *and* participate in creating conditions that are healthier for patients, families, communities, and other nurses.

TRY IT OUT 1.2
Looking Back

Go back in your mind to the situation you were thinking about in Try It Out 1.1. Consider the following questions in relation to that situation:

1. How was concern for patient/family, nurse, and system well-being guiding the situation?

2. Other than this well-being, toward "what" were the actions in the situation oriented? For example, to what extent was short-term efficiency or expediency driving the situation? Available resources and staffing?

3. What do your answers to these questions suggest about what different actions might have been taken?

To get an extended view into the situation you experienced, swap a short description of your experience (not your analysis of it) with a partner (a classmate or colleague). Have that person answer the questions. How does that person's analysis of your situation compare to yours? How was your analysis of his or her situation different/similar?

ENGAGING IN A RELATIONAL INQUIRY PROCESS

In the remaining chapters of this book, we invite you to join us in a *relational inquiry* process to examine the complexities of contemporary nursing practice and to explore and develop ways of effectively navigating through them. We enlist you as active participants with the hope that by engaging in this process, you will develop a conscious, intentional, and responsive way of practicing nursing—one that is relationally oriented, consciously chosen, and grounded in inquiry. As part of this process, we hope to inspire you to scrutinize what is informing your nursing work, how you are living your knowledge, how you are enacting your nursing ideals, and to develop wider possibilities for knowing and responding within your nursing practice.

Throughout the book, we will be asking you to consider this question: What would it mean to practice with the understanding that you are affecting and being affected by everything that is happening around you, in you, among you and others, and in the world? In exploring this question, we will be inviting you to look at how you understand and enact your work as a nurse; how you choose, integrate, and live knowledge; and how you relate with and to people/families, yourself, colleagues, and the health care system in which you work. We will ask you to look with fresh eyes—to be a curious inquirer noticing and paying attention to people and situations to see beyond the everyday routines of health care. For example, what if the nurse in the story that opened this chapter came to see the limitations of her practice as located beyond herself? What if she began to trust her own questioning and to push it even further? What if she had ways of working with her colleagues to more concertedly examine the normative practices that were limiting nursing care? What if she had ways of inquiring *with* her colleagues in the ER? We will explore such possibilities throughout the book and suggest philosophical, theoretical, and practical strategies to support a relational inquiry approach to nursing practice.

Conceptualizing through a Relational Lens

Throughout the book, we will be inviting you to look through a relational lens. By "relational lens" we mean looking at the *connections between* ideas, theories, and situations, considering how patients, families, communities, and health care systems are integrally connected and shaping each other and how the well-being of each is interdependent with the others. As a first step, we direct your attention to the way in which individuals, families, and communities are conceptualized and how these conceptualizations are shaping nursing practice.

Conceptualizing Individuals Relationally

Do you believe that the context in which you grew up and/or the context in which you currently live has shaped you as a person? What about others you have known—can you see how their contexts have shaped them differently from you? Do you think it is possible not to be affected by your contexts? For example, when you made your decision to enter nursing school, although it was a personal decision, did you make it in relation to your world? Did you think about what it would mean in terms of getting a job, being able to travel, and having economic security? Did you take into account the opinions of other important people in your life? In what ways were your own personal thoughts sparked and/or influenced by what you had heard and learned in your relational world? What stereotypes about nursing did you balance in your decision making?

Conceptualizing relationally begins with the understanding that each person has a unique personal, sociohistorical location that affects and shapes that person's identity, experience, interpretations, and way of being in the world. It assumes that the values, knowledge, attitudes, practices, and structures that dominate the sociocultural world within which each person lives are passed on through relational interactions. Subsequently, people's experiences, interpretations, and actions are understood as products of a multitude of interactions occurring at the intrapersonal, interpersonal, and contextual levels. In contrast to a decontextualized view that sees people as distinct entities separate from one another and their worlds, conceptualizing individuals relationally highlights how people are connected and shaped by everyone and everything else in their worlds. Specifically, this means that people are both shaped by and shape other people's responses, situations, experiences, and contexts. Not only nurses but also patients and families, other health care providers, and actors beyond the immediate health care context, such as policy makers and the media, continuously negotiate and shape one another.

TO ILLUSTRATE
A Frustrating Man

Rosa, a friend of mine who started working at a diabetes clinic recently, told me (Colleen) about a young man, Artur, who attends the clinic on an irregular basis. The staff at the clinic told Rosa that Artur is "difficult, frustrating, and noncompliant." He only occasionally attends clinic, and his blood sugars are often high when he does, despite the staff giving him regular warnings and repeatedly explaining his prescribed regimen. Policies require that people who are insulin dependent must obtain a medical certificate in order to purchase needles from the pharmacy, but Artur has not attended the required education session, so the staff cannot issue his certificate. The staff had a team meeting and decided someone should follow up with Artur regarding the choices he has been making. Rosa volunteered.

She reviewed Artur's chart and found that he has had diabetes since he was 11 years old. In addition to dealing with diabetes, Artur had a learning disability and dropped out of school 4 years ago at age 15 years. There is little other information on his chart except lab work, insulin orders, and his dietary prescription. Rosa had difficulty in contacting Artur as the phone number on his chart turned out to be a youth drop-in center. A week later, Artur called Rosa from the drop-in center where he had received the message.

Rosa asked how Artur was doing and told him that the staff were concerned that he had not turned up to get his certificate. Artur explained to Rosa that there was no point in him coming in because his social assistance had been cut off, so he could not afford new needles anyway. He told Rosa that he works at a McDonald's part-time now, so he is "eating better," but his scheduled work hours are the same as the clinic's hours. Rosa asked Artur about his phone number and whether he had somewhere to stay. He explained that he is living with an aunt but that they cannot afford a phone.

This story illustrates the contrast between seeing individuals as autonomous and understanding people and families relationally. The staff who saw Artur as noncompliant and as making bad choices were drawing on liberal individualist ideas of Artur as a rational, autonomous actor. They "know" that following a diabetic regimen is logical and rational and therefore they expect Artur to comply. In concert with that knowledge, the staff focuses on Artur's responsibilities for his own health and health care. When the circumstances of Artur's life come into view, however, his "bad choices" can be seen as being shaped by a network of influences beyond biomedical knowledge of diabetes and beyond his own decision making and choice. For example, it is possible to see how his choices are strongly shaped by policies and economics that limit his access to a phone, to nutritional food, to needles, and so forth. It is possible to see that his "failure" to attend the diabetic outpatient program is connected to his work and life context.

Conceptualizing people relationally is similar to taking what Kleffel (1996) identifies as an "ecocentric" view. Kleffel argues that in order to account for the conditions that compromise health, nurses need an ecocentric view that enables them to approach people with the understanding that "everything is connected to everything else" (Kleffel, 1996, p. 4). People and environments are not separate entities. Rather, people are quite literally constituted by and through the contexts in which they live. That is, sociocontextual experiences intricately shape how people biologically "develop, grow, age, ail, and die" (Krieger, 1999).

Kleffel suggests that nursing theorists such as Parse, Rogers, Newman, and Watson have based their work on such a paradigm. Understanding people from this relational perspective, nurses attend not just to individuals *in* context but also to individuals and families *as continuous with* their social, economic, historical, political, and physical contexts. That is, it is understood that people live within a relational web, and consequently, any health care intervention must not only be offered through this relational understanding but interventions must also be evaluated from that relational vantage point.

A good example of this relational web was recently offered by an anthropology colleague of ours who remarked on how health care practitioners went about measuring the efficacy of Viagra (a medication used in the treatment of erectile dysfunction). Looking through an individualist lens at the efficacy of Viagra with Viagra users, the questions centered on men's physical response to the drug (the men are the objects whose response can be seen and quantified). Looking through a relational lens, the web of social, economic, historical, and political relations becomes clearer. Our colleague commented on the multitude of aspects that were crucial to explore if we were actually to understand the drug's efficacy. For example, what had taking the drug meant for the man? How had the man's *life* been affected by the drug? Was affordability an issue? If the man had a partner, how had this person's life been affected? What had it meant for their relationship? Had there been an impact on how he related in his larger community? Were there sociocultural aspects significant to how the drug had affected him and his life? For example, how does male identity vary in different societies? This example illustrates the way in which conceptualizing people relationally can expand our view of people, health, and nursing action.

Conceptualizing Families Relationally

Although nursing literature offers a range of definitions of *family*, most describe "family" according to structure (who is in the family) and function (what the family provides or does). These definitions offer a conceptualization of family as a configuration of people who are connected in some way. Hanson (2001) offers the following classifications of these connections: legal (relationships through blood ties, adoption, guardianship, or marriage), biologic (genetic, biologic networks among people), sociologic (groups of people living together), and psychological (groups with strong emotional ties).

As the two-parent nuclear family norm has been challenged over the past few decades, new definitions have arisen to expand the conceptual possibilities. Two examples include Wright and Leahey's (2012) definition, "The family is who they say they are" (p. 40), and Hanson's (2001) "two or more individuals who depend on one another for emotional, physical, and economic support. The members of the family are self-defined" (p. 6).

Although these alternative definitions accommodate family diversity, they continue to focus on family in its *literal* form, conceptualizing it as an *entity* that can be demarcated in some way (such as by form, "who they say they are"; or function, "emotional, physical support"). As we have worked with families, however, we have experienced "family" in ways that are not revealed through literal conceptualizations. In particular, we believe what is missing is the conceptual understanding of family as a complex relational experience (Doane, 2003). Given that family is a central organizing structure for society, we are all influenced by family regardless of the extent to which we are involved with a literal family; family is an experiential social reality. This means that by virtue of living in the world, we and our health experiences are highly affected by our family experiences. In conceptualizing family relationally, we highlight how understanding family as a complex process in which economics, emotion, context, and experience are interwoven and multilayered is essential to the promotion of well-being (Doane, 2003).

TO ILLUSTRATE
A Family Experience

The following story of a family experience is not typical of those told in the family nursing literature nor does it reflect how most people usually think of family. It moves beyond the taken-for-granted view and reveals family as a relational living experience.

A number of years ago, I (Gweneth) was asked to be a parent driver for a field trip for my daughter Teresa's sixth grade class. The destination was a drop-in center for people who were homeless and living on the street. During our time at the center, a staff member named John told the children about his experience of "living on the street" for 20 years. As John told his story, he invited the children to ask questions. Because it was close to Christmas, one child asked him how he spent Christmas when he lived on the street. This idea of Christmas suddenly sparked a flurry of questions about family. Didn't he have a family? Where was his family all those years he was living on the street? What was it like to live on the street without your family?

In response, John began talking about how lonely he had felt during that time. He described how people would walk by him as though he didn't exist and how he gradually began to feel invisible. At first, it didn't

continued on page 19

TO ILLUSTRATE *continued*

A Family Experience

really seem as if John was addressing the children's "family" questions. However, as I listened, I realized that he was. John's family experience was one of not mattering to people, of being invisible.

The reason that I had difficulty at first connecting his response to the children's questions was that his experience in no way resembled what *I* expected in response to questions about family. John did not talk about his parents or his brothers and sisters. Rather, he talked about *how family was meaningful to him*. John's relational experience of family had been one of absence, invisibility, and isolation. Over time, this family experience had had a profoundly detrimental effect on his health. He described how his experience of being invisible had provoked a deep sense of isolation and had heightened the gulf between himself and the rest of the world. Concluding the conversation, he told the children how important it was to acknowledge people and to include them. "Even if it seems like they are different or don't care, the most important and caring thing you can do for a person you see sitting on the street is to look them in the eye and say hello just like you would if they were your family."

This story speaks to the importance of conceptualizing family through a relational lens—as a relational living experience. My initial thought that John wasn't addressing the children's questions was really a result of my own limited conceptualization of family. Because *I* knew family to be a configuration of people, I initially had difficulty making sense of what he was saying and more importantly did not immediately understand the significance of his family experience to his overall health and well-being.

Within a relational inquiry approach, the focus moves beyond family in its literal form. That is, whether we are working with a literal family or an individual who has no current ties to a literal family, nursing practice focuses on the *significance* of family and how *all people are meaningfully experiencing family*.

Conceptualizing family nursing in this way has important consequences. First, it is assumed that every moment of practice involves "family nursing." Second, regardless of who your designated patient is, to work effectively and responsively, you need to consider family. Overall, relational inquiry extends the view of family and family nursing and provides a way of "doing" family nursing that is relevant across all contexts and populations. Whether working on pediatrics with a family with a child newly diagnosed with asthma, making a home visit to a new mom, doing discharge planning for a man who has just had a stroke and going home alone, working with a woman who has left a violent partner, or caring for a patient at EOL, when family is conceptualized *relationally*, nurses can work more effectively to promote well-being.

TRY IT OUT 1.3
Think about Your Family

Think about your "literal" family. Thinking of yourself at the center of a web of relationships, take a piece of paper and map out your connections to other people. Then use keywords to describe your *experience* in relation to particular people, both within the literal family and beyond. For example, when I (Colleen) draw my experience of family, the connections I draw go far beyond my "literal" family to people from whom I feel disconnected (I use keywords such as "no contact" or "disappointed" between myself and some) and see the profound connections and influence of people who are literally "friends" but more "family" than those with whom I have kinship. What does pushing your thinking beyond your literal family reveal to you about your understanding of the concept? Of yourself?

Conceptualizing Community Relationally

Like family, community is often conceptualized in literal form. Communities are often defined geographically (e.g., the lower east side), by ethnicity (e.g., the Chinese community), by some other form of identity (e.g., gay, bisexual, lesbian, and transgendered community), or by experience (e.g., the immigrant community). These literal definitions draw attention to the boundaries of communities and miss the way in which those boundaries are shifting, porous, and permeable. Homogeneity and stasis are implied, and the complexity, diversity, and changing nature of communities go unacknowledged. For example, many cities in Western countries have sizable Chinese communities. However, the diversity within such communities often exceeds the differences between the presumed community and the wider society. Further, the differences between such named communities may be extensive. For example, the Chinese community of San Francisco has a unique history, a variety of migration generations, mix of "source" communities, religions, and levels of wealth, even when compared with other similarly named communities in other cities in the United States.

Again, we contend that a relational view of community is required to understand how individuals experience, are shaped by, and shape their multiple communities. Nursing practice grounded in a relational orientation focuses on the significance of community and the living relational experience of community with all people in all situations, and it involves attending to how *all people are meaningfully experiencing community*. Which "communities" are relevant to people at particular points in time? When community is conceptualized relationally, nurses begin to understand the significance of community to health, healing, and EOL experiences.

TO ILLUSTRATE
A Supportive Community

In North America, the dominant culture often perceives so-called ethnic communities as insular but supportive to their members. One consequence of this stereotype is that health care providers who are not members of a given community may assume that a certain level of social support is available to all its members.

In a study I (Colleen) led regarding social system support for women experiencing intimate partner violence, women who were recent immigrants from various countries reported that health care providers and other social service providers assumed that they would receive financial, emotional, and social support from their ethnic communities. However, as other authors have shown (Guruge & Collins, 2008; Guruge, Khanlou, & Gastaldo, 2009), the women's experiences often contradicted this. Contrary to the stereotype, the women variously described being isolated by their partners within the community or being denigrated by their partners to other community members. Describing her experience of how she was seen by her particular ethnic community, one woman said, "I am the bad guy. I am the bad woman. I am the one nobody trusts."

Further, women varied in the extent to which they were accepted within their ethnic communities depending on their behavior, religion, class, and other factors. A woman who identified as a member of the South Asian community said, "I don't know why I couldn't see [the abuse] was happening, see what was happening. I feel it's related somehow to my disability; my health made me feel vulnerable. I was afraid to be alone. I needed support. I also feel it was related to feeling ostracized from my family and community, because I am a lesbian . . . there's nothing to make it safe for me. There's no . . . use. There's nobody in the community I can go to."

A relational orientation to community helps nurses see communities as living relational experiences. Such an orientation leads nurses to inquire how individuals and groups experience the various communities of which they are part. It also leads nurses to inquire as to how communities are situated and constituted within wider contexts.

Engaging as a Relational Inquirer

In and throughout this book, we hope to *engage you as a relational inquirer*—to join us in a knowledge development and inquiry process. As writers, we see ourselves as being in relation with you, the reader. In that spirit, we have chosen to use a conversational style of writing. As we present ideas throughout the book, we share our own experiences, how our thinking has changed over time, and questions we're currently exploring. And we invite *you* to consider your own experiences and ideas in relation to ours. At the same time, we are aware that you are also in relation with many others who will influence and inform your understanding and practice of nursing. We hope that as you work your way through this book, you will use the numerous other relational connections you have to further develop your knowledge and practice.

As learners and teachers, we have come to understand learning not as merely an intellectual activity but a deeply embodied and personal process that requires active and substantial engagement at the experiential level. To become an intentional, competent nurse, you must bring intellectual understanding (e.g., theory) together with embodied, emotional experience (e.g., personal experience, nursing practice experience). We see you in much the same way as we see ourselves. That is, to follow Thayer-Bacon (2003), as people, we each have the potential to learn to be more critical, creative, and constructive. As you read, you may find yourself identifying limitations in our thinking. Rather than being concerned about this, we welcome your differing perspectives and insights. Our intent is to not just present ideas or content for you to read. We want you to *think hard* as you read this book and consider the ideas in relation to what you see happening at point-of-care.

Certain attitudes and capacities will help you reap the most benefit from this book. These same attitudes and capacities will serve you as a nurse since they are ones that support *being a relational inquiring nurse*.

Relating with Curiosity

First, as a reader, you will need to relate with curiosity and be willing to take a *stance of not knowing*. We hope you will be open to the questions that arise within you without rushing to fill in an answer. Bringing an attitude of curiosity enables you to traverse *that relational space between knowing and not knowing*. As learners and teachers, we have found that when people think they know something, they are less likely to see what they do not know and thereby less likely to learn. They lose the curiosity that is the impetus for learning. Therefore, as a relational inquirer, we invite you to step out of a stance of knowing from your life experience and/or prior study, consider other ideas and conceptualizations, and explore previously unthought-of possibilities.

Relating to Complexity and Uncertainty

As a relational inquirer, you also need to engage with complexity. We will be inviting you to enter ambiguous and uncertain situations and develop effective ways of relating within them. We'll ask you to look through new lenses and risk seeing in new ways. Learning is risky business. It is far less risky to carry on with the status quo and do things according to the dominant norms in nursing and health care. Throughout the book, however, we ask you to see patients/families, yourself, colleagues, and the systems in which you practice from vantage points from which you may not have looked before.

Relating to Vulnerability

Relational inquiry brings you face to face with vulnerability—your own and that of others. To honestly look at who you are, discover what you believe and value, and how you are living those values and beliefs in practice, you will need to be willing to be uncomfortable and vulnerable—to be willing to be perturbed and discover things about yourself or your practice that you may not like. We believe that discomfort is an important catalyst for learning. When your solid foundations of knowledge and practice are called into question or you bump up against your own lack of knowledge, it may feel uncomfortable, but this discomfort sparks questions and exploration that have the potential to foster your ongoing development as a competent and compassionate nurse. We encourage you to pay attention to your own discomfort. As you are more directly introduced to the vulnerabilities that patients, families, communities, and other nurses live and experience, you may begin to see how those vulnerabilities are being perpetuated—perhaps by your own contradictory values and/or by some of the normative practices within health care in which you yourself have participated. In inviting you into these vulnerable relational spaces, we encourage you to bring compassion to yourself and to others. Compassion offers a way of being and orienting relationally in the midst of discomfort and angst. It allows us to join and be in our "common suffering" (the root meaning of compassion) as we explore new possibilities for action.

Scrutinizing and Developing Our Habits of Practice

Part of the intent of nursing education is to provide the opportunity for you to develop deeply ingrained ways of being, ways of knowing, and ways of doing that are consistent with the values, ideals, and competencies of the nursing profession—that is, to develop habits of knowing/being/doing that are helpful to and support good nursing care. While we have that educative intent in writing this book, we also want to provide the opportunity for you develop the "habit" of *not* acting habitually. Paradoxically, we want you to develop the habit of scrutinizing your taken-for-granted ways of knowing/being/doing—to see your habits in action so you can more consciously choose and respond in nursing situations.

We Are Our Habits

Habits can be thought of as the taken-for-granted truths and ingrained actions that shape our practice. Taken up in a nonreflective way, these truths become bodily responses and flow through us unconsciously. As patterns of activity, these habits are constantly reproduced by us in a nonreflective way. As we learn to think and act in particular ways, those ways become ingrained in our bodily responses and flow through us unconsciously. Elias (1978, 1982) has clearly described how habitual ways of acting are so deeply integrated that they extend to how we conduct ourselves bodily. People discipline and control their own bodies according to the social groups within which they live and work. The "busy gait" of nurses (Tomlinson, 1988) is an example of embodied habits of conduct. This "busy gait" conveys messages to patients and other staff about how efficient and organized a nurse is and the extent to which a nurse has time, is available, or can be interrupted or asked for help.

Habits Are Helpful

Simply put, we all operate with habits. Dewey (1922) contended that part of the reason habits are so powerful is that they start out as helpful. They provide an expertise and efficiency necessary for daily living. As

Dewey (1922) described, a sailor can be at home on the sea, a hunter in the forest, a scientist in the laboratory. Concrete habits do all the perceiving, recognizing, imagining, recalling, judging, conceiving, and reasoning in such an efficient way that energy and attention can be freed up for other activities and possibilities (Dewey, 1922). Therefore, the mechanism of habit is indispensable. The constant interruption of consciously searching for and intentionally performing each act would make daily life impossible.

Driving is a good example of how one develops and integrates habits. If you drive a car, think back to when you first learned and how everything felt so strange—how each time you got in the car you had to think about starting the car, putting it in gear, releasing the parking brake, and so forth. After a while, however, it is likely that the action of driving has become so habituated that you no longer need to think about what you are doing. In this way, habits are very helpful.

Habits Are Problematic

Nevertheless, habits alone are problematic. "With habit alone, there is a machine-like repetition, a duplicating recurrence of old acts" (Dewey, 1922, p. 180). By themselves, habits are too organized, too insistent, and too determinate. Because they are so adapted to the environment, they no longer need to be analyzed, and if left unchecked, habits end in thoughtless action (Dewey, 1922).

The power of habit was brought home to me (Gweneth) during a trip to New Zealand. Having learned to drive in Canada where the passenger seat is on the right-hand side of the car, as a passenger, I found it amazingly difficult to move beyond the habit of walking to the right-hand side of the car to get in. Unless I paid very close attention, I would inadvertently walk to the wrong side of the car. It is this gap between what we intend and what we habitually do that we will be asking you to notice.

Given that we all operate from habit and those habits can be helpful or constraining, the more awareness we bring to that gap, the more we can align our actions with our chosen values and intentions. Our intention in this book is to help you consciously develop habits of practice that are consistent with nursing values and commitments and will serve you to be effective in your nursing practice.

Orienting to Knowledge and Knowledge Development

This book takes a pragmatic perspective as described by pragmatist philosophers such as William James, John Dewey, Richard Rorty, and Barbara Thayer-Bacon. From a pragmatic perspective, all knowledge is understood to be limited and fallible, and any theory or expert truth is considered to be in need of continual scrutiny. As such, a pragmatic view of knowledge assumes the existence of multiple truths and interpretations and considers knowing to be a relational process. Pragmatists contend that all knowledge is "socially constructed by embedded, embodied people who are in relation with each other" (Thayer-Bacon, 2003, p. 10). Said another way, pragmatists assume that what is known is always shaped by who is doing the knowing. Even "facts" are interpreted by people. Thus, pragmatists reject the idea that objective knowledge is possible. From a pragmatic perspective, it is understood that we can never really separate ourselves from our experiences. This means that the knower is always central to the knowing process (the nurse assessing a patient/family is central to the interpretations and diagnoses that are made).

Three features of the pragmatic perspective inform this book.

Knowledge Is Limited

First, because it is impossible to separate human beings from human knowing, it is impossible to obtain knowledge that is certain and/or universal. As Thayer-Bacon (2003) puts it, "The only truths we have access to are derived through our own error-prone . . . procedures" (p. 63). Because as relational beings, all knowers are limited by their particular location and "embeddedness," all knowledge is understood to be limited in its scope and depth. That is, as socially embedded people, we each bring our *"selective interest"* to any experience or situation. Thayer-Bacon (2003) describes selective interest as the bias or attitude that exists in each thought we have. It is our own attitude or selective interest that determines the questions we ask and even the way we go about answering our questions. Selective interest causes us to notice certain things and not others and to attend to certain experiences and not others.

Even scientists and theorists have been shaped by their social worlds and bring selective interests to their work. Thus, no matter how strong the claims to "objectivity" and truth, research always reflects selective interest. Similarly, any theory or framework offers a particular and selected view of individual/family/community and health care situations. Subsequently, one must always scrutinize how any particular concept, theory, or research finding is shaping (and may be limiting) one's views and knowledge of a particular individual/family/community. For example, think about how conceptualizing family as a literal or relational experience shapes your thinking differently.

Knowledge Is Active

The second important feature of a pragmatic approach to knowledge is the connection of knowledge, experience, and practice. In contrast to other views that separate theoretical knowledge from practical knowledge, pragmatists do not see a deep split between theory, practice, and experience. Knowing is considered to be a relational, experiential action. According to pragmatists, knowing is an action, and all so-called theory is understood to arise from and be grounded in experiences and practices (Rorty, 1999). Subsequently, pragmatists share Berman's (2000) contention that "truth" is a verb; it *happens* to an idea. Ideas become true, are *made* true by events (James, 1907). For example, calling patients "bed blockers" shifts attention from the health care experience of the patients to the effect of the patients on the system. This in turn supports health care providers in engaging with patients as problems to be solved. If a nurse's main engagement with a patient focuses on how to get him or her transferred (and we have heard many interactions that begin with "we've got to get that patient moved"), this has an effect on patients and their well-being, perhaps in ways that delay transfer out of the given unit. As we work with patients/families, we are (often unconsciously) continuously theorizing and retheorizing them. And our theorizing shapes how we see, understand, and relate to them. In this way, knowing (and theory) is a living, active process. Our knowledge and theories shape *how* we relate to and within situations.

Knowledge Is Useful

Third, from a pragmatic perspective, the value of knowledge lies in its pragmatic contribution. That is, knowledge is valued because it enables us to be more effective in the world. While one way of evaluating any conceptualization or theory might be to try to determine how "true" or accurate it is, from a pragmatic perspective, it is assumed that we can never know which theory is truer (since there is no one truth). What is important— what gives any theory its value—is not how true it is but how it fosters increased responsiveness to people. Consider how conceptualizing people as bed blockers or limiting your theorizing of family to the literal family might limit responsiveness. For this reason, pragmatism directs us to approach knowledge by specifically focusing on its usefulness for responsive action. For example, any theories or research evidence guiding nursing must be scrutinized according to how useful they are in enhancing our capacity to respond and practice in ways that promote the health and well-being of particular people, families, and communities in particular moments.

TO ILLUSTRATE
The Truth of Family

To consider how ideas (and knowledge) are limited, active, and used to create "reality," let's think about how we understand family and the way in which those understandings are relationally "made" by the media in Western countries. If one looks closely at media representations of family, it is possible to see particular Eurocentric "truths" of family being promoted. For example, marketing people promoting everything from food to health to real estate enlist the truth of family (usually mom, dad, and the two children) as a warm, nurturing, safe haven. Similarly, politicians seeking election will speak of "getting back to family values," as though all families share the same values (Doane, 2003). Journalists wanting to incite people to listen to their news coverage will use the family truths and images (e.g., smiling faces depicting closeness and safety) to emotionalize stories with headlines that read "Family devastated by . . . "

As we are bombarded by such media and live within these strong value messages, we begin to assume certain things about family. Perhaps the most problematic thing we begin to assume is that these values and images are "true." Worse yet, we begin to expect families to function according to these images and truths. Families who model themselves according to these images are seen as healthy, normal, and well-functioning. Families who do not reflect these stereotypical images are deemed "other" and often "less than."

continued on page 27

TO ILLUSTRATE *continued*

The Truth of Family

Instead of seeing media and social images and truths as problematic and therefore revising the truths to more accurately reflect the reality of family in contemporary society, we begin to see families as lacking and in need of revision. One just has to look at the language of "broken family," "single-parent family," "gay/lesbian families," and so forth to see the "othering" that routinely takes place. These descriptions (many of which have been coined by "experts" in academic fields and have subsequently been taken up and used by nurses and other human service professionals) depict how families are "other than" the norm which usually requires no modifiers—the dual-parent, heterosexual norm. Within this othering is the implicit message that families who do not fit the norm are somehow "less than." This is an example of how taken-for-granted ways of thinking and conceptualizing can constrain our understanding and responsiveness. And since all theory and knowledge is developed by people who have been influenced by ideologies and normative ways of thinking, all knowledge needs to be carefully scrutinized for its impact on action.

Becoming Pragmatic

As a result of our pragmatic location, the truth that governs this book is a truth we hold about the most responsive (and responsible) way to live knowledge. Rather than identifying one particular theoretical framework of nursing for you to learn and follow, *we suggest that the way to foster knowledgeable and competent nursing practice is to develop a more conscious, intentional, and responsive way of living knowledge.* By "living knowledge" we mean "living" as a verb—how you enlist your knowledge as you take action. So, for example, any time you encounter practices that are problematic, rather than just accepting that things "are just the way they are," you can live knowledge differently. The nurse in the opening story illustrates this in the way she was questioning ("*Should we just suck it up?*"). To extend her way of living knowledge, she might inquire further. She might ask, "*I wonder if this is really working for the nurses in Emerg*" or "*I wonder if the managers know how this is affecting patients and families.*" From this pragmatic perspective, theory moves beyond an abstraction that is developed in isolation from everyday practice and becomes a practical activity that is central to every nursing moment. Using a relational inquiry approach, you are able to consciously theorize your practice to determine effective action.

In this book, we employ critical and experiential theories, nursing theories from the human science tradition, and contemporary ethical theories as instruments to aid us. The goal is to develop the habit of engaging in thoughtful inquiry to more intentionally and consciously develop your own theories, truths, and forms of nursing practice.

Relational inquiry is guided by an *ethic of social justice*, in which decisions and actions are not only health-promoting and/or economically viable but are also *socially just*. By social justice, we follow Kirkham and Browne's (2006) explanation that while justice has to do with fairness, "*social* draws our attention to the application of justice to social groups, brings into focus how justice and injustices are sustained through social institutions and social relationships, and highlights the embeddedness of individual experience in a larger realm of political, economic, cultural, and social complexities" (p. 325). Social justice infers collectivism over individualism, including the need for collective action.

Practice guided by an ethic of social justice continually asks "So what?" If I do or do not do this, what may the impact be? Such practice is not idealistic in the sense of "being able to fix things" or in overlooking the limitations of the "real world," but it is practice that is *inspired by ideals*. As nurses, we strive toward the ideals of compassion, respect, equitable relations, and the honoring of life in many forms. Regardless of whether we are able to change a particular situation or fix what is wrong in the world, striving toward these ideals supports us in acting in ways that are respectful, compassionate, and equitable and that leave us feeling that we have somehow "done good."

We view practice as a way-of-being as much as a form of action. Thus, relationships, ethics, health promotion, culture, safety, diversity, power, communication, and economics (ideas we explore in detail later in this book) are all integral to any nursing moment. In a relational inquiry approach, these elements fundamentally shape and determine the how, what, and why of practice. As you read this book, participate in the learning activities, and consider the theories in light of your nursing experiences, our intent is to support you in developing ways of viewing and responding more fully to the people, families, colleagues, and systems with whom you work.

Cultivating Habits to Support Relational Inquiry

Three particular habits that we will be inviting you to develop throughout the book include (a) the habit of knowing/not knowing, (b) the habit of humility, and (c) the habit of looking with fresh eyes, in other words, the habit of conscious inquiry.

Developing the Habit of Knowing/Not Knowing

Perhaps one of the most powerful habits that can limit responsive action in health care is that of "knowing." Fuelled by successes of biomedical science and evidenced-based practice, there is a strong tradition of knowing within nursing and health care. Being knowledgeable is seen as the foundation for safe, competent practice. While there is no question that knowledge is vital and we of course want to practice using the latest research evidence, this habit of knowing can actually serve to limit the types of knowledge that are called upon and/or used to inform clinical decision making and action. It also promotes the idea that knowledge is a certain practice (Hartrick, 2002) and that it is possible to know. Given our pragmatic approach, we will be inviting you to develop the habit of walking in that space between knowing/not knowing—to consciously consider what you know and what you do not know, how you relate as a knower, and to experience how a habit of knowing/not knowing can support more responsive and safe nursing practice.

Developing the Habit of Humility

Closely entwined with the habit of knowing/not knowing, and the openness to curiosity it affords, is the habit of humility. People in societies not steeped in humility as a value may confuse humility with weakness or tenuousness. As professionals, we are schooled to become "experts," and often inherent to that process, we are inadvertently schooled to be arrogantly confident in our professional knowledge and to privilege that knowledge over the knowledge and perspectives of the people for whom we care. Being mindful of the limits of our knowledge is critical to high-quality nursing practice. One of the hallmarks of a good nurse is awareness of his or her limitations. Developing the habit of humility as a knower requires confidence and clarity.

Developing the Habit of Looking with Fresh Eyes

Throughout the book, we will also be cultivating the habit of looking with fresh eyes—to move beyond your selective interests and/or the taken-for-granted views to consciously inquire to see more fully. We begin that process by offering the story below.

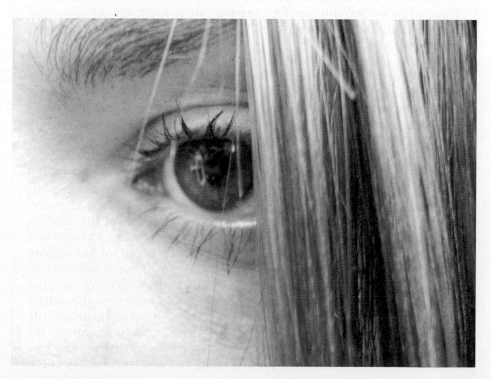

Seeing with fresh eyes.

TO ILLUSTRATE

An Ordinary/Extraordinary Experience

The following is an experience I (Gweneth) had while working with an ethics research team on a medical oncology unit (Hartrick Doane, Storch, & Pauly, 2009; Rodney et al., 2002). As a researcher, I was shadowing a nurse to observe and learn about everyday nursing practice on the unit. Although I had practiced as a nurse for many years and "knew" nursing, as a researcher, I was looking with fresh eyes as I "re-searched" the nursing situation.

We responded to the call bell of an elderly woman who had recently had chemotherapy and was experiencing severe nausea. The woman and her middle-aged daughter, who was in the room with her, were both quite distressed. As it became evident that the woman was about to vomit, the nurse reached for a kidney basin. Looking upset, the daughter stood by, clearly unsure how to help, yet obviously wanting to do something for her mother. Seeing the daughter's distress and her obvious desire to participate, the nurse responded by inviting the daughter to hold the kidney basin. Gently guiding the daughter, the nurse showed her how to position the basin and hold her mother's shoulders for support. With the daughter "in place," the nurse quietly went to a get a damp facecloth and towel. Once again inviting the daughter into the care process, the nurse handed her the cloth and towel and stood by as the daughter gently wiped her mother's face.

On the surface, this was an ordinary, everyday nursing situation. Yet looking with fresh eyes as the "re-searcher," I was able to see the intricacies of the extraordinary relational process that was taking place. The daughter had initially exhibited great anxiety about what to do in response to her mother's nausea. In noticing the daughter's anxiety and also her obvious love and concern, the nurse had responded in such a way as to create the relational space and opportunity for the daughter to express her care in a practical way that was meaningful to both herself and her mother. By *focusing on the relational interplay*, the nurse saw beyond the routine and beyond the surface of everyday occurrence. What made the qualitative difference was the way the nurse addressed the nausea and vomiting by *responding to the whole situation*. The daughter's love and concern as she cared for her mother was almost palpable. Given the woman's prognosis, the significance of this life moment was evident. As I watched, I could clearly see how the nurse orchestrated that moment. While she could have seen the elderly woman as her patient and dealt with the nausea by quickly getting the kidney basin in place herself (showing her expertise and control), *she instead related within the situation as it was meaningfully being lived*. She engaged with the elderly woman, the daughter, and the urgency of the

continued on page 31

> ### TO ILLUSTRATE *continued*
> ## An Ordinary/Extraordinary Experience
>
> nausea all at once. By doing so, she was able to respond in an effective manner to all.
>
> This nurse's action offers an exemplar of relational inquiry practice. With one action, the nurse simultaneously provided physical care to the elderly woman, taught the daughter about how to position her mother to prevent choking or aspiration, offered emotional support to both women, and created a relational bridge through which the daughter and mother shared meaningful time together even in the midst of problematic chemotherapy side effects. At the same time, she explicitly and effectively showed the daughter how she might care for her mother throughout the chemotherapy.
>
> As our team carried on with our research on the unit, we continually witnessed this kind of ordinary/extraordinary nursing practice. Interestingly, at the end of our time on the unit, we were told by many of the nurses that the most valuable contribution of the research had been that it had created an opportunity for *them* to see their own work in new ways; as we pointed things out that we had seen, they started to look with fresh eyes themselves.

The story highlights both the importance of looking beyond habits and consciously choosing our actions. A pressing feature of contemporary health care practice is time. With cuts in staffing ratios, bed utilization strategies, and stretched resources, on the surface, it can seem idealistic to even think it is possible to practice in a relationally responsive way. However, *relational inquiry is not about having the time necessary to practice in the way we ideally would like but rather making conscious choices about how to spend the time we have.* In the above situation, it did not take more time for the nurse to see beyond a nauseated patient on an oncology unit and respond to the particular needs of the people in the situation—and to what might well have been one of the last opportunities a daughter had to express her love and care for her mother. As a skilled practitioner who was very much under time pressures and competing obligations to other patients, the nurse integrated her nursing actions in an adept way to address multiple obligations simultaneously. Ironically, by doing so, she probably ended up actually saving herself time. That is, since the daughter now knew how to respond to her mother's nausea and had a chance to actually experience her ability to do so, it is possible that she would not be calling the nurse for assistance the next time. However, even with that possibility, it is important to distinguish the relational intention. That is, underneath the nurse's action was the clear intention to support the meaningful relational experience of the patient/family which is quite distinct from downloading care to families. It is that distinct intent that made the care relationally responsive.

TRY IT OUT 1.4
Look with Fresh Eyes

The next time you are in practice, observe someone with whom you are working. Try to see this person with fresh eyes. When you see something positive, share your observation with that person. For example, I (Gweneth) remarked on how thoughtful the nurse's action was to the woman and her daughter on the oncology unit and how effective it had been to involve the daughter so skillfully in the woman's care.

Notice what happens. How does your intention to observe with fresh eyes and look for something positive attune you to the situation? Do you see differently than usual? What effect does sharing your observation have?

DEVELOPING YOUR RELATIONAL INQUIRY TOOLBOX

Throughout the book, we will be inviting you to experience relational inquiry as a powerful form of action. By engaging you in a relational inquiry, our intention will be to open the space for you to see each nursing situation with fresh eyes and to cultivate sensitivity to the intricacies of nursing work. It is our hope that in doing so, you will come to know relational inquiry as a form of action through which you can be in and navigate through the complexities of everyday practice, provide high-quality care to patients and families, care for yourself, and also respond to systemic limitations. We also hope it will enable you to, in a deeply meaningful way, experience the extraordinary magic of nursing work.

As you proceed through the chapters in this book, you will have the opportunity to continue considering the ideas put forward in this chapter and to critically look at how you are living knowledge and enacting practice. Whether you are an undergraduate student who has had little clinical experience or are a nurse with many years of practice experience, there are some fundamental questions regarding how one lives knowledge and relationally responds to people and families that must never cease to be asked, questions which we hope to help you cultivate. We are inviting you to join us on a journey of exploration and discovery into terrain that you may not have previously traveled. Similar to when one travels to a foreign country, it is our hope that what you read and experience will not only expand your knowledge and understanding of nursing but also will shake up your thinking about new possibilities for your everyday practice.

We will also be helping you develop a relational inquiry toolbox. Each of the subsequent chapters explores "how to nurse" by examining nursing practice from different vantage points and describes tools (in the form of knowledge, strategies, inquiry frameworks, etc.) for you to enlist in your day-to-day practice. At the end of each chapter, we identify the tools you can add to your relational inquiry toolbox. Chapter 2 focuses on expanding your view and offers two inquiry lenses to add to your toolbox.

Chapter 3 provides direction for discerning your nursing obligations and outlines five capacities (what we call the five Cs) essential to your relational inquiry toolbox. Chapter 4 explores the inseparability of context and culture and how people and their health are constantly shaping and being shaped by them, offering strategies for working across differences. Chapter 5 explicitly focuses on "family nursing as relational inquiry" and offers concrete ways to integrate family into your day-to-day work as a nurse. In Chapter 6, we explore ways of knowing that support relational inquiry and introduce four interrelated modes of inquiry: empirical, ethical, aesthetic, and sociopolitical inquiry. Chapter 7 examines the role of theory in nursing and the value of approaching relational inquiry as a conscious, intentional, theorizing practice. Chapter 8 considers how all nursing action is relational and is shaped by personal values, values that dominate health care, and broader social values. We identify what we call the five Ws of relating that can support more effective nursing action in contemporary health care contexts. Chapter 9 offers four specific relational inquiry strategies and a series of inquiry checkpoints to help you assess whether or not you are putting the strategy into action. Chapter 10 focuses specifically on how to enlist relational inquiry to practice collaboratively within contemporary health care contexts with emphasis on the distinct role that nursing plays within diverse, interprofessional teams. Finally, Chapter 11 explores leadership as a component of every moment of practice and suggests ways in which nurses can lead regardless of whether or not they are in formal positions of leadership.

THIS WEEK IN PRACTICE
Observing the Relational Interplay

To begin to explore a relational inquiry approach, try out this inquiry exercise.

Part 1:
This week when you are in a practice setting (if you are not in practice, you could sit in an emergency waiting room), take a 15-minute window of opportunity to observe. Sit somewhere where you can observe "relationality" in action—that is, where you can watch the interplay of people, situations, and contexts happening (a charting station or waiting room is excellent). Pretend you are reading, studying, or charting so that you don't feel out of place.

Start by noticing the people and their appearances and behaviors. What do you see? Do you find yourself noticing some people over others? What curiosities arise as you watch the different people? Observe the location— the sights, smells, and sounds. Jot down notes on the left-hand half of a piece of paper. Observe the situations that are in play. What are people doing? Who is talking to whom and how? How are the people, contexts, and situations shaping each other?

continued on page 34

THIS WEEK IN PRACTICE *continued*

Observing the Relational Interplay

Notice your own response. What is garnering your attention? Observe yourself—how you are feeling, what you are thinking, what you are wondering, of what you are particularly aware. Begin to analyze what you are seeing and make notes about this as they come to mind on the right half of the paper.

Part 2:

When you are away from the context, complete your analysis. Start by thinking intrapersonally. For example, how did you find yourself interpreting the behavior you observed? Did you find yourself experiencing some people's actions more favorably than others? Why might that be, and what does that tell you about your own thinking?

Then, think interpersonally. What was going on among people? How were they influencing one another? Does anything surprise you? What questions come to your mind? This will raise more intrapersonal questioning—for example, why did you notice what you noticed about the interactions?

Expand your thinking to consider how the context was shaping the interplay. How does the physical setting (space, equipment, lighting) influence what happens? If, for example, you are in a long-term care setting, does it look more institutional or home-like, and what influence do you think this has? Can you infer any "rules" or policies at play? Were there signs conveying certain messages? How did you see the people, context, and situations shaping each other?

Again, this will raise questions about your own thinking. What contextual features stood out for you and why? Putting it all together, can you see any habits or selective interests that shaped your observations? Did you feel uncomfortable about any of your observations or responses? Did you notice yourself making any judgments that surprised you? Did you find yourself averse to certain people? What might you want to explore further?

REFERENCES

Berman, M. (2000). *Wandering god: A study in nomadic spirituality*. Albany, NY: State of New York Press.

Dewey, J. (1922). *Human nature and conduct*. New York: Henry Holt.

Dickoff, J., & James, P. (1968). A theory of theories: A position paper. *Nursing Research, 17*(3), 197–203.

Doane, G. A. (2003). Through pragmatic eyes: Philosophy and the resourcing of family nursing. *Nursing Philosophy, 4*(1), 25–32.

Doane, G. A. (2004). Being an ethical practitioner: The embodiment of mind, emotion and action. In J. Storch, P. Rodney, & R. Starzomski (Eds.), *Toward a moral horizon: Nursing ethics for leadership and practice* (pp. 433–446). Toronto, Ontario, Canada: Pearson.

Duchscher, J., & Myrick, F. (2008). The prevailing winds of oppression: Understanding the new graduate experience in acute care. *Nursing Forum, 43*(4), 191–206.

Elias, N. J. (1978). *The history of manners: The civilizing process* (Vol. 1). Oxford, United Kingdom: Blackwell.

Elias, N. J. (1982). *State formation and civilization: The civilizing process* (Vol. 2). Oxford, United Kingdom: Blackwell.

Guruge, S., & Collins, E. (2008). *Working with immigrant women: Issues and strategies for mental health professionals*. Toronto, Ontario, Canada: Canadian Center for Addictions and Mental Health.

Guruge, S., Khanlou, N., & Gastaldo, D. (2009). Intimate male partner violence in the migration process: Intersections of gender, race and class. *Journal of Advanced Nursing, 66*, 103–113.

Hanson, S. M. H. (2001). *Family health care nursing*. Philadelphia: F. A. Davis.

Hartrick, G. A. (2002). Beyond polarities of knowledge: The pragmatics of faith. *Nursing Philosophy, 3*(1), 27–34.

Hartrick Doane, G. A. (2002). Am I still ethical? The socially mediated process of nurses' moral identity. *Nursing Ethics, 9*(6), 623–637.

Hartrick Doane, G. A. (in press). Cultivating relational consciousness in social justice practice. In P. Kagan, M. Smith, & P. Chinn (Eds.), *Philosophies and practices of emancipatory nursing: Social justice as praxis*. NewYork: Routledge.

Hartrick Doane, G. A., Stajduhar, K., Bidgood, D., Causton, E., & Cox, A. (2012). End-of-life care and interprofessional practice: Not simply a matter of more. *Health and Interprofessional Practice, 11*(3), EP1028.

Hartrick Doane, G. A., Storch, J., & Pauly, B. (2009). Ethical nursing practice: Inquiry-in-action. *Nursing Inquiry, 16*(3), 232–240.

Hartrick Doane, G. A., & Varcoe, C. (2005a). *Family nursing as relational inquiry: Developing health-promoting practice*. Philadelphia: Lippincott Williams & Wilkins.

Hartrick Doane, G. A., & Varcoe, C. (2005b). Toward compassionate action: Pragmatism and the inseparability of theory/practice. *Advances in Nursing Science, 28*(1), 81–90.

Hartrick Doane, G. A., & Varcoe, C. (2007). Relational practice and nursing obligations. *Advances in Nursing Science, 30*(3), 192–205.

Hartrick Doane, G. A., & Varcoe, C. (2008). Knowledge translation in everyday nursing: From evidence-based to inquiry-based practice. *Advances in Nursing Science, 31*(4), 283–295.

James, S. M. (1907). *Pragmatism. A new name for some old ways of thinking*. New York: Longmans, Green & Company.

Kirkham, S. R., & Browne, A. J. (2006). Toward a critical theoretical interpretation of social justice discourses in nursing. *Advances in Nursing Science, 29*(4), 324–339.

Kleffel, D. (1996). Environmental paradigms: Moving toward an ecocentric perspective. *Advances in Nursing Science, 18*(4), 1–10.

Krieger, N. (1999). Embodying inequality: A review of concepts, measures, and methods for studying health consequences for discrimination. *International Journal of Health Services, 29*(2), 295–352.

Labonte, R. (1993). Health promotion and empowerment: Practice frameworks. *Issues in Health Promotion Series No. 3*. Toronto, Ontario, Canada: Center for Health Promotion.

Rodney, P., Hartrick, G. A., Storch, J., Varcoe, C., & Starzomski, R. (2002). *Ethics in action: Strengthening nurses' enactment of their moral agency within the cultural context of health care delivery*. British Columbia, Canada: Social Sciences and Humanities Research Council, University of Victoria.

Rorty, R. (1999). *Philosophy and social hope*. London: Penguin.

Stajduhar, K., Hartrick Doane, G. A., Cook, H., Butcher, C., Cruikshank, S., Bidgood, D., et al. (2008). *Knowledge translation in action: Improving the quality of care at the end of life*. British Columbia, Canada: Canadian Institutes of Health Research.

Thayer-Bacon, B. (2003). *Relational "epistemiologies."* New York: Peter Lang.

Tomlinson, A. (1988). Communication skills. *Nursing, 3*(27), 1006–1009.

Varcoe, C., Doane, G., Pauly, B., Rodney, P., Storch, J. L., Mahoney, K., et al. (2004). Ethical practice in nursing: Working the in-betweens. *Journal of Advanced Nursing, 45*(3), 316–325.

Walker, M. U. (2003). *Moral contexts*. Lanham, MD: Rowman & Littlefield.

World Health Organization. (1984). *Health promotion: A discussion document on the concept and principles*. Geneva, Switzerland: Author.

World Health Organization. (1986). *Ottawa charter for health promotion*. Geneva, Switzerland: Author.

Wright, L. M., & Leahey, M. (2012). *Nurses and families: A guide to family assessment and intervention* (6th ed.). Philadelphia: F. A. Davis.

2 Using Theoretical Lenses to Support Relational Inquiry

LEARNING OBJECTIVES

By engaging with the material in this chapter, you will be able to:

1. Describe the importance of relational inquiry at the point-of-care.

2. Explain how hermeneutic phenomenologic (HP) and critical lenses can expand the quality of your perceptions in nursing.

3. Describe how hermeneutic phenomenologic and critical lenses work in concert and support the relational inquiry process.

4. Demonstrate an ability to examine nursing situations and nursing practice from several vantage points.

I n this chapter, we introduce two lenses, the hermeneutic phenomeno-logic (HP) and critical lenses, that serve to expand relational consciousness and guide the inquiry process toward effective nursing action.

ENGAGING IN RELATIONAL INQUIRY

Engaging in a relational inquiry enables you to both expand and deepen your views of health/illness situations. It enables you to focus your attention as a nurse, discern what is most important in any situation, and work between what you know and what you do not know. Moreover, it enables you to move beyond an individualist orientation and your own selective interests and purposefully look at any situation from multiple vantage points.

TO ILLUSTRATE

Inquiry into the Living Experience of COPD

A number of years ago, I (Gweneth) worked with a group of nurses who wanted to develop their health-promoting practice for people living with chronic obstructive pulmonary disease (COPD). The nurses expressed great frustration. For example, one nurse said that after 20 years

continued on page 37

TO ILLUSTRATE *continued*

Inquiry into the Living Experience of COPD

of work, she had reached the point of wondering "what the point was." No matter what she did, people didn't seem to respond. Not only did they not show up for their appointments at the outpatient clinic where she worked, but they also continued with behaviors (such as smoking) that were obviously detrimental to their health. As an example, she described a woman for whom she felt that all of her time and hard work had been "for nothing."

In response to the nurses' frustration, I suggested that we undertake a relational inquiry into their nursing challenges by simulating a clinic visit. To help the nurses gain more insight into what might be happening for their patients, I suggested that the nurse who had mentioned the particular woman she'd tried to help take that patient's role in the simulation. My intent was that the inquiry would provide an opportunity to *inquire into the nursing situation*—to examine what was happening for the woman with COPD, for the nurse, and between them that was significant to the provision of nursing care.

Within a couple of minutes of beginning the simulation, "the patient" became more and more resistant to the nurse with whom she was interacting. A few more minutes passed, and suddenly the nurse who was in the patient role stopped and exclaimed, "This is horrible! It's not that I don't want to comply with the treatment; I just find it so hard to even think about doing what you're asking me to do. It's so overwhelming to think of making the changes you are telling me I need to make. You have no idea how it will change my life, and I am not sure I want my life to change in that way." She then turned to the rest of us with a look of total amazement on her face exclaiming, "It is so clear to me now why people have not responded—what I am telling them is what is important to *me* as a nurse, not necessarily what is important to *them*!"

Seeing beyond Your Own Selective Interests and Blind Spots

Seeing the experience of COPD from another vantage point, the nurse had recognized that her narrow view was at the center of her nursing difficulty. Looking only from the vantage point of her nursing concerns, she had failed to see the wider picture of the woman's life and what her nursing interventions might actually mean for the woman. The nurses were asking the patients not merely to change a few behaviors. The changes would require the patients to fundamentally alter their lives. However, because the nurses were interpreting the patients' behaviors through their own limited understanding, interests, and concerns, they were blinded to the magnitude of their requests. In their eyes (and clinical judgment), the patients were simply "noncompliant."

To move beyond their limited understanding and approach, three levels of inquiry were needed. First, intrapersonal inquiry was needed to consider what might be happening for patients beneath the surface. For example, what was most important to patients in their everyday lives, and how did the illness and treatment protocols factor into that? How were the patients' concerns and values similar and/or different from the nursing concerns and values? Once the nurses gained insight into this intrapersonal disjuncture, they could more effectively orient themselves interpersonally. They were able to see that, rather than collaboratively working toward the goal of supporting a meaningful life *with* their patients (remember the socio-environmental perspective of health from Chapter 1), they had been working from their own personal assumptions about what a full and meaningful life might be (e.g., to get well physically). Their nursing assumptions about how best to create a full life with COPD (e.g., give up smoking and fully comply with the COPD program) had dominated. Looking contextually at how current health care systems privilege physical health and biomedical intervention, it is possible to see how the nurses' intrapersonal and interpersonal imperatives arose and how they came to reduce their patients' health experience to a "problem" that needed "fixing." That is, it is possible to see how contextual values shaped the focus of their care toward that end. Most importantly, this oversight prevented the nurses from asking their patients what was of particular meaning and concern to them. In essence, the simulation allowed the nurses to shift *from an individualist orientation to a relational orientation*. In so doing, it enhanced their ability to respond effectively.

In order for the nurse in the above story to nurse effectively, she needed to expand her view and see beyond her own blind spots. This is where relational inquiry is of value. Together, the two components of relational inquiry (relational consciousness and inquiry) enable you to extend your view to see the relational interplay that is shaping everyone and everything in the situation; offer a more expansive vantage point through which to know and practice as a nurse by orienting attention toward the intrapersonal, interpersonal, and contextual levels; provide a fuller picture of people's and families' health and illness situations and attune you to what is most significant; and tailor your nursing interventions to correspond with and affect well-being at all levels.

Expanding the Quality and Focus of Perception

I (Gweneth) am a budding photography enthusiast. In attempting to develop my knowledge and skill in photography, I have realized how similar the process of photography is to the process of relational inquiry. At its heart, good photography requires one to develop an expansive way of relating to the world that extends the perceptual quality of engagement. It involves developing the ability to see widely and fully yet simultaneously focus so one can select, from a vast array of visual stimuli, the particular elements and details that are significant in a picture.

Relational inquiry rests on the premise that effective, competent, high-quality nursing practice is oriented to the living experience of people and families and purposefully extends the view to consider what is shaping the living experiences within, between, and around any patient/family or health care situation. For example, although a number of women may be going through treatment for breast cancer, as unique beings who live particular lives in particular contexts, the meaning of the illness and the best treatment will vary. Moreover, the decisions they make about treatment will depend upon the concerns that are significant to *them* within their own particular lives. Similarly, the treatment options they have available to them and their access to those options is dependent on their context—for example, their geographical locations, economic resources, social/familial support systems, and so forth. To practice effectively, therefore, nurses must extend their view to see how all of these elements and levels are interrelated and informing nursing care.

TO ILLUSTRATE

Seeing beyond the Microscopic Slide

The importance of looking beyond selective interests and expanding perceptions was highlighted by a physician during a forum on breast cancer that I (Gweneth) attended a number of years ago. Speaking to an audience of physicians from various specialities, nurses, psychologists, and professionals from other health-related fields, he began his presentation by putting up a slide of a microscopic view of breast cancer cells. Putting the slide on the screen, he commented that if he were to ask the oncologists in the room about how best to treat the particular type of breast cancer represented on the slide, although there might be slight variation, a fairly standard treatment would likely be agreed upon. Next, the speaker put up a slide that pictured a woman standing in a garden of flowers with her husband and pointedly stated, "This is the woman whose breast cancer you just saw, and this is where the treatment changes." What the physician was pointing to was how vitally important it is to look beyond our own selective interests as health professionals, in this case the medical diagnosis and disease state. The physician was illustrating that even the treatment of physical disease must be located within the personal and contextual elements of people and their everyday lives.

When looking at a health/illness situation then, your perception needs to be wide enough to encompass people's life experiences and honed enough to recognize the significant details. Relational inquiry enables you to perceive situations in this way. It is similar to how good photographers employ a repertoire of knowledge (e.g., learning about light, composition, Photoshop techniques, etc.) and tools (lens, filters, light, shutter speed, etc.) to both sharpen their perceptual skills and enable them to access and compose a picture that expresses the living experience of what they are attempting to express. Comparably, relational inquiry is supported by developing particular ways of being and relating to the world and by employing knowledge and tools that can expand and sharpen the perceptual quality of your nursing view and engagement—tools that enable you to see widely and yet hone in and select what is most significant and relevant. Two perceptual tools that are particularly helpful and that are central to relational inquiry practice are a hermeneutic phenomenology (HP) lens and a critical lens.

Theoretical lenses are similar to lenses on a camera. By intentionally enlisting specific lenses, you are able to view nursing situations and nursing practice from different vantage points, see different angles, hone in on specific elements, or get a wide-angle view. Hermeneutic phenomenology focuses on people's living experiences and how those experiences are meaningful and interpreted; a critical lens focuses on how the power-laden contexts of people's lives shape their experiences and interpretations. Combined, these two lenses expand what you see when you look at

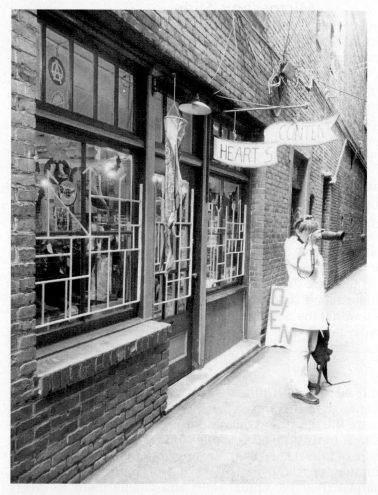

Looking through different lenses. (Photograph by Gweneth Doane.)

people/situations/contexts and thus serve to extend your knowledge and understanding as well as your options for nursing action. In concert with a pragmatic approach in which theories are seen as tools that can enhance our knowing and response to people/families, relational inquiry enlists the HP and critical lenses as pragmatic tools to expand relational consciousness and guide the inquiry process. Table 2.1 can assist you in translating the description of the lenses we present below and identify how they can be used in practice. The table highlights the questions for inquiry prompted at different levels by the HP and critical lenses. Use the table as a guide as you read.

Table 2.1: Lenses

Lens		Intra personal	Interpersonal	Contextual
Hermeneutic Phenomeno-logical Interpretive Analysis		How are people making meaning of their situations? How are different people interpreting situations differently?	How are different interpretations shaping situations and interpersonal relations?	How are people variously situated and constituted?
Critical Power Analysis		How do relative positions of power shape understanding?	How are power dynamics shaping each interpersonal relationship?	How are social structure and arrangements shaping people, situations and interpersonal relationships?
	Critical feminist	How do gender, race, class, age, ability, size, and other forms of social positioning shape understanding?	How do gender, race, class, age, ability, size, and other forms of social positioning shape each interpersonal relationship?	How are gender, race, class, age, ability, size, and other forms of social positioning shaping people and situations?
	Post colonial	How do history, colonial relations and racism shape understanding?	How do history, colonial relations and racism shape each interpersonal relationship?	How do history, colonial relations and racism shape social structures and arrangements?
	Post structural	How doe language shape understanding?	How does language shape each interpersonal relationship?	How does language shape social structures and arrangements?

SEEING THROUGH A HERMENEUTIC PHENOMENOLOGIC LENS

Originating in philosophy, hermeneutic phenomenology has been quite influential within the nursing world, influencing nursing theory, nursing education, nursing research methodologies, and also informing models of nursing practice (Burhans & Alligood, 2010; Earle, 2010; Gerow et al., 2010; McCloughen, O' Brien, & Jackson, 2011). Below, we offer a brief description of some of the central concepts of HP that we have drawn upon to create a lens that is helpful to relational inquiry practice. It is by no means a full description of hermeneutic phenomenology as a philosophy or methodology. A summary of the key concepts, assumptions, and questions within our HP inquiry lens are included in Box 2.1.

TO ILLUSTRATE

A Disobedient Boy

A neighbor once told me (Gweneth) about an experience her son had at school. The school had decided to put on a live theatre production of one of Charles Dickens' stories. All children in her son's class were expected to participate. My neighbor described how distressed her 10-year-old son was at what he saw as violent parts in the story. He had grown up in a family where strong concerns about the condoning of violence in our society were regularly expressed. To him, participating in this play was comparable to participating in a violent act. As a result, he refused to be involved in the play. His teacher viewed his refusal as uncooperative behavior, which she interpreted as disobedience. The school principal viewed the problem as an educational concern, in that by not participating in the play, the boy would miss an essential learning experience. In relating this story to me, the boy's mother was expressing her pride in her son's obvious ability to make his own decisions and assert himself with authority figures.

From this description, it is easy to see how the living experience of each person in this situation was unique and the way in which the living experience of each person arose through the individual interpretations of the situation. Enlisting the earlier photography analogy, it becomes evident that whoever takes the picture (interprets the situation) will determine what is highlighted in the picture. If the mother was taking the picture, it would look quite different (and tell a different story) than if the teacher was taking it. The teacher interpreting the behavior would offer a picture of a disobedient boy, but for the mother, the same behavior was evidence of an assertive boy who acted based on his convictions. Each person's interpretation arose from his or her own personal concerns, interests, and contextual location. As individuals, they each interpreted this situation in different ways, thus experiencing the situation differently.

This story illustrates many of the central features of an HP lens and how it can be helpful to your nursing practice. First, the HP lens draws attention to how our experiences are shaped by our own interpretations (and who is holding the camera). Thus, it draws attention to how the same situation can be experienced differently because different people will interpret and assign meaning based on their own particular locations and concerns. The picture of a patient/family that I (Gweneth) might take and communicate (for example, when I am charting or giving report) is not necessarily the same picture another nurse or the patient might take. This illustrates how any picture offers a somewhat limited view. The HP lens also highlights that the interpretations we make as nurses and how we know and experience particular patients and/or health care situations is dependent on who we are and how we see and interpret. This is because, according to HP, a person is not an individual who merely lives in an environment; he or she is situated in and constituted by that environment.

We Are Situated in the World

Situated means that people do not just live in their environments but they are embodied in their respective worlds (Benner, 2000; Benner & Wrubel, 1989; Lyon, 2009; Robbins & Aydede, 2009). As situated beings, we live in a meaningful world that is informed by our experiences with family, culture, school, work, friendships, and a myriad of other influences. Our everyday smooth functioning in the world is facilitated by sharing a common language and understanding customs and practices. An HP lens focuses on the relationship of the person "in" the world, not separate from it. "World" in this sense goes beyond the physical environment to include the meaningful sets of relationships, practices, and languages that we have by virtue of being born into cultures (Leonard, 1989). From this perspective, it is impossible not to be influenced and shaped by the world because we are an integral part of it, and it is integral to us. People and their worlds are one.

A simple example of how we are situated is how, as nurses, we function in the world of health care. Having been situated in the routines and geography of health care for many years, touching the naked body of a complete stranger is experienced as a normal, everyday occurrence. However, remembering my (Gweneth's) first bed bath as a nursing student on a male urology unit, that same experience had a different meaning. It would be an understatement to say that I felt "out of my element." However, by the time I was finished my nursing program and was "well-situated" in the world of health care, I had become embodied in and by it. That is, how I interpreted and made meaning of experiences was shaped by the years I had practiced as a nursing student and my current location as a nurse. I was at home in the customs and practices and had begun to take them for granted. I have been reminded of just how much I take for granted when friends or family members have been admitted to the hospital and I listen to them describe their experiences and try to make sense of what is happening to and around them in the health care setting.

BOX 2.1

Hermeneutic Phenomenologic Lens

Part A: Underlying assumptions:

- People are not separate from their worlds but are situated in and constituted by them.
- The world influences and shapes people since we are an integral part of it, and it is an integral part of us.
- People have life experiences that are unique in meaning and at the same time have shared meanings with others.
- People can only be understood in relationship to their worlds, for it is only within their contexts that what people value and find significant is visible.

Part B: Enlisting an HP lens to expand your perceptual field and develop relational consciousness:

- How is the person/family situated and constituted?
- What is of particular meaning and concern?
- What is in the picture at the intrapersonal, interpersonal, and contextual levels?
- What is being ignored or overlooked?
- What might be important about their sociohistorical background and location?
- How am *I* framing the living experience of this person/family?
- What in me is shaping my interpretations and the picture I am taking of this person or family?
- How might I expand my perceptual field to know this person or family more fully?

Part C: Enlisting an HP lens to sharpen your focus:

- What is happening for the person or family in this situation?
- What is it like for them to be in this situation?
- What seems to really matter to them (e.g., what do they repeat, what do they emphasize, when does their voice convey that something is important)?
- What do they find challenging or difficult?
- What strengths and capacities do they have?
- What impact is this situation having on their lives?
- What contextual factors are influencing their experience (e.g., resources, lack of resources)?
- What is most important to them in this moment, at this time?
- Given this particular person or family, their living experience, and the contextual realities of this situation, how might I act most effectively and responsively?

We Are Constituted by the World in Us

An HP lens also views people as *constituted*. People become who they are as a result of their sociohistorical experiences, as well as the teachings handed down by previous generations (including cultural do's and don'ts and family norms and standards). Just as we embody the genetic biology of our parents, as we live in the world, we begin to embody the evolving sociocultural norms of our society. We take up experiences, knowledge, and teachings bodily, and they become part of us. Overall, the notion of "constituted" refers to the world that is in us—the world that we have taken up and that has become an integral part of us.

The young boy in the To Illustrate story had grown up situated in a family that abhorred violence. Being situated in his particular family, he had become constituted as a person who was deeply concerned about violence. How he was situated "in" the world (e.g., in his particular family who abhorred violence and in a society that condoned violence in the media) and how he was constituted by the world that was "in" him (for example, the family values and attitudes that had become a part of him) directly shaped the meaning he made of the Dickens play, how he experienced the school project, and how he was compelled to act. Similarly, how his teacher and the school principal were each situated and constituted gave rise to different meanings and truths about the same situation.

TRY IT OUT 2.1

Examine Nursing as Situated and Constituted

Think back to the earlier story of the nurses in the COPD clinic. Can you see how being situated in the health care world that is dominated by the biomedical imperatives of treating disease shaped their interpretations of their patients? Can you see how the values and norms they practiced within became embodied to the point that they shaped their own emotional responses? How they were situated and constituted shaped not only their nursing interpretations and assessment (the woman was interpreted as a noncompliant patient) but also their own nursing experiences (they felt frustrated, ineffective, and perplexed).

Nursing is situated within and constituted by the larger social world, and as we will explore throughout this book, it is shaped by multiple competing influences. We have already pointed to the influence of individualism and biomedicine. To illustrate the HP lens and the idea of being situated and constituted, let's look a bit further at some of the other dominant influences shaping nursing and what you as a nurse are situated in and being constituted by.

TO ILLUSTRATE
Seeing the Impact of Eurocentrism and Racialization

Nursing is situated in the larger world in which race and cultural privilege are social structures that shape how people think and act. Subsequently, these social structures influence how nurses think and act as they go about their work. We select this example because Western nursing has been profoundly shaped by Eurocentric ways of thinking and by white cultural privilege ("whiteness") (Allen, 2006; Gustafson, 2007; Puzan, 2003; Wilby, 2009).

Eurocentrism is the ideology that assumes European and North American values and technologies are superior to those of others (Hall, 1999). It is not simply values, beliefs, and practices enacted by people descended from white Europeans. Rather, it has been globally promoted. Western health care in particular has been infused with Eurocentric views and practices. Simple examples of the influence of Eurocentrism include the normative practices in terms of the diet menus in hospitals, how visiting hours are structured, how visitors are treated, and so forth. Similarly, whiteness (privileging whiteness) is not just a set of practices enacted by "white people." Rather, being situated in a world that is shaped by race relations, we are all affected (becoming constituted by them). For example, within the dynamics of "white privilege," describing someone as a "white person" is less common than identifying people with other skin tones by "race." Have you ever observed how health care providers tend to use racial and/or ethnic descriptors more with people who do not have a white skin color or are of non-European descent? Consequently, some people, including nurses, are more likely to be *racialized*—a process of assigning racial categories in which a person's apparent "race" becomes an important feature and associated with social characteristics (e.g., "whites are selfish").

Enactment of these dominant views has been perpetuated in nursing by the fact that historically, nursing has primarily been a "white" profession. Despite the ethnic diversity of people entering nursing today, in many countries, the nursing workforce and/or leadership is predominantly white. Indeed, nursing leaders in most Western countries have been calling for greater ethnic diversity in nursing, in part to better reflect the populations served and in part in hopes that people marginalized by racial and ethnic discrimination will be better served.

Regardless of the ethnic composition of the nursing workforce, because nursing is situated in the larger world, these dynamics continuously influence nurses' educational experiences and their experiences within the workforce and their practices. For example, Ryan's research (2007) highlights how racialization and Eurocentrism work together in nursing contexts. Ryan explored how Irish migrant nurses working in Britain were positioned ambiguously as both white, European insiders (relative to "other" ethnicities) as well as cultural outsiders. Similarly, in a study of Polish nurses working in Norway, van Riemsdijk (2010) found that Europeanness and Norwegianness were constructed in complex, shifting forms in relation to changing notions of whiteness and that the partial inclusion of certain migrants more fully excluded migrants of color who were not able to benefit from white privilege. She argued that ideas of "whiteness" in nursing which have been developed based on whiteness studies from the United States are not adequately nuanced to account for national and ethnic specificities. The researcher proposes that notions of variegated whiteness are needed to investigate differential inclusion. Thus, which nurses are more or less racialized and interpreted as "others" in their educational and work experiences depends on context (where and how they are situated). Think of your own educational or work context. Who is usually racialized, and who is not usually racialized? What is the impact of this racialization?

Eurocentrism and white privilege also shape nursing education. These entities dominate nursing theory (Allen, 2006), curricula (Hagey & MacKay, 2000), the composition of faculty (Hassouneh, 2008), educational experiences (Scammell & Olumide, 2012), and textbooks (Byrne, 2001). These factors shape what students learn and believe about nursing. Racialization relies on racial categories, and because racial categories are constructed as different and unequal in ways that lead to social, economic, and political effects (Galabuzi, 2001), nurses who are racialized are often treated differently in both educational and practice settings from those who are not. Moreover, since these racialized practices are embedded within their education, students come to see them as normal; they see and experience themselves and others in that way.

Racialization can lead to ineffective and at times detrimental action. When teachers, fellow students, and those in practice racialize students as "others," student success can be impaired (Jackson et al., 2011; Markey & Tilki, 2007; Martin & Kipling, 2006). For example, in the hospitals where I (Colleen) teach students, it is common practice for staff to identify some students as "Chinese" or "South Asian," whereas students who are visibly white are not identified in any racialized way. Sometimes, staff members make assumptions about racialized students; for example, they assume that they might speak certain languages, but of course, a person's physical appearance or last name doesn't convey linguistic skill or nationality. As a clinical teacher supervising students in a range of clinical settings, I have had to work against the tendency for nurses to racialize certain students and assign those students to patients who the nurses thought were of the "same" ethnicity. The nurses often intended to promote better care for patients through what they assumed would be the student's language skills or familiarity with the patient's culture. However, first, this did not necessarily serve the student's learning needs (that were usually focused on providing care related to particular health issues or using particular skills). When the student *did* speak a language in addition to English that was similar to that of the patient's first language, the student ended up spending more time interpreting than learning nursing. Second, it almost never served the patients well. Broad categories such as "Chinese" or "South Asian" encompass an incredible diversity of people. For example, in Canada, there are multiple generations of people descended from hundreds of countries, speaking hundreds of languages and dialects, so there was rarely a match even on these dimensions. Further, these practices elevated racialization to a central process in care for certain students and patients. Occasionally, time was saved for the staff, albeit at the expense of the student's learning and/or responsive patient care.

The negative effects of Eurocentrism, white privilege, and racializing processes on nurses' health and well-being do not end with their educational experiences. They can also affect nurses' career advancement (Allan, Larsen, Bryan, & Smith, 2004; Hagey et al., 2001; Kovner, Brewer, Wu, Cheng, & Suzuki, 2006; Shields & Price, 2002). For example, in the United States, echoing wider social dynamics, the history of black nurses has been a constant struggle against racism (Grypma, 2003; Johnson, 2008) with evidence of significantly higher stress and moral distress for contemporary black nurses compared to others in their workplaces (Corley, Minick, Elswick, & Jacobs, 2005; Kovner et al., 2006; Ulrich et al., 2007).

While these dynamics have particularly negative effects on those who are racialized, we all have a relationship to white privilege. The dynamics of racializing and enacting white and Eurocentric privilege serve to shape us at the intrapersonal, interpersonal, and contextual levels. Intrapersonally, these ways of thinking and interpreting are internalized as people become constituted by them. That is, people begin seeing and relating to themselves according to these values and norms; they begin thinking of themselves respectively in better or lesser ways (often unconsciously). Interpersonally, these discriminatory practices become habits of interpretation and conduct. Contextually, whole social systems operate to keep such dynamics in place. For example, a study in Canada showed how many within health care settings had a vested interest in denying racial discrimination so that nurses who made complaints experienced reprisals (Turrittin, Hagey, Guruge, Collins, & Mitchell, 2002). Regardless of your own self-identity, your way of thinking about yourself and others always occurs *in relation* to Eurocentrism and racial categorizing since these aspects are practiced widely in health care environments.

As a nurse, you will be practicing in contexts influenced by the dominance of whiteness, Eurocentrism, and racializing processes. Whether in any given context you are racialized as "other," seen as part of the dominant group, or both, you need to thoughtfully decide how to practice in relation to these dynamics as you move between contexts. Trying to be "colorblind" or "treat everyone the same" just makes room for "usual practice," which typically supports normative patterns of dominance. Whether you aim for this neutrality, actively reinforce normative patterns, or actively resist and work to change them, you are relating to them in some way.

An HP lens can bring attention to how you and the patients/families you care for are situated within these broader social systems and, as such, how you are being constituted by them, including how your own identity and nursing action is informed through them. Using an HP lens highlights and helps us see how our own views are limited and how our interpretations are being shaped by our own locations and backgrounds. As we expand our consciousness using an HP lens, we can form allegiances across various differences to promote equality and social justice with colleagues as well as with individuals and families to whom we provide care. Attention is drawn to the interpretations we are making about people, ourselves, and our experiences and what is shaping those interpretations. We are also guided to inquire into meaning—both shared and unique meanings and interpretations.

We Have Shared and Unique Meanings

The HP lens also draws attention to shared and unique meanings. This idea of shared and unique meanings is important. A simple example is the experience of having a cold. The actual course of the illness for each of us is unique (e.g., what exact symptoms we get and how they affect us) and what the cold means for us varies (it might give us a valid reason to get some much needed rest, or it might mean missing out on something we really wanted to do). As well as unique meanings, each of us shares an understanding of what it is like to have a cold. Having had the experience, we are sensitized to what it is like to have a headache, runny nose, cough, and fatigue. However, a vital distinction is that we can't really know what it is like for another person in a particular moment of time unless that person tells us of his or her experience.

Given this understanding that situations have unique meanings for people and those unique meanings shape their experiences, it is important for nurses to inquire into how people are *meaningfully experiencing* an illness or disease condition. The same physical illnesses, injuries, risk factors, or other health issues, and the way people engage with health care professionals and/or "adhere" to treatments, will be determined by their own particular concerns and what is meaningful and significant to them in their lives at that particular time within those particular circumstances. Importantly, given how people and families are constituted and situated differently, a patient's or family's concerns might differ from our own nursing concerns since what they value might be different from what matters to us as health care providers.

We Have Different Values and Concerns at Different Times

Depending on how people are situated and constituted, their meaningful experience of events, actions, and situations result in different concerns and priorities. The HP lens draws attention to what is of particular value and concern to people at different times. For example, once again thinking of the experience of having a cold, within that same experience, different things will be of concern and significance to different people. For a mother with a new baby, giving the cold to her baby might be of particular concern; for a mother situated in a low-paying job without paid sick leave, being unable to work might be of greatest concern. If a patient visits a physician for treatment, the physician's particular concern might be preventing the cold from turning into pneumonia. For the woman in prison, a cold might be of little significance in contrast to her other concerns. For this reason, in relational inquiry, an HP lens is used to gain an understanding of people in relation to their world, for it is only within those contexts that what people value and find significant is visible.

For example, I (Gweneth) had a back injury in my early 20s. At the time of my injury, I was working in psychiatry. Given that the physical aspect of my nursing work was not too onerous, after recovering from surgery, I was still able to work. The most significant meaning of the injury was that it limited my physical activity and my engagement in regular recreational sports. When I moved the following year and started working in emergency, my back injury took on a whole new meaning. I found lifting patients and moving heavy stretchers challenging. This concern led me to see an exercise physiologist so I could learn how to care for my back as I worked. A few years after that, following the birth of my first son, probably due to hormonal changes, my back flared up to the point that I was flat in bed for a couple of weeks. My biggest concern at that point was how I was going to care for my son. I went to physiotherapy and diligently did the exercises and procedures the physiotherapist suggested to address the inflammation because I urgently needed to be functional again in my life and be able to care for my son.

My back experience offers an example of how, as people, our lives are ordered by our own networks of concerns. It also highlights how a patient or family's concerns might be different from our own concerns as nurses. Given those differences, we can enlist the HP lens to (a) inquire into what is of particular meaning and concern to the patients and families for whom we are caring, (b) identify how those concerns might differ from our own health care provider concerns, and (c) look for the connection between people's concerns and our nursing care. For example, in the case of my back injury, the nursing action could be targeted specifically to what was meaningful to me at a particular time. By working with me to address my primary concern at a particular point in time (e.g., get back into sports, be able to work a 12-hour shift in the ER, be able to care for my young son), as the patient, I would be motivated to engage in any treatment protocols, and the nursing care could not only be more targeted but more meaning-ful. This idea *of targeting nursing action in meaningful ways to connect across differing concerns* is an important concept that we will continually revisit throughout the book.

TO ILLUSTRATE
Visiting Hours

To illustrate meaning, values, and concerns as shared, unique, and tempo-ral, let's further consider how everyday nursing practices can be influenced by Eurocentrism and racializing processes. A few years ago, I (Colleen) was asked to work with an acute care hospital to help them integrate the idea of cultural competence. I was asked to give a talk about the ideas to nurses from many different settings. I gave a short talk and then asked the nurses to talk about how they saw culture as relevant to their practice. The hospital is located in a community that has grown exponentially over the past few decades, shifting from being composed primarily of descendants of people who emigrated from European countries (mostly the United Kingdom, Germany, and Holland) to the majority being new immigrants primarily from India (referred to as the South Asian community). The nurses (mostly from the former group) immediately brought up the "problem" of visitors. Many expressed considerable frustration that families of recent immigrants had so many visitors all the time. In some units, the nursing staff had instituted "tougher" visiting hours and set limits, such as "two visitors per patient," and they wanted similar policies hospital-wide.

continued on page 51

TO ILLUSTRATE *continued*

Visiting Hours

I asked what their concerns were. They listed a range of issues. First, they could not get care done because family members were in their way. It was obvious that their concerns were specific to getting their nursing work done. Each time I addressed an issue, a new one would be raised. For example, when I asked how the nurses handled this with non-South Asian families, they responded that they were "comfortable" asking such visitors to step out when they wanted to do care, and perhaps they could do so with South Asian families, except language barriers were problematic. When I addressed possible solutions for language barriers, they said, yes, but when direct care wasn't being done, the patients could not get enough rest, other patients were disturbed by the noise, and so on.

One nurse angrily said, "They seem to think that every member of the temple [referring to Hindu and Sikh places of worship] has to visit!" I tried using the example of my mother who had recently been hospitalized for acute pancreatitis. At least two to three different members of her Bible study group visited her daily, and friends and family had "come out of the woodwork" to visit. I thought she was exhausted and asked her to cut back her visitors. She said she would rather be exhausted and have the comfort of her priest and other visitors; further, the nurses had moved her to a private room. Some of the nurses in the group could see the parallels, but others were visibly angry at the comparison.

For me, this experience directly illustrated how different values, meanings, and concerns play out within the dominance of Eurocentrism and racializing processes. The issue of visiting hours is often contentious, and this is rooted in health care traditions that focus on the individual as separate from his or her context and family and on the control and responsibility for care resting with professional health care providers. While all the nurses wanted to provide good nursing care, they varied in the extent to which they could see the similarities and differences between themselves and their patients and families, particularly when the latter were racialized as "other."

TRY IT OUT 2.2

Look for Racialization

Think back to the practice setting in which you did your observations for "This Week in Practice" in Chapter 1. Review the notes you made. What evidence did you see of racializing processes during your observations? Intrapersonally, were you more likely to notice the race or ethnicity of some people and not others? Interpersonally and contextually, did you notice any patterns? For example, do certain roles (e.g., technician, nurse, janitor, physician, food services staff) tend to be filled by any ethnic groups? What do you think supports these processes or patterns or the lack of them?

Enlisting the Hermeneutic Phenomenologic Lens to Target Nursing Action

The HP lens can be used to help us (a) consider how we are absorbing dominant values and normative practices and how they are shaping how we think and feel about ourselves and about others; (b) orient to and understand illness as a meaningful, temporal experience in which people will bring differing concerns and values; and (c) more effectively target our nursing action. The HP lens guides us to inquire into particular concerns and priorities and to ask what is important and significant at different points in time. Understanding the unique meanings and concerns enables us to target our nursing actions in specific ways.

TO ILLUSTRATE
Relational Inquiry in Asthma Care

A number of years ago, I (Gweneth) was asked by administrators from a large acute care hospital and a public health agency to conduct education sessions with a multidisciplinary team of health practitioners working with families and children living with asthma. The focus of the educational sessions was socio-environmental health-promoting practice. In conjunction with the education, I conducted an educative-research project (Hartrick, 1998a) to document the shifts in practice that occurred when the team members intentionally moved their practice from a medical individualist-based approach to a socio-environmental relational one.

The most predominant finding in the research was how, in concrete and pragmatic ways, the team's focus of care moved from their overriding emphasis on reducing the children's asthma to focusing on enhancing the families' health experiences and their capacity to live with and manage asthma in their everyday lives. Through their experiences, the team developed an appreciation for the complexity of people's lives and how this influenced families' experiences of asthma. As they began to see and inquire into the families' experiences and respond to what was meaningful and significant to them, the team members' practice changed in several ways. First, the team moved from thinking of themselves as experts in asthma care to seeing themselves as facilitators of health. They came to see health through a socio-environmental perspective and began focusing their attention on the families' ability to realize their aspirations and live meaningful lives. This change is reflected in the following quotes. The first quote exemplifies the descriptions of the participants during the initial interview at the beginning of the project.

> I'm the one that has the knowledge, and I want to make sure that they can learn from that. Their role is first of all to learn something about their disease process and how to prevent it, or make it worse, or how to recognize signs when it is getting worse ... just to recognize, not to be in so much denial about it.

continued on page 53

TO ILLUSTRATE *continued*

Relational Inquiry in Asthma Care

The next quotes are characteristic of the descriptions given during the final interviews and reveal the shift in their practice focus that took place.

Going to people and finding out what they need to know is the best way to go for it to succeed.

Rather than having concrete goals, the goals are more nebulous now, and the families are coming in when they want to; it's like a dance almost. You're trying to get them on this health promoting dance ... they dance alone when they want to, or dance away ... I'm trying to make sure that the floor isn't slippery, they're not going to fall off the edge, that kind of stuff.

A second change involved moving from focusing on asthma to focusing on children and families. For example, rather than focusing on giving asthma information and therefore giving the information that they thought families needed to know, the nurses began to inquire into the needs of particular families. As one nurse describes:

In the beginning, I used to go with my big pile of papers and go in there, and they'd barely say hello, and do you want a coffee, and I'd go into my thing about their asthma. And now I'm more relaxed about just letting them tell me what their needs are, and where I can help them, and not just giving them information they need for the asthma part ... listening to where they're coming from.

Another fundamental shift was how the team members moved from an "outsider" to an "insider" perspective of illness. According to Conrad (1987), an outsider perspective of illness views illness from outside the experience. An insider perspective focuses directly on the subjective experience of living with and managing an illness. An insider perspective includes understanding the meaningful experience of the illness as well as knowledge of the disease process. As the team members strove to become more health promoting, they became aware of the significance of the personal meaning in people's health and illness experiences. Consequently, their care became focused on responding to the meaningful experiences of the families living with asthma.

This shift to an insider perspective meant that the team members moved from a stance of telling to one of inquiring. For example, rather than providing standard information to all families, the members began asking about the families' experiences and providing information and teaching based on the context of those experiences.

My beliefs have come around a different way, ... and it wasn't until I realized that they weren't really listening to me ... I could see where I wasn't looking at them as people. I was looking at them as a client, and I had to give this asthma information, and now I just feel totally different about it, I don't know how to explain it, I just feel totally different.

continued on page 54

TO ILLUSTRATE *continued*

Relational Inquiry in Asthma Care

One of most predominant changes was the profound shift that occurred for the team members with regard to their views of health and health promotion and how that change in perspective shifted the way they targeted their actions. During the final interviews, they all referred to social determinants of health and the importance of looking at "the bigger picture." They had moved from thinking of their work as individual-focused to realizing the "power of bringing people together." They had come to see how a socio-environmental perspective that focuses on enhancing peoples' sense of empowerment and choice was conducive to concrete outcomes such as decreasing the number of hospital admissions. And they saw how focusing on families' living experiences and what mattered to them in their everyday lives could not only be more effective in helping families manage asthma but also contribute to a decrease in hospital admissions.

It is important to highlight the focus and effort it took on the part of the asthma team members to actually affect such shifts in their practice. For some of the members, the move to a socio-environmental perspective of health promotion and relational inquiry required a complete reconfiguration of their practice. No longer the "expert," they had to learn to look beyond their own preconceived ideas and knowledge to seek out the knowledge the family had to offer. They needed to learn how to inquire into what mattered to families and not just follow their own professional agendas. Their learning involved figuring out how to "collaborate with" rather than "do to" and "do for" families.

TRY IT OUT 2.3

Looking through an HP Lens

Reread the quotes from the educative-research project in the To Illustrate box as you look through an HP lens. Look at the pre-education quotes. How are the nurses seeing and interpreting health? How did their own nursing concerns shape how they initially worked with families? Next, look at the quotes from the nurses at the end of the education. How did their nursing concerns change during the educative-research project? Can you identify some specific examples of how they expanded their perceptual fields and became more relationally conscious? What did they start seeing and looking for as their views expanded? How did their expanded views change their nursing actions?

SEEING THROUGH A CRITICAL LENS

While an HP lens points to the social context as important to understanding meaning and living experience, a critical lens focuses attention on the contexts themselves—how the social, political, historical, economic, and linguistic features of the world are shaping lives and our nursing practice. Within what we are calling a critical lens, we include three overlapping elements or perspectives—the feminist, the postcolonial, and the poststructural—to focus attention on power and the social context. Using a critical lens draws explicit attention to power, inequities, and structural determinants of health. *Structural* refers to basic structures in society such as local, state, and global political economies, globalization, racialization, and institutions such as health, legal, educational, and government systems (Browne, 2001). *Inequities* refers to differences that arise from social arrangements that are unfair (Whitehead & Dahlgren, 2006). A critical lens helps us examine how structural conditions and inequities shape people, health, and health care, aligning with a socio-environmental view of health.

A critical lens directly focuses attention on power, oppression, culture, economic conditions of life, social change, and emancipation. This lens is a fairly wide-angle view that is informed by and encompasses many perspectives and sociologic theories—all of which are aimed at challenging and disrupting what is taken for granted ("the status quo") by digging beneath the surface of society and examining the assumptions that shape our understanding of how the world works. Using the photography analogy once again, the critical lens helps us look beyond the surface features to examine the multiple layers beneath. A critical lens helps you both take a wide-angle view (so that you can see how broad social structures, inequities, power dynamics, language, etc. operate generally) and to take a close-up view (so that you can see how these same social structures, inequities, power dynamics, language, etc. shape the health and health care experiences of particular individuals, families, and communities).

Continuing with the example of the woman with breast cancer we described earlier in the chapter, a critical lens would assist you in considering how the structural conditions of the woman's life would shape her experience. For example, how have social norms and corporate objectives related to breastfeeding shaped her risk? How do economics and geography (e.g., living in a remote rural village, an urban inner city, suburbs) shape her access to treatment? And how does the woman's social location (e.g. income, ethnicity, age) influence the power dynamics related to her care?

A critical lens always draws attention to power. Often, power is thought about as a "top-down" hierarchy, in which some people "have" power and others do not. However, the view of power that we take is that power operates at all levels; all acts involve power (Foucault, 2003). Power can most easily be seen in its *effects* rather than in the deliberate or conscious intentions of those individuals or institutions that wield power. Thus, a critical lens helps you focus on the effects of power in all acts and to understand yourself, your colleagues, and your patients as acting within relational webs of power with effects at intrapersonal, interpersonal, and contextual levels. For example, in a knowledge translation research study focused on improving end-of-life care that I (Gweneth) and a team of colleagues undertook, we found power shaped how interprofessional team members communicated with each other

(Hartrick Doane, Stajduhar, Bidgood, Causton, & Cox, 2012). Functioning within a taken-for-granted power hierarchy, physicians preferred to talk with the charge nurse even though the RNs had more direct knowledge of the particular patients, and the interchange of that knowledge would have probably enhanced care of the patients. This power dynamic also determined how a particular team member's questions or input was received and how it was valued and/or used. For example, one nurse described how her hands were tied in providing appropriate pain control to patients saying "some people have a hard time even bringing pain control up with the docs . . . they simply blow it off" (Hartrick Doane et al., 2012, p. 7).

When we look at health through a critical lens, we are compelled to question the everyday *taken-for-granteds* (ideologies) that shape us and our understanding of health and that shape people's health and health care experiences. For example, a taken-for-granted ideology can be seen in Chapter 1, when the ER nurse says, "No, we don't do that down here," and the nurse on the medical unit reports that her colleagues say of similar situations, "That's just how things are." These ideas operate at all levels, and compliance is required at all levels to keep them in place. For example, although policies may be set at an organizational level (for example, length of stay for a given procedure, standards for time to be seen such as "door-to-doctor" policy in ER), the individuals and groups throughout an organization either support them or they don't. For example, if ER nurses believed (intrapersonal) that transferring a person in his last dying hours was unacceptable, they might decide to do differently (interpersonal) and take issue with that practice by addressing it with the manager (contextual).

Donning a critical lens positions us to expose the underlying *sociopolitical structures* that advantage some people and disadvantage others. For example, the hierarchy of health care is not built exclusively around the well-being of patients but also around the well-being of corporate systems (i.e., to produce profit for pharmaceutical, biotechnology, and information technology corporations), and the well-being of health workers in a complex set of power relations that *differentially* advantage cleaning staff, executives, physicians, nurses, and others. For example, doctors are typically more advantaged than cleaning staff; executives more so than nurses, and so forth. A critical lens reminds us that these kinds of *social conditions* are not natural or constant and that existing structures (e.g., health care structures) may need revising in order to be more *equitable* and responsive to people, families, groups, and communities, particularly to those who do not or cannot conform to dominant values.

While the HP lens draws our attention to how people are situated and constituted and thus experiencing and being shaped by social conditions, the critical lens draws our attention to the sociopolitical, economic, and language contexts within which people are situated and constituted. A critical lens helps you more carefully analyze the contextual elements and relate to them more consciously. For example, in Chapter 1, we used a critical lens to show how Rosa and the other nurses related differently to taken-for-granted ideas about choice (intrapersonally), to point to how structural conditions, such as socioeconomic policies affected Artur's health and health care (contextually), and how Rosa practiced from a relational inquiry perspective to consider these dynamics. A summary of the key concepts, assumptions, and questions within our critical lens are included in Box 2.2. As with an HP lens, we offer only the most basic ideas that are fundamental to the critical lens we offer as a tool for relational inquiry practice.

TO ILLUSTRATE
Seeing Class and Liberal Individualism

To illustrate the usefulness of a critical lens, again, consider nursing. As we enlist a critical lens, our attention is directed to two key elements that shape nursing: class and liberal individualist ideology. In Western countries, nursing has primarily been seen as a middle-class profession and as a profession of upward mobility, particularly for women (Allam et al., 2004). The values that dominate nursing characterize it as middle class. That is, regardless of your own socioeconomic class, how you think of and relate to yourself as a nurse is shaped by middle-class values, one of which is economic upward mobility. Similarly, middle-class values dominate health care overall. For example, middle-class values shaped the perspectives of the nurses in the diabetic clinic Artur attended; they never questioned his socioeconomic situation or whether he had the financial resources to follow a diabetic diet and treatment regime.

Nursing is also shaped by liberalism. Liberalism is a political ideology that arose with the breakdown of feudalism and the rise of the free market or capitalist economy (Browne, 2001). To a large extent, liberalism still characterizes most contemporary economies. The concepts of individualism and equality are at the heart of liberalist ideology. That is, people are assumed to be individuals who have equal opportunity and free choice. This explains how the nurses saw Artur's failure to attend clinic as his choice. Given the liberalist ideology that dominated and shaped the nurses' understandings (that everyone has the same opportunities and can make free choices), the inequities that hindered Artur's attendance (lack of phone, money) were not taken into consideration.

Liberalism assumes that people's choices are driven primarily by desire for economic gain. The world is seen primarily as a free market economy in which supply and demand function to determine the value of goods and services, and power is held by people competitively selected according to their talent or ability (meritocracy) (Browne, 2001). Writing from a Norwegian context, Hanssen (2004) writes that liberalist, individualistic societies focus on the "I" consciousness—on autonomy, independence, individual initiative, self-reliance, right to privacy, and universalism. In contrast, collectivistic societies tend to focus on "we" consciousness—collective identity, emotional interdependence, group solidarity, duties and obligations, and group decisions. Hanssen writes that independence and self-reliance are so central to Western character, and their positive aspects are so taken for granted, that it is difficult for members of such societies to conceive of any other kind of self-concept. Even those members of Western societies who also are influenced by more collectivist communities (think of any number of faith-based communities, for example) are influenced by these ideas. Indeed, because of globalism and colonialism, although all societies have their own dominant ideas, Western ideas are influential. Throughout the world, individuals and groups *relate to* Western ideas in various ways, ranging from uncritical embrace to armed rejection.

BOX 2.2
Critical Lens

Part A: Underlying assumptions:

- All forms of social order (e.g., communities, families, groups, organizations) involve forms of domination and power.
- All knowledge is shaped by socially and historically shaped power relations.
- Facts (or "truth claims") can never be separated from values or ideologies; there is no foundational knowledge that can be known outside of human consciousness, values, and history.
- Belief systems presented and treated as "facts" can act as barriers to conscious action and freedom.
- A critical lens helps to see through taken-for-granted relations to examine underlying structures and social relationships.
- Mainstream practices generally maintain and reproduce (perhaps unwittingly) intersecting systems of race, class, and gender oppression.
- Certain groups in any society are privileged over others; oppression is most forcefully reproduced when people who are subordinated accept their social status as natural, necessary, or inevitable.
- Language is central to developing knowledge and creating meaning.
- Critically oriented knowledge serves as a catalyst for action with a goal of transforming the status quo, including enlightenment, empowerment, emancipation, and social change.
- Individual experiences occur within multiple social structures (e.g., organizations, policies) and webs of power (Browne, 2001; Browne et al., 2011; Hankivsky et al., 2010; Kincheloe & McLaren, 2000).

Part B: Enlisting a critical lens to expand your perceptual field:

- What are the common power dynamics within your society and within and among the communities, health care organizations, groups, and families within and for which you provide care? How do your values and practices align with these dynamics?
- What key historical, economic, and political forces predominantly influence the communities and groups for whom you provide care?
- Which groups tend to be privileged over others in your society, communities, and health care organizations?
- What are the most common race, class, and gender dynamics within your society, communities, and health care organizations?
- What key taken-for-granted beliefs predominate in your areas of practice?
- What are the common labels and stereotypes in your health care organization and/or area of practice?

continued on page 59

> **BOX 2.2** *continued*
> ## Critical Lens
>
> - How do you relate to (think about, practice in relation to) these dynamics, ideas, labels, and stereotypes?
> - What changes in the status quo can you see that would benefit multiple recipients of care?
>
> Part C: Enlisting a critical lens to sharpen your focus:
> - What structural conditions and inequities are advantaging/disadvantaging the health and health care experiences of *this* person/family/community?
> - What power dynamics are most advantaging/disadvantaging the health and health care experiences of this person/family/community?
> - What stereotyping and labeling practices might be affecting this person/family/community?
> - What changes in the "status quo" (structures, ideas, and practices) can you see that would benefit this person/family/community?
> - How can you related to these conditions, dynamics, and practices?

So how are these political ideas of class, liberalism, free market economy, and supply and demand relevant to you as a nurse? Of particular importance to nursing is the way in which liberalist ideology assumes that the world is a "level playing field," on which every person can compete and succeed if they try hard enough. This way of thinking overlooks disadvantages that are beyond individual control (such as illness, physical or mental disability for individuals, or poverty for whole communities) and unrealistically suggests that these disadvantages can be overcome with effort. It also overlooks the network of social relations in which a person is embedded (such as the advantages or disadvantages offered by a person's family) and the many motivations that fuel people's actions other than economic gain (such as compassion, pleasure, or enlightenment).

This matters to nursing because individualism has become central to the character of nursing in Western societies, encouraging nurses to see people as individuals who can make "free choices" and to overlook the life circumstances and relationships that shape these possibilities and choices. One can see this ideology at play in the way nurses are schooled to think of themselves as autonomous agents whose competence rests on their knowledge and skillfulness as individual practitioners. Similarly, nurses are often encouraged to think of their role as being there to support patients to make "healthier choices," without necessarily considering what choices are indeed possible given their life contexts. It also directs nurses to make decisions about who is deserving and/or undeserving of nursing care and ultimately to see the nurse's responsibility to particular individuals as "the driving force of nursing care" (Hanssen, 2004, p. 32). A critical lens draws your attention not just to the contexts of people's lives, but also to the way in which those contexts shape our interpretations.

Seeing How Structural Conditions and Inequities Shape Health and Health Care

A critical lens draws attention to structural conditions (basic structures in society) and inequities (unfair social arrangements). Basic structures in society such as government systems and institutions such as health care are embedded within political and economic systems (Browne, 2001). Economic structural conditions and inequities are key determinants of health and thus are of particular concern to nursing. In most Western countries, income inequities are widening with more wealth concentrated among fewer people at the top of income brackets (Beddoes, 2012) and with the effect of widening health inequities (Coburn, 2004; Raphael, 2007). Unlike a liberal individualist view, which suggests that each person has an equal chance of achieving positive health outcomes, economic security, or even prosperity, using a critical lens to develop your relational consciousness helps you to attend to how the lives and health of individuals, families, and groups are shaped by structures and structural inequities such as variable life circumstances stratified by gender, racism, geography, and other factors. This makes some more vulnerable to poverty and poor health.

Relative and absolute poverty are among the most significant determinants of health (Conroy, Sandel, & Zuckerman, 2010; Marmot & Bell, 2012; Raphael, 2010). However, those of us living in reasonably wealthy countries can often be lulled into overlooking the profound effects of poverty and the ways that the effects of poverty are translated into poor health. Inequities in access to material and immaterial resources (e.g. social support, child care) are substantial even in wealthy countries with generous social welfare arrangements (Mackenbach, 2012). Further, people who have higher social positions in societies are able to benefit more readily from nonmaterial resources such as lower levels of stress and cleaner environmental conditions.

TO ILLUSTRATE
An Irresponsible Daughter

Recently, Bulbir, a nurse on a medical-surgical unit of a small urban hospital, told me (Colleen) about a kerfuffle on her unit. The staff members were furious with the daughter (Lena) of a woman who had been recently discharged following a hip replacement. The 82-year-old woman was readmitted with bedsores, was dehydrated, and was in severe pain. Bulbir had been working on the day the woman had been discharged and recalled that at the time, her daughter had said clearly that she could not look after her mother. However, the staff had insisted that her mother "had to go" as there were other patients awaiting admission, and thus there was no bed for her. Both at discharge and on readmission of the woman, various staff members expressed considerable anger, wondering "what kind of daughter" would refuse to care for her mother.

continued on page 61

TO ILLUSTRATE *continued*

An Irresponsible Daughter

Bulbir said that the daughter, Lena, was very upset at the staff and their treatment of her. Lena felt guilty about her mother's condition and felt even guiltier in the face of the staff's anger (expressed both indirectly with accusatory glares and head shaking, as well as directly, when one staff member asked, "How could you let this happen?"). Bulbir asked Lena what was going on for her. She explained that they live in a small mobile home but that the rent is quite high. They need to live in the area because Lena's son (age 43) has schizophrenia and has been doing well at a day program nearby. Lena has a weekend housekeeping and caregiver job in a wealthy community two bus rides from her home (ironically caring for her employer's elderly family member). The job requires Lena to stay overnight, and during the weekend, her mother's condition deteriorated.

To nurse effectively, a critical lens becomes crucial for Bulbir. Most obvious is how the family's immediate economic circumstances are shaping their experience. Less obvious perhaps is how the structural conditions of the health care system are shaping how the nurses are practicing, the resources they are able to offer (or not), ultimately the family's experience, and how these health care structures and expectations will affect different people and families differently (and thus unfairly). It is not just about how the nurses (and others) are pressured to discharge Lena's mother that shapes the experience but also what is available to support care of Lena's mother at home and for the son living with schizophrenia. If you look more broadly still, you will see how other structural conditions and inequities are at play.

Lena and her family are living inequities shaped by global, national, and local political economies, with Lena providing housekeeping (generally low-paying work) for a presumably wealthier family. As the story of Lena's family illustrates, lack of employment with provisions for paid leave and lack of access to caregiving support can translate directly into poorer health. As their story also illustrates, various forms of inequity, advantage, and disadvantage overlap.

Using a Critical Feminist Filter: Seeing How Inequities Are Gendered and Intersect

To follow the photography analogy, a critical lens with a feminist "filter" draws attention to how power and inequity are gendered and how gender relations are socially produced. Lena, for example, is caregiving for both her elderly mother and her adult son, and this caregiving is influencing her employment possibilities. Again, unlike a decontextualized individualist view, a critical lens using a critical feminist filter helps you to see that rather than being a "choice," caregiving (or not) is "structured" by income and gender. People with more advantage (e.g., employment with paid leave for caregiving, high-income earners) can afford greater support in a wide range of ways, including caregiving, and these advantages are gendered. A critical lens also extends your view to see that what is happening for Lena locally is affected by larger forces. For example, there are global persistent gender wage gaps (e.g., Alksnis, Desmarais, & Curtis, 2008; Blau & Kahn, 2007; Hausmann, Tyson, & Zahidi, 2012). Arulampalam et al. (2007) analyzed 11 European countries (see Box 2.3) and found persistent gender wage gaps, especially in the private sector. Hence, women tend to have lower earning power. Further, in most countries, women do the majority of caregiving and household work. For example, in the United States, women perform approximately twice as much household labor as men (Blair, 2013), and there is evidence that this is linked to persistent gender wage gaps (Albanesi & Olivetti, 2009).

BOX 2.3
Gender Wage Gap Dynamics in 11 Countries

"The raw average gender wage gap in the public sector was in excess of 20% in Britain, Finland, and the Netherlands, in Belgium, Italy, and Spain it was under 10%, and indeed in Italy it is found to have been insignificantly different from zero. In contrast, in the private sector, the raw average gender gap exceeded 13% in all countries, and in Britain and Austria it was close to 30%. In France, Germany, Ireland, the Netherlands, and Spain the gap was around or over 20%.

"In summary, we find that in both the public and the private sectors there was a tendency in some countries for the gender wage gap to be higher at the top of the wage distribution than in the middle region, hinting at a possible "glass-ceiling" effect. However, the gender wage gap was wider at the bottom end, too, for public sector workers in five countries (Austria, Britain, Denmark, France, and Spain) and for private sector workers in four countries (France, Germany, Italy, and Spain). This hints at a "sticky floor" effect in some countries" (Arulampalam, Alison, & Bryan 2007, p. 167–168).

Using a critical feminist perspective draws explicit attention to the gendered contexts of people's lives, helps you pay attention to the subtle ways that dominant societal values proscribe gender roles and responsibilities, and helps you explore the power of these gender roles. For example, a feminist critical lens highlights how families can be prime sites for continually reproducing relations of domination and subordination between the sexes. Mandell and Duffy (1995) describe how women have contradictory and socially prescribed relationships to "family" as "chief family laborer, as principal victim of family violence, as embodiment of family sentimentality and romance" (p. 2). A critical feminist lens highlights how men's and women's roles are gendered within the family, the workplace, and social life more generally and how such gender roles are shaped by larger social forces. This is important for nursing because nurses need to understand how such dynamics operate and decide how to participate in relation to them—blindly supporting, actively reinforcing, or neither.

Nurses can subtly and often unwittingly participate in reinforcing gender dynamics and inequities. For example, recently, I (Colleen) was part of a conversation between a charge nurse and a "bed utilization coordinator" (a person who allocates patients to beds trying to maintain a hospital at as close to 100% capacity as possible). They were reviewing the list of patients in a "temporary holding unit" for patients who did not require emergency care but required either admission to the hospital or long-term care or further assessment. Most of the patients were elderly and had been in the unit more than three days. The two staff members were reviewing each patient trying to determine where each could be discharged. On the list (on a whiteboard) was a column entitled "family." As I listened, they reviewed the potential in each column, quickly skipping those who had "no family." Those patients with a "daughter" or "wife" were explored in depth and followed up, whereas those with "son" or "husband" were usually dismissed as having little or no caregiving potential.

Looking at health from a critical feminist perspective draws attention to the way in which health *is a gendered experience* and the way *power* within a health care encounter is gendered. In Chapter 1, we defined health from a socio-environmental perspective as being the capacity and power of people to live a meaningful life. Looking through a critical feminist lens, it is possible to see how gender roles and inequalities shape different people's possibilities for living meaningful lives. Gender roles and inequalities are played out in families, groups, communities, and health care encounters in ways that are continuous with the wider fabric of society. Therefore, gendered roles and experiences are not merely "choices" made by individuals, but rather are enactments of wider social values, expectations, and ideologies. People decide that they want to have children, care for elders, pursue certain jobs, and so forth in relation to gendered expectations and possibilities that are reinforced on a daily basis in many small ways.

When we look at health and health care from a critical feminist perspective, we are compelled to question how gender shapes our understanding (intrapersonal), how we participate in shaping (interpersonal), and how our worlds (contextual) shape us. This perspective assists us in questioning how gendered assumptions shape our practices and how those practices might reinforce gendered inequities. For example, research has consistently shown that caregiving has a tremendous impact on women's health. Researchers such as Stajduhar (2003) and Wuest (1997, 2001) have shown that health care providers reinforce expectations that women are caregivers, often overlooking the burden of that care, and this can create and intensify problems for caregivers. A simple example is a sign with visiting instructions on a wall in a unit for children with eating disorders. The top two lines of the sign read, "Moms! No food from home." In subtle and not so subtle ways, gendered expectations are conveyed. These expectations advantage and disadvantage both women and men.

Gendered expectations don't simply oppress women and advantage men. Gendered expectations shape the lives of and advantage and disadvantage people of all genders. For example, Stajduhar and her colleagues (2011) described how one home care nurse arranging palliative care believed that a "son caring for his father would not attend to his father's needs because he was male, and the two 'lived more of a bachelor kind of situation'" (p. 282). Further, socially proscribed gender roles are not reinforced by nurses in a vacuum. Rather, we all participate together in relation to such roles and expectations.

Using a relational inquiry approach with a critical feminist lens draws attention to the intricacies of gendered power dynamics and how such dynamics shape each moment. As nurses, our role is not to impose a new set of expectations that defy dominant expectations but rather to inquire as to the expectations of others and more consciously participate. For example, in relation to caregiving, it is not merely a matter of nurses trying not to hold gendered expectations for women to provide caregiving. Rather, it is a matter of seeking to inquire as to the expectations and possibilities and to best support the well-being of all within those expectations and possibilities.

For example, Wuest has shown that rather than caregiving being seen as either a burden or fulfillment, caregiving can be *both* destructive and renewing (Wuest, 2001). People of all genders bring their understanding of what a good child, partner/spouse, parent does—and these understandings shape what happens "relationally" within families, among family members, and between nurses and family members. Taking a relational view allows a nurse to see gender at play, dynamics which may not be at the forefront of a particular family's view. Rather than simply aligning with dominant expectations, the nurse can open up a range of possibilities bringing that knowledge to extend the view beyond proscribed gender roles and invite individuals and families to consider a range of possibilities that might be workable for them. Think for a minute where you might see gendered expectations playing out, and then think how they might be broadened.

Western feminism (or certain forms of feminism, often labeled "liberal white feminism") is often critiqued as focusing on gender as though gender is experienced in the same manner by all women. However, all women are not equally disadvantaged, and many men, depending on racism, sexual orientation, class and so on, are more disadvantaged than many women. Other feminists, notably those who sometimes call themselves "black feminists" such as hooks (1984, 1990), Collins (1986, 1990, 1993), and Brewer (1993) have offered analyses of power and oppression that distinguish feminist perspectives which foreground gender from those that emphasize the "intersectionality of oppressions." Intersectionality refers to the interaction between forms of oppression (e.g., racism, classism, sexism) in ways that magnify one another (Brewer, 1993; Collins, 1993). That is, for example, the experience of being poor (or subjected to racism, disabled, or aged) is not simply an "added" form of oppression for a woman; rather, being poor magnifies the oppression inherent in being a woman. Similarly, being subjected to racism amplifies poverty, as does disability, heterosexism, and so on. Think, for example, about how the socioeconomic circumstances of Lena's family intersect with disability as it affects both her elderly mother and her son. Intersectionality addresses the ways in which various forms of oppression reinforce each other and interact (Hankivsky et al., 2010). Thus, for example, a family whose members cannot find employment because of racism is forced to remain poor, and so on. This form of feminism overlaps with a postcolonial perspective, which draws particular attention to the continuing legacy of colonialism and to the impact of ongoing neocolonialism.

Using a Postcolonial Filter: Seeing How Inequities Are Structured by Colonialism and Race

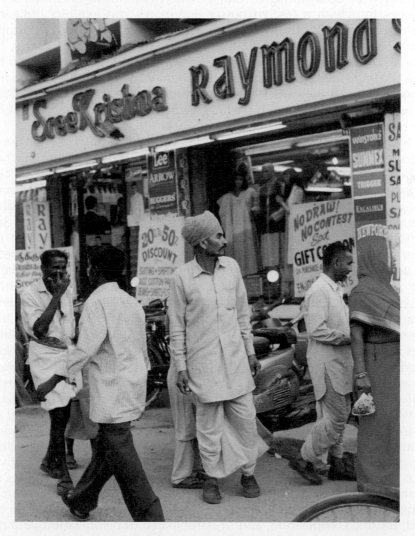

Postcolonial. (Photograph by Len Budiwski.)

While some strains of feminism draw attention to forms of inequality beyond gender, postcolonial or decolonizing theory helps us bring our attention to the social conditions occasioned by colonialism and its constant companion, *racism*. Such theory draws attention to the history of social conditions and draws attention to people who have been and continue to be marginalized by colonialism and racism. Smye and Browne (2002) explain that the "post" in postcolonial does not mean the notion of "after" colonialism but rather refers to the importance of engaging in a purposeful examination of colonialism as it existed and continues to exist both locally and globally. Drawing on the work of Bhabha (1994) and Quayson (2000), Smye and Browne (2002) explain that postcolonialism takes us back and forth between ideas of the past to solutions in the present and the structures that create them. Actively working against the ongoing effects of colonialism is referred to as "anticolonial" or "decolonizing."

All people around the world are affected by colonialism, some more advantaged or disadvantaged than others. Colonialism encompasses the processes by which a foreign power dominates and exploits indigenous groups and more specifically refers to these processes enacted by European powers between the 16th and 20th centuries (Henry & Tator, 2006). Neocolonialism refers to similar domination and exploitation, but rather than being accomplished through physical settlement and military domination, as was the case in the earlier European colonialist expansion, neocolonialism is accomplished through trade agreements and diplomacy backed up with military threat.

Today, because of economic globalism, colonial and neocolonial dynamics shape the entire world economy. For example, most clothing purchased in North America is produced through the labour of people in other countries where pay is often below subsistence. Similarly, fruits and vegetables throughout North America are largely cultivated using low-waged labour, often of undocumented and/or migrant farm workers in the United States and Canada. These dynamics produce wealth for corporations and their owners and shareholders, keep produce prices within reach for some people, and keep others in poverty with everyone being affected by colonialism, most negatively the farm workers themselves (Cason, Nieto-Montenegro, Chavez-Martinez, Ly, & Snyder, 2004; Inouye, 2012; Perry, 2012; Pysklywec, McLaughlin, Tew, & Haines, 2011; Ramirez & Villarejo, 2012; Walia, 2010). A postcolonial perspective extends the idea that people, families, and communities are constituted and situated by drawing attention to particular social, historical, political, and economic conditions. A postcolonial perspective also focuses attention upon the ways in which our own experiences of power and privilege based on nation and "race" shape our understanding and practice.

When you use a postcolonial filter in your critical lens to consider your nursing practice, it can deepen your understanding and shift your practice in multiple ways. Importantly, such a view expands your understanding of history and how it affects the communities, groups, families, and individuals to whom you provide care. The history of your country and its relationship to colonization has shaped the health and well-being of different groups of people differently. Each country around the globe has been colonized, resisted colonization, and/or participated in colonization, and these dynamics continue to play out everywhere on a daily basis. For example, each country has its own history of internal migration, migration out, and migration in, creating layers and layers of different experiences.

Imagine you are a nurse providing care in the United States to a family who emigrated from Mexico (people commonly referred to as Latino, although this label encompasses diverse Spanish-speaking people of various national and ethnic origins). While each family will be unique, having a knowledge base of US-Mexican colonial relations will provide a starting point from which you can inquire with this particular family. Your own history and knowledge provides this staring point. For example, if you have descended from indigenous North American people, you may have a different starting point than if you have descended from people who emigrated from Europe many generations ago or if you recently immigrated yourself. What would be important to consider? When did this family immigrate? Did they immigrate many generations ago, prior to the drawing of the current boundaries? More recently? What economic conditions shaped their immigration? What "push" economic factors (e.g., poverty in Mexico) and "pull" factors (e.g., demand for cheap labor in the United States, a job opportunity for one family member as an executive in an oil company) influenced their immigration, and how in turn did colonial structures shape these? For example, trade agreements between countries are constantly shaping the fortunes of individuals, families, groups, and entire communities, but these are often overlooked in the tendency to construct people's decisions as individual choice. Importantly, a nurse in the United States would know to inquire as to the family member's citizenship status. Indeed, throughout the United States, entire health care programs and systems have been set up in attempts to provide health care to people with illegal citizenship status who otherwise have to avoid health care (Campbell, Sanoff, & Rosner, 2010; Dolgin & Dietrich, 2009; Fields et al., 2001; Marrow, 2012). How does a family's citizenship status and socioeconomic status interrelate? How are these dynamics affecting their health?

At a population level in most countries, the poorer health of immigrants in part can be tied directly to poorer socioeconomic status. In the case of Latino people in the United States, their poorer health as a population can be tied both to their poorer health, and for those who have illegal citizenship, to the stress, precarious housing, food insecurity, limited access to health care, and so on, associated with such status (Rodríguez & Vega, 2009; Vega, Rodriguez, & Gruskin, 2009). These dynamics are supported by laws, policies, and practices, including stereotypical thinking that maintains that certain people deserve more than others.

But how does this play out for a particular family or individual? And why does it matter to the nurse? First, the better the nurse (intrapersonally) understands history and economics at a population level, the better that nurse will be able to critically analyze and decide how to relate to dominant assumptions and stereotypes that allow inequities to go unchallenged. Think about how jokes, cartoons, costumes, media, and advertisements encourage thinking in certain ways about certain groups—in this case, Latino people. Second, with greater understanding, a nurse is less likely to impose (interpersonally) a liberal individualist view in practice. If, for example, the nurse is providing perinatal care to the family, the nurse will be able to understand the family's access (or lack thereof) to previous prenatal care as arising from the intersection of socioeconomics and colonial dynamics.

Third, when you approach people with greater understanding, fewer errone-ous assumptions, and a stance of inquiry, you foster your own approach-ability. Fourth, when you take such an approach to your practice, you can more effectively integrate contextual knowledge into your practice. A sug-gestion of nutritional supplements will require different contextual knowl-edge when made to a wealthy Latino family with full US citizenship than when made to a family of Latino migrant farm workers without.

Peter Stephenson's (1999) example of a newspaper article about a 5-year-old girl who died of chicken pox in the United States illustrates how a liberal individualist view can overlook the dynamics of colonialism. The little girl's parents were "undocumented" immigrants from Mexico who did not speak English, did not have money, and did not know where to go for help. Thus, they did not seek care until too late to prevent her death. However, the reporter asked what it was about Mexican *culture* that led them to delay treat-ment, effectively overlooking the socioeconomic and colonial conditions of their lives and placing responsibility on the family for the child's death. Can you imagine if a nurse caring for the family during the child's death shared the reporter's view? Can you imagine if a nurse acting within a relational inquiry approach had better understood the family's situation?

TRY IT OUT 2.4

Looking through a Postcolonial Lens

Think about your own family history through a postcolonial lens. How has your family history been shaped by colonial conquest, war, and migration? How have socioeconomics been an integral part of these dynamics? What ideologies have supported these dynamics? For example, when I (Colleen) think about a small slice of my family history, I can see how the many men of my family who fought in WWII (in both Europe and Asia) were part of larger dynamics to protect the financial interests of Canada and large cor-porations. Although my family's participation in the war was constructed as being about loyalty, service, and protecting freedom, it was also shaped by the fact that in the late 1930s and early 1940s, for many men, global eco-nomics had left few employment opportunities other than military service.

Racism is a constant companion to colonialism because assumptions of racial superiority are used to justify and facilitate domination of indigenous peoples and "others." Throughout the history of colonialism, colonizers have seen indigenous peoples as "backward," "savage," less civilized than the colonizers, and in need of taming, education, or civilizing. The values and practices of the colonizers were (and continue to be) imposed as supe-rior, and cultural hegemony, as well as political, economic, and military dominance by Europeans was achieved throughout much of Africa, Asia, and the Americas (Henry & Tator, 2006).

One of the most notorious examples is that of the residential schools imposed on Aboriginal people in Canada. Over many decades, Christian churches in concert with the state have forced Aboriginal families to send their children to residential schools. In addition to separation from community and family, as well as loss of language and culture, these children were often subjected to emotional, physical, and sexual abuse. Today, lawsuits related to such abuse are widespread throughout Canada and are ongoing. Such domination by Western powers continues today through neocolonialist practices, fueled again by racism. A current example is the trafficking of women from countries such as the Philippines, a country laboring under enormous foreign debt. The economy of the Philippines is such that many citizens migrate around the world in search of income with which to support their families. Some women (often educated as nurses) immigrate to Western countries (including Canada, the United States, Britain) to work as nannies and caregivers, whereas many others are marketed as "brides" or as sex trade workers in these same countries.

When a nurse has a sense of how racism intertwines with colonialism, he or she can better decide how to relate to assumptions of racial superiority or inferiority. Such assumptions routinely play out in relation to people's health and health care. For example, in my (Colleen's) area of research, I have observed that violence is routinely racialized in health care. Violence is associated with particular groups identified by ethnicity or race: "native women are vulnerable to that sort of thing [violence];" "South Asians are prone. . ." Often, "culture" is used as a proxy for ethnicity or race and is associated with assumed inferiority (e.g., being more violent, more willing to accept violence, more vulnerable). Health care providers ask me, "What is it about their [referring to any number of groups'] culture that leads the women to stay with abusive men?" Or they tell me that "[violence] is in their culture." These assumptions, if uncritically held, lead health care providers and others to think that violence is "natural" for some groups and therefore unchangeable and somehow "deserved."

Because "race" is *not* a biologic phenomenon (UNESCO released its first statement on race in 1951 dispelling its validity as a biologic category; there is only one human race), all racial, ethnic, or cultural assumptions are social constructions that self-perpetuate. Understanding how racism functions to sustain notions of superiority/inferiority and thus deservingness, privilege, and advantage/disadvantage helps nurses decide how to relate to racism. Think about any given racialized group you know (or of which you may be part). What negative stereotypes exist, and how do they function? For example, in Canada, one of the most pernicious negative stereotypes affecting health for Aboriginal people (a term that encompasses diverse indigenous First Nations people who speak over 50 different languages, Inuit people, and Métis peoples) is the stereotype of the "drunken Indian" (somehow, the mistaken belief of early European colonizers that they had reached India has been perpetuated in the use of the term "Indian" in law, policy, and common parlance). This stereotype is ascribed to individual people, (a) failing to take into account how alcohol was widely used to pacify indigenous populations as a tool of colonization; (b) overlooking how contemporary policies and practices continue to do so (e.g., alcohol pricing policies, tax policies, and liquor store bylaws that continue to market alcohol differentially to indigenous people); and (c) ignoring evidence that counters such stereotypes. For example, in the Canadian province where we (Gweneth and Colleen) live, evidence shows that despite a greater concentration of alcohol outlets in neighbourhoods dominated by Aboriginal people, they consume less alcohol per capita than the rest of the population (Kendall, 2001, 2009). Yet the stereotype continues to affect health care. For instance, in research in both community and emergency contexts in our area, Aboriginal people report health care providers routinely making erroneous assumptions about their alcohol consumption (Browne et al., 2011; Smye, Browne, Varcoe, & Josewski, 2011; Varcoe, Browne, Wong, & Smye, 2009), and I (Colleen) have observed nurses incorrectly assuming alcohol intoxication in the presence of neurologic symptoms. Recently, a young Aboriginal woman with a postpartum cerebral hemorrhage was misdiagnosed as being intoxicated (she had never consumed alcohol, but despite her family's protestations, this was disbelieved by hospital staff).

A postcolonial lens draws your attention to history and economics as they intertwine to advantage some people and disadvantage others. It provides you with a basis from which to inquire, to tailor your care to history and contexts, and to be more effective in promoting well-being.

TO ILLUSTRATE
Pap Smears in Reserve

A group of nurses in a remote community recognized that Aboriginal women had very high rates of cervical cancer. They discovered that the women typically did not have Pap smears done routinely or sometimes ever. Rather than adopting a finger-wagging, blaming sort of approach ("You *must* have a Pap smear every year, my dear"), the nurses realized that, given the history of the church school in the area, many of the women may have been sexually abused. They also considered that the history of race relations in the community had not created an atmosphere of trust between the Aboriginal women and the predominantly white nurses. Accordingly, they sought the input of female elders and offered a women's clinic where Pap smears were only suggested as a possibility after dealing with a range of other issues that the women raised. The elders were enlisted as healers/supporters during the exams, and although some women continued to decline to have Pap smears, the number of women doing so tripled within a year.

A postcolonial lens reminds us that we are situated and constituted not only within an immediate local culture, but also within a global culture and within a historically determined context. As illustrated in the above example, such a lens draws our attention to the ways in which power and privilege associated with nation and "race" have shaped families and individuals and continue to shape them. By donning a postcolonial lens, our attention is drawn to historical locatedness and a consideration of how existing practices and policies may be colonizing rather than decolonizing in their consequences. As evidenced in the above example, a postcolonial lens encourages us to better understand and therefore counter specific instances of local oppression.

TO ILLUSTRATE
No Fighting

Many years ago, I (Colleen) was in an emergency unit doing research on how nurses deal with violence against women (Varcoe, 2001). As I arrived one day, a number of the staff greeted me excitedly. "We've got one for you," said one of the physicians. The staff pointed out a young woman who was in with paralysis and aphasia. The staff said that she had been admitted before and that both organic and psychiatric explanations for her paralysis and aphasia had been ruled out. The staff said they suspected her husband was violent toward her, because during the woman's previous admission, the husband had been angry, shouting, and abusive toward the psychiatric nurse who was doing an assessment, and on this admission, he seemed angry and hostile toward the staff. Relevant to this situation was the fact that the family was from a particular group whom many of the staff identified by race and previously told me that they saw as more violent than the majority (white) population. The woman (I will call her Fatima) was accompanied by two men, her husband and brother-in-law.

Partly because the staff indicated the woman to me, the brother-in-law approached me. He was frustrated with the staff for not having any explanations for his sister's condition and for assuming violence was an issue. I asked him what he thought was the problem. I had a little difficulty following his English. He told me that Fatima had paralysis and quit talking before and explained that she was afraid of ghosts. The nurse with whom I was working joined us and asked him if anything happens at home prior to her becoming paralyzed. A wary light shone in his eyes, and he said defiantly, "It has never happened. No fighting." I asked what he meant, and he said, pointing to the nurse, "That's what she means, fighting at home." He went on to explain that the last time they were here, his brother (the woman's husband) became very angry, and now everyone thinks that it is "fighting" that causes her behavior.

Stop for a minute and think about this situation. As a nurse, what stands out for *you*? Certainly, if we don an HP lens, we can see how different people are making meaning of the situation in different ways. From an HP view, it is obvious that what is of meaning and concern to the nurses is different from what is of meaning and concern to the family. Yet they both have the welfare of Fatima at the forefront of their concerns. A critical lens can help us understand what is giving rise to such strong differences, and the gendered filter and postcolonial filter illuminate certain features.

One of the first things that becomes apparent is how the staff are seeing the family in terms of their racial and ethnic background and applying stereotypical beliefs (e.g., how violence is a norm in a particular group of people). Based on these stereotypical beliefs, they reached the conclusion (or should we say, jumped to the conclusion) that the husband is abusive toward his wife. In dealing with Fatima, the staff drew on the idea of race to identify Fatima and her family, thus engaging in the process of racialization.

The story of Fatima's experience illustrates how a postcolonial perspective draws attention to certain features of the situation as nursing concerns. For example, nurses using a critical postcolonial perspective would be concerned with how racialization is constraining Fatima and her family's experience in the emergency department. Using a postcolonial perspective, a nurse would also be concerned about how stereotypical thinking might shape understanding of family. For example, drawing on a Eurocentric understanding of "family," the nursing staff said that they thought it was "weird" that Fatima's brother-in-law accompanied her to the hospital, and the nurses seemed to interpret this as further evidence that something wasn't right here, that something sinister was being covered up.

Fatima's situation also points to the importance of inquiring and acting at all levels. Intrapersonally, how is each person seeing the situation? Where are the disjunctures? How are these different understandings playing out interpersonally? How might inquiry help the nurses be more responsive? Beyond this particular situation, what might be done contextually to counter stereotypical assumptions based on race and the dominant power dynamics in operation? For example, as a nurse observing this situation, I (Colleen) felt compelled to question the basis of the staff's assumptions and address the way the family members were at a particular disadvantage in relation to the health care providers because they were brown-skinned people who spoke little English in a community dominated by white-skinned people with medical knowledge. I did so by asking the staff why they thought the family members were angry and sharing what I had been told, and this provoked further conversation with the family members.

When we use a postcolonial perspective, we consider how colonization has shaped and continues to influence us all around the globe. Through colonial rule, many cultures have had to cope with the imposition of Christian-European norms and with the values of colonizers. For example, although forms of family practiced by people in Asia, Africa, and the Americas often were not compatible with the imposed ideals of the heterosexual male-dominated family, colonized peoples responded to such imposition by using a wide variety of family forms (Potthast-Jutkeit, 1997). Today, for example, many new immigrants to Western countries continue to live in extended groups with several generations and families of adult siblings living together in the same home. Former colonial powers in turn have been exposed to this greater variety of family forms, particularly through immigration from their former colonies. Thus, diverse forms of family have persisted despite colonial and neocolonial dominance. A postcolonial perspective further directs us to challenge the ways in which colonialism is enacted through theory and question the use of theories grounded in Eurocentric norms as a basis for practice with people in multicultural societies. For example, the idea of "self-esteem," a common construct in Western countries, has been based on

Eurocentric norms and may have limited relevance to many people. What about the idea of "sibling rivalry?" What meaning might this have for a family whose culture is deeply rooted in ideas of filial piety, such as traditional Chinese cultures influenced by Confucian thought?

A postcolonial perspective helps us pay particular attention to the ways in which racial categories and associated assumptions and stereotypes function in our thinking and practice. For example, the term "extended family" is sometimes used only in relation to people who are racialized. That is, the family form signaled by "extended family" is seen as related to "race" or ethnicity, rather than seeing habitation as an extended family arising from particular economic, social, and historical conditions. This example highlights the importance of language to a critical lens.

Using a Poststructural Filter: Seeing How Language Shapes Experience

A critical lens helps us pay attention to how language is being used and the effects language use has on people's experiences of health and health care. This, in turn, helps us see what taken-for-granted ideas (ideologies) are operating. A poststructural perspective within a critical lens specifically helps us focus on language in action and how language is integral to how power operates. A poststructural perspective highlights how language *creates* social reality as opposed to reflecting or describing it. Language is not a neutral tool we use to describe something. Rather, describing is an act of power; there arc meanings and rules embedded within language that limit the meaning a person can make and subsequently communicate (Cheek, 2000). For example, phrases such as, "Don't cry like a girl," or "She's a real tomboy," give clear messages to children about what boys and/or girls are. A rugby coach criticizing boys by yelling, "You're playing like a bunch of *girls*" reinforces these ideas and implies certain gendered values. People are "spoken into existence" as they participate in the everyday language and discourse of their cultures (Alex & Whitty-Rogers, 2012; Davies & Harre, 1990; Fairclough, 2001, 2004; Fleitas, 2003; Weedon, 1981, 1997). Similarly, applying racializing labels to describe people brings ethnicity and race into the foreground and invites any accompanying assumptions to be activated.

Language Practices Shape Our Experiences of Ourselves and Others

By using and joining in with the ways of using language and the meanings embedded within that use (discursive practices) of any given society, each person experiences what it *means* to be a person and how to *be* as a person. As people acquire language, they learn to give meaning to their experience and to understand it according to particular ways of thinking and believing that are embedded within existing discourses. In Western culture, for example, by participating in and integrating the discourses about mothering, women are provided with specific and select options for how they become and live as mothers. The specific ways of talking about mothers (social discourses) such as, "You must be so thrilled to be a new mother," "There is no more important work than raising children," "A woman's true fulfillment is through motherhood," "When are you planning to start a family?" and "How could a mother let her children run around so unsupervised?" provide women with specific information about what it means to be a mother, what being a mother should look and feel like, and how to enact the role of mother (Hartrick, 1998b; Varcoe & Hartrick Doane, 2007).

Discourses are so powerful because as people participate in the discursive practices of their culture, they forget that the discourses are separate from *who* they are (Bakhtin, 1981). So, for example, I (Colleen) have been struck when working with people who use injection drugs by how readily they label themselves as "addicts." Similarly, Weedon (1987) provides the example of how certain discourses of motherhood can spark feelings of inadequacy for a new mother. The embedded messages that a new mother receives from existing discourses of motherhood tell her that "she is supposed to meet all the child's needs singlehanded, to care for and stimulate the child's physical, emotional, and mental development, and to feel fulfilled in doing so" (Weedon, 1987, p. 34). The language and discourse surrounding motherhood shape, constrain, coerce, and potentiate a new mother's experience, the meanings she assigns to the experience, to her new child's behavior, and to herself and the actions she takes as a mother (Davies, 1990). It is little wonder that feelings of inadequacy often accompany new motherhood!

Language practices both shape how people experience themselves, how we may see others, and how we approach and work with them. For example, the label "appendectomy patient in room 5" shapes how we see and relate to that person. People are well-schooled as patients to assume the identities or labels that we give them and to perform their parts. At least, most people are. When they don't perform according to the language script, we find another label or identifier, such as "demanding patient," "emotional patient," and so forth.

Gender roles offer an example of how paying attention to language can alert us to societal norms that may be subtly constraining people and families. The tradition of women's responsibility for domestic labor and childcare and men's responsibility in the world of work are views that are embedded within discursive practices. For example, we often speak of men "helping out" with household chores or "babysitting" their children when their "wives" are out somewhere, while women dominate the covers of magazines such as *Parenting* and *Good Housekeeping*. Or, to take another example, the language of "parenting" can be seen as gender-neutralizing language that obscures the gendered work of "mothering." At the same time that these practices support and reproduce certain gender roles, they reinforce the idea that heterosexism is unquestionably the norm (heteronormativity), excluding people who are not partnered, are celibate, or who have same-sex partners.

Poststructural theory offers a view of how people and their experiences are spoken into existence by the everyday discourse in which each of us participates (Fairclough, 2001, 2004). This perspective highlights the power of language in actually shaping not only what people experience but how they understand those experiences. As we look from this vantage point, we can see the potential in moving beyond taken-for-granted understandings to listen to how particular people and families are "languaging" their experience. At the same time, we can create opportunities for people to disrupt dominant discourses that are constraining them. The poststructural perspective also reminds us as nurses to pay attention to how we are speaking people's experiences into existence—how what we say to people is enhancing their capacity of choice or perpetuating stereotypical norms and expectations.

For example, in the intervention study that I (Colleen) am working on currently, our research team has had considerable conversation about the ethics of offering the women money to participate beyond the research interviews. We have talked about an "honorarium" or offering bus tickets. The women are living in extreme poverty, and even the smallest amount of money can make a big difference in their lives and thus can coerce them into participating in research. In fact, there is an entire "research industry" in the area (Bungay, Johnson, Varcoe, & Boyd, 2010), such that people vie with each other to participate in research for the small amounts of money offered as compensation. I suggested that because we are looking for the women's expertise in advising us as researchers, we should think and talk about the women as "consultants." When we shifted to talking about women as "paid consultants" rather than "focus group participants," our view of the women shifted dramatically. When we asked the women if we could "hire them as consultants," they expressed a completely different orientation, thinking about the opportunity as much more meaningful and respectful work. It is important to emphasize that this is not about semantics. It is about being relationally conscious of how language is used, how people are being spoken into existence, and ensuring that the way you are narrating someone through your way of speaking is supporting your intention, not undermining it.

TRY IT OUT 2.5

Looking through a Poststructural Lens

Look at a "parenting" magazine.

If you live in Canada or the United States, *Parenting* and *Parenting Magazine* are available at supermarkets and newsstands. *Little Treasures Magazine* or *Kiwi Parent* are available at the similar places in New Zealand, or if you are in Australia, you could pick up *Practical Parenting*, "Australia's favorite parenting magazine," or *Junior*. Other publications such as *Redbook* target women more generally but have a subemphasis on parenting. Some publications target certain groups. For example, *Christian Parenting* is billed as a "magazine that targets real needs of the contemporary family with authoritative articles based on fresh research and the timeless truths of the Bible." *Essence* is described as the "magazine for today's black woman. Edited for career-minded, sophisticated, and independent achievers. Highlights career/education opportunities, fashion, beauty, money management, fitness, parenting, and home décor."

Pick any one of these magazines and examine the cover, the table of contents, or an article that relates to gender roles. What does the magazine convey through the language and underlying narratives? What taken-for-granted ideas can you see? What "truths" do the images and text convey? What stereotypes are reinforced? What is conveyed as meaningful and significant? What would fall outside of the images, stereotypes, ideas, and truths?

Seeing How Language, Discourses, Ideologies, and Belief Systems Operate in Nursing Work

A critical lens with its emphasis on structural conditions, inequities, and language can help you see how language, discourses, ideologies, and belief systems operate to shape and constrain people's health and health care experiences and can help you interrupt and counter such constraints. Belief systems presented and treated as "facts" by those in power can be constraining. For example, in Lena's situation, the staff's assertion that her mother "had to go" is an example of belief systems in action. The staff apparently took for granted that Lena should take care of her mother and did not question whether Lena could financially afford to take care of her mother or what consequences might ensue.

In addition to being in a position of power (relative to their patients) due to their professional status, in Western countries, health care providers often have a greater income and more education than their patients. Thus, health care providers often operate on assumptions that do not match the reality of patients' lives. Assumptions that reflect mainstream, middle-class, white, Eurocentric, heterosexual "norms" can serve as barriers to people, families, and communities who do not fit those norms. In the face of the staff's directive that her mother must go home, and despite her misgivings, Lena took her mother home and then felt guilty at being unable to care for her properly. This example points to another idea within critical perspectives, that *oppression is most forcefully reproduced when people who are subordinated accept their social status as natural, necessary, or inevitable.*

By examining how our nursing practice is socially produced through taken-for-granted norms and stereotypes, a critical lens helps us identify and then reject all forms of "truth" that may be subordinating human consciousness and action (Giroux, 1983). A critical lens helps us expand our relational consciousness as we go about our nursing work and thereby affords us greater opportunity and freedom to choose the "truth" that we will follow more consciously. For example, a critical lens draws our attention to the authority that we are giving to any theory and/or to predetermined assessment tools and leads us to question how those theories and tools may lead us to overlook the patient's own perspectives and constrain our ability to be responsive to what is meaningful and significant to people.

TO ILLUSTRATE
A Critical Look at Caregiving

In a program of research on palliative caregiving, Stajduhar and her colleagues have used a critical perspective that encompasses a feminist perspective to analyze family caregiver experiences within a larger sociopolitical and economic context. This program of research illustrates how a critical perspective can enhance nursing practice by promoting understanding of how power operates at all levels. Throughout their research, they show how

continued on page 77

> ## TO ILLUSTRATE   *continued*
> ## A Critical Look at Caregiving
>
> family caregiver experiences are shaped by broader sociopolitical influences. For example, they show how family caregivers' experiences and their experiences of caregiving burden are shaped by multiple determinants of health, including gender, income and social status, working conditions (primarily within paid employment for caregivers), and health and social services (Crooks et al., 2012). In her early work, Stajduhar (2001, 2003) showed how caregivers did not necessarily choose to engage in home-based palliative care but that their engagement often stemmed from an obligation to care, especially if they were women. She showed how health care providers reinforced the taken-for-granted assumptions that women would make this choice freely and that they were available and able to take up the caregiving role. The research team's work continues to show how deep-rooted gender roles and expectations in family caregiving continue to operate (Crooks et al., 2012). Stadjuhar also found that health care providers and families uncritically took up the narrative of family as a safe haven in the shared ideology that home is the best place to be and die. Health care providers assumed that families wanted to and were obligated to provide this safe haven. This assumption worked in concert with pressures arising from the health care system such as health care reform and rationing of resources. Ultimately, it meant that families felt pressured to provide home care to their dying relatives and that family caregivers felt that health care providers exploited their sense of family obligation.
>
> Throughout their research, these investigators also show how nursing work is conducted within and constrained or supported by broader socioeconomic and political contexts. For example, they have illustrated how the health care system, driven by cost containment and efficiency models, reinforces the idealization of dying at home, leaving the caregivers feeling pressured to conform, disadvantaging many, particularly women and other marginalized groups. In one study (Stajduhar et al., 2011), the researchers showed how home care nurses work within a system in which the health authority allocates how much time will be required for each palliative care visit. These times are based either on an estimate from the previous nurse who visited or on a nurse in an office. The research showed that such practices "have the potential to exacerbate overall workload constraints and reduce schedule flexibility with implications for access and decision-making, particularly as palliative care needs are often unpredictable" (p. 283).
>
> Stajduhar and her colleagues (2011) also show how language and taken-for-granted ideas can operate. For example, they found that home care nurses "invoked reference to common practice ideals (e.g., 'knowing the family'), perceptions of their role (e.g., expertise), and approaches to care (e.g., 'empowerment' or 'caution') as justification for decisions" about the amount and type of service to provide to families caring for people dying at home (Stajduhar et al., 2011). They show how nurses used ideals of empowerment and "promoting independence" to shift responsibility for

continued on page 78

TO ILLUSTRATE *continued*

A Critical Look at Caregiving

particular care tasks to clients and family caregivers at home (Funk, Stajduhar, & Purkis, 2011; Stajduhar, Funk, Jakobsson, & Ohlén, 2010). Finally, this program of research shows how a critical lens assists nurses to make changes—both changes to improve care with specific families and changes that have the potential to enhance care for an entire population of clients. For example, their critical analysis of the idea of empowerment shows how nurses use the idea of "choice" in a very narrow way, confined to choice about the timing and frequency of home visits (Funk et al., 2011). The research shows how nurses used the practice ideal of empowerment as a way of mitigating their own feelings of helplessness related to being unable to effectively help palliative clients and families and to support the shift of caregiving tasks as described above. They suggest that nurses need to be supported to have a more critical analysis of the ideal of "empowerment." Their research helps nurses see when such discourse is being used to bring patients and families into line with nursing goals and to impose "responsibilization" discourses (liberal individualizing discourse of choice and responsibility) that leave families with "no choice but to fill the gaps themselves, inadvertently rendering the effects of cost constraints invisible within the private spaces where care is conducted" (p. 74). Alternatively, they suggest that nurses need to reframe practice with an understanding of the structural roots of practice dilemmas such as cost constraint and gender.

More broadly, these researchers have used their research to make recommendations for improving public health policy related to palliative care in Canada, recommendations that they advise would be useful in other jurisdictions seeking to develop programs to support caregivers based on labor policy strategies and legislation (Crooks et al., 2012; Williams et al., 2011). Importantly, they show that developing public awareness of programs and benefits (particularly for families) is a crucial complement to formal policy, awareness that nurses can be instrumental in facilitating.

Using a Critical Lens to Create Change

A central idea of critical theory is that *knowledge should be used toward social change and for emancipatory political aims*. This lofty sounding ideal does not mean that nurses are responsible for rectifying all the inequities in the world. It does not mean, for example, that nurses can change people's economic circumstances. However, it does mean that nurses can *understand* people's economic circumstances and *not judge them negatively* for their circumstances. It also means that nurses can *take people's circumstances into account* when planning care, offering advice, or intervening in other ways, and that nurses should find ways *to affect circumstances that are beyond individual control*. For example, the home care nurses in the research by Stajduhar and her team might work toward changing the practice of preallocating their time for home visits. Rather than using "empowerment" discourse to mitigate their own feelings of inadequacy, they could act more directly on some of the factors constraining their care.

To take another example, in Chapter 1 we asked what might happen if the nurse who cared for the dying man and his wife had ways of working with her colleagues to more concertedly examine the normative practices that were limiting nursing care. That is an example of how a critical lens might be employed. Using a critical lens, the nurse in the situation might have felt more empowered. Rather than feeling distressed and feeling responsible but unable to affect end-of-life care, a critical lens would have helped the nurse take a wider and deeper look into the situation to see and name the factors that might need to be addressed at the intrapersonal, interpersonal, and contextual levels.

Critical thought must be combined with critical action (praxis) to bring about change in what we critique. Osmond (1987) explains that "critical sciences aim to both understand the world and to change it" (p. 107). The goals of a critical perspective are to provide a critique of the societal status quo and to effect social change. Critical theorists argue that knowledge should be used toward the alleviation of social problems and draw attention to families, communities, and health care organizations as social, political, and economic units. This matters in nursing in every moment of care.

Bulbir used a critical lens to "dig beneath the surface." She inquired about the context of Lena's and her family's lives and thus surfaced how economic conditions (among other things) were shaping their experiences of health and health care. In doing so, she helped show that what appeared to be common sense (that a daughter should care for her elderly mother) was an idea that was being *socially produced*, not just by the nurses in the immediate situation, but by the health care system and the wider society and its dominant belief systems. On the surface, to some of the staff, the family's "reality" was an uncaring, neglectful daughter refusing to take on her social and familial responsibilities. What is not so readily evident (until you use a critical lens) is that the staff's assumptions (about what a family and a good daughter are) are wider social expectations that work with health care system policies (such as length of stay for a hip replacement) to create this detrimental situation.

From Bulbir's story, it is clear that simply discharging Lena's mother back home into the same set of circumstances will not be health promoting. A critical lens and its emphasis on emancipatory political aims work at both the level of the individual and at a social level. For example, at the individual level, Bulbir might share her understanding of Lena's family with the rest of the staff to help broaden their understanding of this particular family. In turn, the staff might be less judgmental of Lena and seek better ways to support her. The staff might then see if some home support or alternative care is possible for Lena's mother. At the contextual level, they might challenge the discharge rules that dictate a proscribed length of stay regardless of the patient's condition or the availability of suitable care after discharge. Thus, a critical lens promotes action at the intrapersonal level (e.g., examining and modifying values and beliefs), the interpersonal level (e.g., sharing understanding, decreasing negative judgments based on untested assumptions), and contextual levels (e.g., changing rules and policies, developing alternative practices).

TRY IT OUT 2.6
Looking through a Critical Lens Using Multiple Filters

Part 1: Inquire at the contextual level:

Pick a specific community to whose members you will be providing care. Try to select a community *with which you are not very familiar*. For example, I (Colleen) work with many different Aboriginal communities and have worked with multiple rural communities. Any time I work with a community, I try to learn as much as I can about that community. In Box 2.4, see an example of a short community profile of Bella Coola that helped my research team contextualize the maternity care experiences of people there (Brown, Varcoe, & Calam, 2011; Varcoe, Brown, Calam, Harvey, & Tallio, 2013). Use literature, media, the Internet, and other resources to answer the following questions:

■ What key historical, economic, and political forces predominantly influence this community (think about migration in and out of the community, wars, settlement, and economic recessions)?

■ Which groups tend to be privileged over others in this community?

■ What are the most common race, class, and gender dynamics within this community?

■ What key taken-for-granted beliefs, "labels," and stereotypes might be operating in relation to this community?

■ What changes in the status quo (think structures, inequities, and taken-for-granted thinking) can you see that might improve health and health care for this community?

Part 2: Inquire at the contextual and interpersonal levels:

Pick a specific person or family from that community:

■ What structural conditions and inequities are advantaging and/or disadvantaging the health and health care experiences of *this* person or family?

■ What power dynamics are most advantaging and/or disadvantaging the health and health care experiences of this person or family?

■ What stereotyping and labeling practices might be affecting this person or family?

■ What changes in the status quo can you see that would benefit this person or family?

Part 3: Inquire at the intrapersonal level:

Think about your own inquiry process

■ What differences and similarities do you see between yourself and this community and person or family?

■ Which of your values, beliefs, assumptions, and practices are confirmed or challenged as you inquire?

■ How might you relate differently at the intrapersonal, interpersonal, and contextual levels?

BOX 2.4
An Example Community Profile

Located in the middle of the Bella Coola Valley on the Bella Coola River in Northern British Columbia, Bella Coola is home to the Coast Salish Nuxalk people. Before colonization, the Nuxalk people had a vibrant commerce, trading along the historic Nuxalk-Carrier "Great Road" or "Grease Trail" (named for the versatile oolichan grease), making seasonal rounds that included a vast shrimp and oolichan fishery, hunting, and trading with interior people (Birchwater, 1993; Kennedy & Bouchard, n.d.). In 1793, the Nuxalk people, who were experts in their knowledge of the geography and trails, guided the European explorer Alexander MacKenzie over the Grease Trail to the ocean. Contact with other Europeans followed quickly, and in 1862–1863, the smallpox epidemic killed over 70% of the people. The Hudson's Bay Company established a post in Bella Coola in 1867, and the fur trade shifted people away from their traditional work and the seasonal "round." The hospital was established in Bella Coola in 1908, and by 1928, the United Church assumed responsibility. Church and government officials took Nuxalk children from their families and sent them to residential school, primarily to St. Michael's School in Alert Bay (over 200 km away), which ran from 1929 to 1975. Throughout Canada, Aboriginal children endured multiple forms (physical, sexual, emotional, mental, cultural, and spiritual) of abuse in residential schools, with profound ongoing negative effects on health and well-being for subsequent generations (Bombay, Matheson, & Anisman, 2011; Elias et al., 2012; Smith, Varcoe, & Edwards, 2005).

In just over a century, the population of the Aboriginal people in the area had been decimated, the way of life changed radically, the children removed, and the oolichan gone. These policies and actions continue to shape the lives of Nuxalk people today, including their economics, politics, and their health and well-being. As in other areas, the colonizing Europeans brought their ideas of health and health care and imposed their ideas and practices on the Nuxalk. The hospital, established in 1908, was taken over by the United Church at the same time that children were taken away from their families to residential school. As elsewhere in Canada, women were gradually discouraged from giving birth at home and were expected to give birth at the hospital, further disconnecting people from their children (Brown et al., 2011; Varcoe et al., 2013).

HOW TO ENLIST THE HERMENEUTIC PHENOMENOLOGIC AND CRITICAL LENSES TO INFORM YOUR NURSING PRACTICE

Paterson and Zderad (1988) describe nursing in its highest form as "an experience lived between human beings" (p. 3). The HP and critical lenses are tools that you can enlist to both expand your view and understanding of people's experiences of health and illness and also to guide you in your nursing experiences and actions. In many ways, the lenses overlap. For example, the notion of being "situated" that is part of the HP lens is similar to the focus on social context that is emphasized in the critical lens. *Both are offering a relational view of how people, situations, contexts, environments, and processes are integrally connected and shape each other.* As you undertake your nursing practice as a relational inquiry, the lenses can be used to look at the relational interplay of individuals and/or contexts, individuals in contexts, and contexts shaping communities, groups, families, and individuals. You can use each lens to look at all levels (intrapersonal, interpersonal, and contextual), and each will help you bring different things into focus. Or you may use each lens for specific purposes.

The HP lens can help you examine the interpretive realm—how people are making meaning and how you as a nurse are interpreting the people and families for which you care. It can also help you consider what in *you* might be leading to those interpretations and how you might expand your perceptual field. An HP lens can help you work across differences (e.g., when you and a colleague interpret a situation or person differently) and use interpretive differences as windows into a fuller view. In this way, the HP lens is a helpful tool at the intrapersonal, interpersonal, and contextual levels.

A critical lens similarly can help you inquire at the intrapersonal, interpersonal, and contextual levels. In concert with an HP lens, a critical lens can help you consider how structural conditions (e.g., economics, racial dynamics, gender) shape your thinking so that you can more consciously expand your perceptual field, test your assumptions, and make more informed choices. For example, a person isn't "racist" by virtue of being "white"; rather, a person, regardless of his or her own racial or ethnic identity can critically examine racializing practices and choose how to participate (embracing, ignoring, or countering). A critical lens is central to helping you work across difference interpersonally because it draws explicit attention to difference, including differences that arise from social arrangements and are unfair (inequities). Finally, a critical lens helps you fully consider the contextual elements that are both shaping people's interpretations (yours, your colleague's, and your patient's) and the experiential realities of people's lives. For example, a critical lens will help you draw attention to power, social inequities, and structural determinants that are shaping the care a patient is receiving or not receiving, or the structures that are shaping interactions (where physicians and nurses are constructed as expert knowers and patients are supposed to "comply").

The important thing in terms of the lenses is not to worry too much about distinguishing between them but to understand how helpful they can be when consciously used to support good nursing practice. We invite you to practice with them just like you might play with a new camera. Decide to enlist a critical lens one day when you go to work just to see what happens. What comes into the picture? How does the critical lens help you frame the picture of a particular person or family in a different way? How does it help you expand the picture? How does it help you hone in on what is important? Then shift to an HP lens, and notice if your attention goes to other places. Play with how things can look and be understood differently depending on the lens through which you look (e.g., wide-angle, telephoto) and the kind of picture you are taking (portrait, landscape). When you play with this awhile, you will begin to realize that, given your own selective interests, you always have a partial view. Moreover, you will realize that any understanding you may have of a patient/family or nursing situation is only a snapshot in time. Because people are living beings, to know and work effectively with people requires that we continually adjust our view.

Bringing the lenses together and bringing them to bear on nursing practice can be facilitated by (a) using the practice of reflexivity and, through reflexivity, (b) examining some of the practices and habits that keep an individualist, decontextualized approach firmly in place.

Use Reflexivity to Enlist the Lenses

Reflexivity is central to relational inquiry and involves a combination of observation, critical scrutiny, and conscious participation. It involves paying attention to who, how, and what you are being/doing/feeling/thinking in the moment (intrapersonal inquiry), being aware of and critically scrutinizing how you are relating to and with other people, and how they are relating to you (interpersonal inquiry) while considering the contextual elements you are in the midst of and that are shaping what is happening in the situation (contextual inquiry). For example, after observing themselves through HP and critical lenses over the course of a few days, some of the nurses I (Gweneth) have taught who work in critical care areas have noticed an emphasis on (or one might say culture of) control in their work context. The monitors that are part of the physical architecture (heart monitors and other technology used to track certain physiologic levels in patients) are like a symbol of what happens interpersonally in their units. As they more carefully observe the inner workings of their units, they begin to see patterns they did not see previously. For instance, some have noticed a professional stance of monitoring and control that plays out in the way the interprofessional staff speak to each other, relate around emotions (the norm being to relate by "not being emotional"), filter what they say to families, and how they guard the parameters (who is allowed in, who speaks to whom, etc.). They also begin to notice how this interpersonal practice is affecting them and the way they relate to the patients and families for whom they provide care. Some have described how surprised they were to realize that they carried such tension in their muscles and how their facial expressions and body language reflected that tension. They also noticed how they carried this bodily and interpersonal demeanor into their interactions with patients and families. Their controlled, instrumental approach provided a protection from the deeply emotional experiences they faced—the pain and suffering they witnessed daily. At times, they could see how it was also serving as a barrier to providing good care for patients and families living through crucial life and death experiences and feeling a range of emotions such as joy, pain, celebration, and sadness.

Orienting relationally, *enlisting the lenses*, and *consciously inquiring* into their everyday practice enabled the nurses to more clearly see what was happening at the different levels. It also enabled them to work more consciously within those realities. Ultimately, taking a relational inquiry approach enabled them to see and make new choices about how they could relate more effectively. They could be both instrumental in terms of monitoring and treating the physiologic elements and simultaneously more human in their responses to the emotions and suffering (of patients, families, themselves, and their colleagues) that are part and parcel of critical care nursing.

Examining how *you* think about and relate to others is an essential part of relational inquiry. Intrapersonally, there are some things that are specific to you as a person that influence how you think and relate interpersonally: factors such as your own particular sociohistorical background and location, past experiences, how outgoing or shy you are, how comfortable you are in a particular situation, and so forth. A number of contextual elements also shape the way you think of others and relate interpersonally. As in the critical care example above, the normative structures and practices within health care settings explicitly and implicitly shape the way nurses practice interpersonally in all settings. For instance, compare how nursing is oriented to a 72-year-old patient in an intensive care unit (ICU) with how nursing is oriented to exactly the same patient in a long-term care (LTC) setting. What different values operate? How is time used differently? These contextual elements can influence how you engage as a nurse, how you see patients and families, who and what dominate your attention, how you interpret people in different situations, how you respond, and so forth. These elements also influence what you do *not* relate to, notice, and/or think. Reflexivity used in concert with the lenses provides the tools to examine common practices that hamper the pursuit of well-being and social justice in nursing.

Examine Some Common Practices

In discussing the HP and critical lenses, we described how as people, we come to embody the norms and practices within which we are situated. Three common practices nurses tend to embody include the practice of privileging individual choice, the practice of categorizing, and the practice of differentiating. Like all normative practices, they develop from our social, political, cultural, historical, and economic environments, often to the point at which they become naturalized and invisible. Because these practices can serve to sustain inequities and interfere with promoting well-being, it is crucial that we enlist the HP and critical lenses to see when we are inadvertently enacting those practices.

The Practice of Privileging Individual Choice
Although an *individualist, decontextualized* view of people is incongruent with the relational complexities of most contemporary nursing situations and insufficient to working within those complexities, individualist ideology often plays a central role in how we think of people (both ourselves and others) and how we relate. While it is important to look individually at people to relate to them as unique beings with particular needs, lives, and aspirations, to *only* see individually is problematic.

An individualist ideology can lead us to privilege individual choice to the extent that we fail to see and understand how the circumstances of people's lives influence the choices they make and/or the choices available to them (think of Artur or the people at the COPD clinic). When we see people as autonomous and self-determining, we assume they are able to make free choices, regardless of their environments. We forget that those choices are always made within relational circumstances. For example, we might view John's time of living on the street (Chapter 1) as a personal "choice," rather than a result of complex relational, historical, economic, and political circumstances. Similarly, think back to the story of Artur, the young man with diabetes. When we consider the contextual realities of Artur's situation, we immediately see that he does not have the same choices as we (Gweneth and Colleen) might have. We cannot respond to Artur's behavior as if it were a manifestation of individual "choice."

The story opening Chapter 1 shows how privileging individual choice limited the nurse who was caring for her dying patient. Although the nurse was aware of the way her practice was constrained by the contextual realities within which she worked, she still interpreted the situation through the individualist lens—seeing herself as an autonomous moral agent with choice and an obligation to ensure a good death. Thus, the story she told herself and told us as researchers was how she had failed to give good nursing care. In her story, it is also possible to hear how her colleagues had used an individualist understanding to narrate their nursing realities. They told her that was "just the way things were." Feeling powerless (as individuals without choice), they saw no other option in terms of how they cared for dying patients.

Overall, liberal individualism has led nurses to assume that people (including themselves) are autonomous and that their behavior and choices are independent of their relational, economic, historical, and political worlds. This perspective blunts nurses' abilities to know and respond to people in ways that are relational and health promoting. For example, liberal individualism often leads nurses to put the responsibility for health on the individual without really considering how the person's context may be constraining his or her choices as an individual. Understanding autonomy as "relational" draws attention to constraints and supports for choice (Sherwin, 1998). As we further expand on the relational inquiry approach throughout the book, we will be further distinguishing a relational approach from an individualist, decontextualized approach and illustrating how a relational inquiry approach seeks to understand, honor, and attend to people in context, *viewing choice as a relational act that is profoundly shaped by contextual resources and constraints.*

The Practice of Categorizing
While categorizing is a dominant practice in health care and can be helpful, it can also be detrimental. For example, categorizing patients on the basis of acuity can be helpful to nursing in prioritizing care. However, categorizing can also serve to limit our view and care. Each time you apply one category to a person, situation, or issue, you draw attention to certain features and not to others. Using the HP and critical lenses, you can see how the categories are drawn through your own interpretations shaped by normative values and structures.

For example, in her study of women with cardiac symptoms, Russell (2012) showed how the use of the Canadian Triage and Acuity Scale (CTAS) in emergency shaped thinking in certain ways. Emergency staff is mandated to use the CTAS system to categorize patients in one of five levels, ranging from Level 1 (resuscitation) to Level 5 (nonurgent). Use of the CTAS is mandatory in Canadian hospital emergency units. Russell showed that the CTAS score kept nurses focused on biomedical criteria. "With every assessment, with every CTAS score specified by the nurses, was an orientation and reorientation to this biomedical perspective through their assessments and again through their written documentation. Each patient during their stay would be referred to in terms of their CTAS score, so the identity of the patients became, to a large extent, a product of this scoring technique" (Russell, 2012, p. 89).

At the same time, the score drew attention away from other features of the patients' situations. For example, Russell described how although the CTAS score for an elderly man with angina was high enough to warrant putting him on a stretcher, his elderly, frail wife had to "steal" a wheelchair to steady herself to get to the parking lot to go home. No one took into account the woman's well-being or the effect on the man from worrying about his wife. Paying attention to how you enlist categories, how others use categories, why, and the effects helps you to be more conscious, purposeful, and selective in categorizing and helps you to mitigate unintended consequences.

Social categories are always operating. Categorizations of age, gender, size, class, race, ability, and language (among others) are always operating. From our earliest social encounters we learn to differentiate, for example, on the basis of age and to attach value differently to various categories. We learn that in general, power and control over one's life increases from infancy through adolescence to adulthood. In most Western societies with free market economies which value individuals according to their economic productivity and competitiveness, power and control tend to decline in older age.

These categorizations are never neutral; they always impact how we see and relate. By their essence, categorizations are value-laden and imply both theoretical understandings and practical implications for nursing. For instance, how we think about children matters in nursing because it shapes how we approach children and their families and how we try to influence health care programming. In Western societies, children are seen as "incomplete," as "adults in the making" who are to be developed to contribute to the economic well-being of society through their productivity (Castañeda, 2002). Einboden, Rudge, and Varcoe (2013) show how these ideas are so entrenched that they seem self-evident, shaping ideas about how early childhood development should be measured and supported. Unfortunately, seeing children primarily in terms of their potential as economically productive adults means that those children with limited potential for such productivity are seen as "threats to the economy." Einboden and colleagues use the example of the Human Early Learning Partnership, designated by the World Health Organization as the Global Knowledge Network for Early Childhood Development (ECD), which argues that only support for ECD will limit the threat to the economy posed by "the future human capital losses that result from high child vulnerability today" (Kershaw, Anderson, & Warburton, 2009, p. 4). Einboden and colleagues show how this way of thinking can construct some children as "waste."

To take another example, elderly people and aging itself are often seen in terms of decline. Even the idea of "successful" aging implies resisting decline and encourages us to condemn as failures those who are unable to do so. These ways of thinking matter. Seeing a child as an incomplete adult or a frail, elderly person as a failure to age well will shape your approach differently than seeing either as full humans shaped by a multiplicity of factors.

Another important aspect of categories is that they do not operate in isolation from one another. That is, although one category and label may be prominent at any moment, others are always operating as well. That is, when you encounter another person, whether or not you are conscious of doing so, you are seeing the person as a certain age, gender, size, class, race, ability, and so on, and the associated social values are informing you. As we have said, it is impossible to be "neutral" or "colorblind." Thus, to the extent that you remain unconscious of the dynamics of categorization, you will be susceptible to unexamined influences.

TO ILLUSTRATE
A Slow Code

I arrived about 15 minutes early for night shift. As I opened the door to the open-heart recovery unit, I immediately saw that there was a resuscitation in progress in the first stretcher bay, the one reserved for the most acute cases. A small white form lay in the centre of the adult-sized stretcher, and there was evidence of chaos all around, plastic wrappers from IV bags, syringes, medication packaging, discarded lines, and the crash cart still sat by the bed. However, there was a curious calm, at odds with the evidence of an emergency situation that littered the space. "Varcoe," said the senior nurse, "Can you put on some tea?" I was stunned. As I took the scene in, I saw that she was doing cardiac massage on the small person, but without seeming to pay attention to what she was doing. A resident was nearby writing in a chart, but other staff members were busy with other patients and not paying attention to the scene. "We're just doing a slow code," explained the nurse. I was struck by her seeming lack of emotion and the apparent lack of concern by the other staff as they continued about their work as a child lay dying. Usually, a dying child was devastating. One of the other nurses explained. The little girl had Down syndrome (trisomy 21, which often includes cardiac anomalies).

That scene has stayed with me, contrasting starkly with the valuing of children usually evident in the actions and demeanor of the open heart staff. At that time, I was a very junior nurse (as suggested and reinforced by the command to make tea) and thought that I likely needed to toughen up. However, I was dismayed at how the child's life was apparently so devalued because of the very health problem being treated. The categorizing problem became worse, however. The next night when I arrived for my shift, a newspaper article on the door displayed a picture of

continued on page 88

TO ILLUSTRATE *continued*

A Slow Code

the little girl who had died. The previous spring, at age 4, she had been the child host for "Timmy's Telethon," a television fundraising campaign, capturing the hearts of audiences everywhere. Suddenly, the child's value seemed to change in the eyes of the staff, and I felt vindicated in my dismay. I remained angry, particularly at the senior nurse and what I saw as her casual and callous approach. It took me years to see that I too had valued the child differently when I learned of her "contribution" and talent.

TRY IT OUT 2.7

Examine the Practice of Categorizing

Pick up a newspaper or get online and look at your favorite news link. Peruse the stories and look for how people are being categorized. For example, how are people being identified (by nationality, religion, gender, age, socioeconomic status, role, professional status, physical status, etc.)? Pick one story, and as you read, pay attention to how your own thinking is being influenced by these categorizations. For example, do you think or feel differently when you read about the death of a 60-year-old in an accident versus that of a 21-year-old? Can you see any associations being made between the categories? For example, do you see religion being associated with nationalities or particular kinds of news events? After your inquiry, talk about your findings with a couple of your classmates or colleagues, and compare the patterns you observed in yourself and in the newspaper stories.

The Practice of Differentiating

Categorizing, particularly categorizing people, functions to differentiate oneself from others and among others. At the same time, categorizing also serves to make certain associations, so if one thing is different from another, it is also more similar to something else. Describing someone using categories is a social act that has consequences (e.g. "a white child with Down syndrome"). The social act of categorizing a person identifies what features are important at that moment at the same time as it differentiates those features from others (not black, not fully abled), including features not mentioned. As Allen (2006) asserts,

> . . . description is the creation of difference; difference entails classification and classification involves power. Describing something is a *performance*, a purposeful *social action* that requires (1) establishing boundaries ('what' is being described); (2) attributing qualities (what is it 'like'); and (3) attribution requires the application of pre-existing criteria. (p. 66)

Thus, how we differentiate and how we understand difference matters. Because nurses are often in positions of power relative to others, nursing acts of describing and categorizing can have significant consequences. Nurses have the power to influence how patients are seen by others through the categories they apply and the differences they highlight. Several habits of differentiating can be problematic including the habit of considering differences as "natural" and the habit of considering differences as a "choice." Both habits promote an individualized, decontextualized view of people.

Some "differences" are seen as naturally occurring. Take size, for example. Certainly, biology plays a role in determining a person's size. However, even a person's height is shaped by social factors. For example, studies comparing children born in certain countries with children born to parents from those countries when they immigrated to wealthier countries reveals that the determinants of stature are complex, associated with gender, economics, nutrition, acculturation, and privilege (Cernerud, 1994; Franzen & Smith, 2009). Similarly, studies within countries illustrate multiple social influences on height. For example, a study in Argentina (Salvatore, 2004) found that differences in skills, education, and social standing translated into significant differences in stature.

Krieger (2003) draws on multiple examples of the interplay of genetics, biology, and environment. For instance, adrenal glands are larger in those who have lived in poverty because of increased cortisol production, which likely results from living with chronic stress rather than from biologic difference. As another example, the risk of obesity, hypertension, and diabetes among people of West African decent is increased not because of race, as genetically constituted, but because of the influence of environmental factors on gene expression. Krieger (2003) raises concerns for the way epidemiologic understandings of "race" have used this biologic/genetic understanding of race to explain health inequities. Krieger argues that "simplistic divisions of the social and biological will not suffice. The interpretations we offer of observed average differences in health status across socially delimited groups reflect our theoretical frameworks, not ineluctable facts of nature" (p. S21).

In line with individualism, in Western societies, the dominant view is that individuals have free choice. Thus, many forms of difference—weight, class, educational level, language fluency, and so forth—are seen primarily as choices. For example, we are encouraged to think of our educational accomplishments as individual, personal achievements. Indeed, your education requires individual effort, and personal achievement is a component. However, multiple factors shape the possibilities for achievement, stretching back many generations. Was education valued in your family? Did you have preparation for school, such as adequate nutrition in childhood and being taught to read? Did you have access to books and primary school? Did you have a home to live in as a child? If so, was it safe and conducive to studying?

Differences are important and must be taken into account. While attending to difference, nurses must always understand differences as

- Reflecting certain theories (e.g., child as a presocial or fully human; height as natural versus height as socially determined)
- Implying value judgments (e.g., taller is better)
- Arising in context (e.g., education or poverty as socially determined)

THIS WEEK IN PRACTICE
Analyze an Interaction

Think back to the most recent interaction you had with a patient. Write down everything you can remember. Where did you stand or sit in relation to the patient? What were you and the patient wearing? What was your purpose (were you there to learn something, to "do" something "to" or "for" the patient)? What was happening around you at the time?

Thinking about that interaction, ask:

- What categories did you apply to that patient? What differentiating effect did those categories have?
- What gave you power in the relationship (e.g., physical position, professional position, clothing)?
- What was your goal in the interaction, and what shaped that goal (e.g., were you told, assigned, or expected to do something)?
- How were you presenting yourself (e.g., knowledgeable, compassionate, understanding, in charge, efficient)?
- What stance did you take toward the patient, and what influenced you to do so (e.g., rules, policies, expectations, norms)?
- Was there any pressure for you to coerce the patient into "complying" with your wishes (e.g., to do something at a certain time or speed) or those of others or the organization? If so, from where did that pressure arise?
- What stance did the patient take? To what extent did the patient seem to be playing the role of "the good" patient? What do you think shaped the patient's stance?
- What did you know about the patient's goals and wishes? What did you know about his or her life circumstances?
- What barriers to the patient's goals and wishes can you identify?
- What was the role of choice in this interaction?

As we progress through the book, we will continue to examine how a relational consciousness not only expands your view but hones it. That is, we will illustrate how as you think about, inquire into, and develop an understanding of these wider influences, your nursing practice becomes more targeted and effective. We suggest that each time you are assigned a new patient in your clinical area, you try enlisting a relational consciousness to see how it can enlarge your understanding of the patient, family, and health care situation.

YOUR RELATIONAL INQUIRY TOOLBOX

Add the following tools to your relational inquiry toolbox.

■ Enlist the HP lens to attune to living experiences.

■ Enlist the critical lens to look for how power dynamics are affecting health and health care.

■ Enlist a critical feminist filter to see how gender dynamics are intersecting with other forms of oppression and affecting health and health care.

■ Enlist a postcolonial filter to see how the dynamics of history, race, and economics are affecting health and health care.

■ Pay attention to how practices of individualizing choice, categorizing, and differentiating are constraining health and health care.

REFERENCES

Albanesi, S., & Olivetti, C. (2009). Home production, market production and the gender wage gap: Incentives and expectations. *Review of Economic Dynamics, 12*(1), 80–107. doi:10.1016/j.red.2008.08.001

Alex, M., & Whitty-Rogers, J. (2012). Time to disable the labels that disable: The power of words in nursing and health care of women, children and families. *Advances in Nursing Science, 35*(2), 113–126. doi:10.1097/ANS.0b013e31824fe6ae

Alksnis, C., Desmarais, S., & Curtis, J. (2008). Workforce segregation and the gender wage gap: Is "women's" work valued as highly as "men's"? *Journal of Applied Social Psychology, 38*(6), 1416–1441.doi:10.1111/j.1559-1816.2008.00354.x

Allam, S., Blyth, S., Fraser, A., Hodgson, S., Howes, J., Repper, J., et al. (2004). Reframing the nurse's role through a social model approach: A rights-based approach to workers' development, editorial. *Journal of Psychiatric & Mental Health Nursing*, pp. 365–373. Retrieved July 15, 2013, from http://search.ebscohost.com/login.aspx?direct=true&db=a9h&AN=13104585&login.asp&site=ehost-live

Allan, H. T., Larsen, J. A., Bryan, K., & Smith, P. A. (2004). The social reproduction of institutional racism: Internationally recruited nurses' experiences of the British health services. *Diversity in Health and Social Care, 1*(2), 117–126.

Allen, D. G. (2006). Whiteness and difference in nursing. *Nursing Philosophy, 7*(2), 65–78. doi:10.1111/j.1466-769X.2006.00255.x

Arulampalam, W., Alison, L. B., & Bryan, M. L. (2007). Is there a glass ceiling over Europe? Exploring the gender pay gap across the wage distribution. *Industrial and Labor Relations Review, 60*(2), 163–186. doi:10.2307/25249069

Bakhtin, M. (1981). *The dialogical imagination: Four essays* (M. Holoquist, Trans.). Austin, TX: University of Texas Press.

Beddoes, Z. M. (2012, October 13). Special report: The world economy. *The Economist.* Retrieved from http://econ.st/QNGakg

Benner, P. (2000). The roles of embodiment, emotion and lifeworld for rationality and agency in nursing practice. *Nursing Philosophy, 1*(1), 5–19. doi:10.1046/j.1466-769x.2000.00014.x

Benner, P., & Wrubel, J. (1989). *The primary of care, stress and coping in health and illness.* Menlo Park, CA: Addison-Wesley.

Bhabha, H. (1994). *The location of culture.* London: Routledge.

Birchwater, S. (1993). *Ulkatcho stories of the Grease Trail told by Ulkatcho and Nuxalk elders.* Quesnel, British Columbia, Canada: Spartan Printing.

Blair, S. (2013). The division of household labor. In G. W. Peterson & K. R. Bush (Eds.), *Handbook of marriage and the family* (pp. 613–635). New York: Springer.

Blau, F. D., & Kahn, L. M. (2007). The gender pay gap: Have women gone as far as they can? *Academy of Management Perspectives, 21*(1), 7–23. doi:10.5465/AMP.2007.24286161

Bombay, A., Matheson, K., & Anisman, H. (2011). The impact of stressors on second generation Indian residential school survivors. *Transcultural Psychiatry, 48*(4), 367–391. doi:10.1177/1363461511410240

Brewer, R. M. (1993). Theorizing race, class and gender: The new scholarship of Black feminist intellectuals and black women's labour. In S. M. James & A. P. A. Busia (Eds.), *Theorizing black feminisms: The visionary pragmatism for Black women* (pp. 13–30). London: Routledge.

Brown, H., Varcoe, C., & Calam, B. (2011). The birthing experiences of rural Aboriginal women in context: Implications for nursing/Les expériences d'accouchement des femmes autochtones en région rurale, mises en contexte: Les implications en matière de soins infirmiers. *Canadian Journal of Nursing Research, 43*(4), 100–117.

Browne, A. J. (2001). The influence of liberal political ideology on nursing science. *Nursing Inquiry, 8*(2), 118–129.

Browne, A. J., Smye, V. L., Rodney, P., Tang, S., Mussell, W., & O'Neil, J. (2011). Access to primary care from the perspective of Aboriginal patients at an urban emergency department. *Qualitative Health Research, 21*(3), 333–348.

Bungay, V., Johnson, J. L., Varcoe, C., & Boyd, S. (2010). Women's health and use of crack cocaine in context: Structural and "everyday" violence. *International Journal of Drug Policy, 21*(4), 321–329. doi:10.1016/j.drugpo.2009.12.008

Burhans, L. M., & Alligood, M. R. (2010). Quality nursing care in the words of nurses. *Journal of Advanced Nursing, 66*(8), 1689–1697. doi:10.1111/j.1365-2648.2010.05344.x

Byrne, M. M. (2001). Uncovering racial bias in nursing fundamentals textbooks. *Nursing and Health Care Perspectives, 22*(6), 299–303.

Campbell, G. A., Sanoff, S., & Rosner, M. H. (2010). Care of the undocumented immigrant in the United States with ESRD. *American Journal of Kidney Diseases, 55*(1), 181–191. doi:10.1053/j.ajkd.2009.06.039

Cason, K., Nieto-Montenegro, S., Chavez-Martinez, A., Ly, N., & Snyder, A. (2004). *Dietary intake and food security among migrant farm workers in Pennsylvania.* Chicago: Harris School of Public Policy Studies, University of Chicago.

Castañeda, C. (2002). *Figurations: Child, bodies, worlds.* Durham, NC: Duke University Press.

Cernerud, L. (1994). Are there still social inequalities in height and body mass index of Stockholm children? *Scandinavian Journal of Social Medicine, 22*(3), 161–165.

Cheek, J. (2000). *Postmodern and poststructural approaches to nursing practice.* London: Sage.

Coburn, D. (2004). Beyond the income inequality hypothesis: Class, neo-liberalism, and health inequalities. *Social Science & Medicine, 58*(1), 41–56.

Collins, P. H. (1986). Learning from the outsider within. *Social Problems, 33*(5), 14–32.

Collins, P. H. (1990). *Black feminist thought: Knowledge, consciousness, and the politics of empowerment.* (2nd ed.). New York: Routledge.

Collins, P. H. (1993). Toward a new vision: Race, class and gender as categories of analysis and connection. *Race, Sex, & Class, 1*(1), 23–45.

Conrad, P. (1987). The experience of illness: Recent and new directions in the experience and management of chronic illness. *Research in Sociology and Health Care, 6*, 1–31.

Conroy, K., Sandel, M., & Zuckerman, B. (2010). Poverty grown up: How childhood socioeconomic status impacts adult health. *Journal of Developmental & Behavioral Pediatrics, 31*(2), 154–160.

Corley, M. C., Minick, P., Elswick, R. K., & Jacobs, M. (2005). Nurse moral distress and ethical work environment. *Nursing Ethics, 12*(4), 381–390. doi:10.1191/0969733005ne809oa

Crooks, V. A., Williams, A., Stajduhar, K., Robin Cohen, S., Allan, D., & Brazil, K. (2012). Family caregivers' ideal expectations of Canada's Compassionate Care Benefit. *Health & Social Care in the Community, 20*(2), 172–180. doi:10.1111/j.1365-2524.2011.01028.x

Davies, B. (1990). Positioning: The discursive production of selves. *Journal for the Theory of Social Behavior, 20*(1), 43–63.

Davies, B., & Harre, R. (1990). Positioning: Conversation and the production of selves. *Journal for the Theory of Social Behaviour, 20,* 43–63.

Dolgin, J., & Dietrich, K. (2009). When others get too close: Immigrants, class and health care debate. *Cornell Journal of Law and Public Policy, 19*(2), 283.

Earle, V. (2010). Phenomenology as research method or substantive metaphysics? An overview of phenomenology's uses in nursing. *Nursing Philosophy, 11*(4), 286–296. doi:10.1111/J.1466-769X.2010.00458.x

Einboden, R., Rudge, T., & Varcoe, C. (2013). Producing children in the 21st century: A critical discourse analysis of the science and techniques of monitoring early child development. *Health.* Advance online publication.

Elias, B., Mignone, J., Hall, M., Hong, S. P., Hart, L., & Sareen, J. (2012). Trauma and suicide behaviour histories among a Canadian indigenous population: An empirical exploration of the potential role of Canada's residential school system. *Social Science & Medicine, 74*(10), 1560–1569. doi:10.1016/j.socscimed.2012.01.026

Fairclough, N. (2001). The dialectics of discourse. *Textus, 14,* 231–242.

Fairclough, N. (2004). Semiotic aspects of social transformation and learning. In R. Rogers (Ed.), *An introduction to critical discourse analysis in education* (pp. 225–235). Mahwah, NJ: Lawrence Erlbaum Associates.

Fields, W. W., Asplin, B. R., Larkin, G. L., Marco, C. A., Johnson, L. A., Yeh, C., et al. (2001). The Emergency Medical Treatment and Labor Act as a federal health care safety net program. *Academic Emergency Medicine, 8*(11), 1064–1069. doi:10.1111/j.1553-2712.2001tb01116.x

Fleitas, J. (2003). The power of words: Examining the linguisitic landscape of pediatric nursing. *Advances in Nursing Science, 28*(6), 384–388.

Foucault, M. (2003). Governmentality. In P. Rabinow & N. Rose (Eds.), *The essential Foucault: Selections from essential works of Foucault 1954–1984* (pp. 229–245). London: The New Press.

Franzen, L., & Smith, C. (2009). Differences in stature, BMI, and dietary practices between U.S.-born and newly immigrated Hmong children. *Social Science & Medicine, 69*(3), 442–450. doi:10.1016/j.socscimed.2009.05.015

Funk, L. M., Stajduhar, K., & Purkis, M. E. (2011). An exploration of empowerment discourse within home-care nurses' accounts of practice. *Nursing Inquiry, 18*(1), 66–76. doi:10.1111/j.1440-1800.2010.00502.x

Galabuzi, G. E. (2001). *Canada's creeping economic apartheid: The economic segregation and social marginalization of racialised groups.* Toronto, Ontario, Canada: Centre for Social Justice Foundation for Research and Education.

Gerow, L., Conejo, P., Alonzo, A., Davis, N., Rodgers, S., & Domian, E. W. (2010). Creating a curtain of protection: Nurses' experiences of grief following patient death. *Journal of Nursing Scholarship, 42*(2), 122–129. doi:10.1111/j.1547-5069.2010.01343.x

Giroux, H. A. (1983). *Theory and resistance in education: A pedagogy for the opposition.* South Hadley, MA: Bergin & Garrey.

Grypma, S. J. (2003). Profile of a leader: Unearthing Ethel John's "buried" commitment to racial equality, 1925. *Nursing Leadership, 16,* 439–447.

Gustafson, D. L. (2007). White on whiteness: Becoming radicalized about race. *Nursing Inquiry, 14*(2), 153–161. doi:10.1111/j.1440-1800.2007.00365.x

Hagey, R., Choudhry, U., Guruge, S., Turrittin, J., Collins, E., & Lee, R. (2001). Immigrant nurses' experience of racism. *Journal of Nursing Scholarship, 33*(4), 389–394.

Hagey, R., & MacKay, R. W. (2000). Qualitative research to identify racialist discourse: Towards equity in nursing curricula. *International Journal of Nursing Studies, 37*(1), 45–56.

Hall, J. M. (1999). Marginalization revisited: Critical, postmodern, and liberation perspectives. *Advances In Nursing Science, 22*(2), 88–102.

Hankivsky, O., Reid, C., Cormier, R., Varcoe, C., Clark, N., Benoit, C., et al. (2010). Exploring the promises of intersectionality for advancing women's health research. *International Journal for Equity in Health, 9,* 1–15.

Hanssen, I. (2004). An intercultural nursing perspective on autonomy. *Nursing Ethics, 11*(1), 28–41. doi:10.1191/0969733004ne664oa

Hartrick, G. A. (1998a). A critical pedagogy for family nursing. *Journal of Nursing Education, 37*(2), 80–84.

Hartrick, G. A. (1998b). Living the question of family nursing. *Journal of Family Nursing, 4*(1), 8–20.

Hartrick Doane, G. A., Stajduhar, K., Bidgood, D., Causton, E., & Cox,

A. (2012). End-of-life care and interprofessional practice: Not simply a matter of more. *Health and Interprofessional Practice, 11*(3), EP1028.

Hassouneh, D. (2008). Reframing the diversity question: Challenging Eurocentric power hierarchies in nursing education. *Journal of Nursing Education, 47*(7), 291–292. doi:10.3928/01484834-20080701-03

Hausmann, R., Tyson, L., & Zahidi, S. (2012). *The global gender gap report 2012*. Geneva, Switzerland: World Economic Forum.

Henry, F., & Tator, C. (2006). *The colour of democracy: Racism in Canadian society* (3rd ed.). Toronto, Ontario, Canada: Nelson Thomson.

hooks, b. (1984). *Feminist theory: From margin to center*. Boston: South End Press.

hooks, b. (1990). *Yearning: Race, gender and cultural politics*. Boston: South End Press.

Inouye, K. (2012). Conditional love; representations of migrant work in Canadian newsprint media. *Social Identities, 18*(5), 573–592. doi:10.1080/13504630.2012.692895

Jackson, D., Hutchinson, M., Everett, B., Mannix, J., Peters, K., Weaver, R., et al. (2011). Struggling for legitimacy: Nursing students' stories of organisational aggression, resilience and resistance. *Nursing Inquiry, 18*(2), 102–110. doi:10.1111/j.1440-1800.2011.00536.x

Johnson, S. A. (2008). *Healing in silence: Black nurses in Charleston, South Carolina, 1896–1948*. (Ph.D.), Medical University of South Carolina. Retrieved July 15, 2013, from http://search.ebscohost.com/login.aspx?direct=true&db=c8h&AN=2010544023&login.asp&site=ehost-live

Kendall, P. (2001). The health and wellbeing of Aboriginal people in British Columbia: Report on the health of British Columbians - Provincial Health Officer's Annual Report, 2001. Victoria, British Columbia, Canada: Office of the Provincial Health Officer, Province of British Columbia.

Kendall, P. (2009). *Pathways to Health and Healing: 2nd Report on the Health and Well-being of Aboriginal People in British Columbia*. Victoria, British Columbia, Canada: British Columbia Ministry for Health Living and Sport.

Kennedy, D., & Bouchard (no date). R. Nuxalk (Bella Coola). *The Canadian Encyclopedia*. Retrieved June 3, 2007, from http://thecanadianencyclopedia.com/index

Kershaw, P., Anderson, L., & Warburton, B. (2009). Executive Summary 15 by 15: A comprehensive policy framework for early human capital investment in BC. Vancouver, British Columbia, Canada: Human Early Learning Partnership.

Kincheloe, J. L., & McLaren, P. (2000). Rethinking critical theory and qualitative research. In N. K. Denzin & Y. S Lincoln (Eds.), *Handbook of qualitative research* (pp. 279–313). Thousand Oaks, CA: Sage.

Kovner, C., Brewer, C., Wu, Y.-W., Cheng, Y., & Suzuki, M. (2006). Factors associated with work satisfaction of registered nurses. *Journal of Nursing Scholarship, 38*(1), 71–79. doi:10.1111/j.1547-5069.2006.00080.x

Krieger, N. (2003). Does racism harm health? Did child abuse exist before 1962? On explicit questions, critical science, and current controversies: An ecosocial perspective. *American Journal of Public Health, 98*(Suppl. 1), S20–S25.

Leonard, V. W. (1989). A Heideggerian phenomenological perspective on the concept of person. *Advances in Nursing Science, 11*(4), 40–55.

Lyon, M. (2009). Emotion, embodiment, and agency: The place of a social emotions perspective in the cross-disciplinary understanding of emotional processes. In H. J. Markowitsch & B. Röttger-Rössler (Eds.), *Emotions as bio-cultural processes* (pp. 199–213). New York: Springer.

Mackenbach, J. P. (2012). The persistence of health inequalities in modern welfare states: The explanation of a paradox. *Social Science & Medicine, 75*(4). doi:10.1016/j.socscimed.2012.02.031

Mandell, N., & Duffy, A. (1995). *Canadian families: Diversity, conflict and change*. Toronto, Ontario, Canada: Harcourt, Brace & Company.

Markey, K., & Tilki, M. (2007). Education and development. Racism in nursing education: A reflective journey. *British Journal of Nursing, 16*(7), 390–393.

Marmot, M., & Bell, R. (2012). Fair society, healthy lives. *Public Health, 126, Supplement 1*(0), S4–S10. doi:10.1016/j.puhe.2012.05.014

Marrow, H. B. (2012). Deserving to a point: Unauthorized immigrants in San Francisco's universal access healthcare model. *Social Science & Medicine, 74*(6), 846–854. doi:10.1016/j.socscimed.2011.08.001

Martin, D. E., & Kipling, A. (2006). Factors shaping Aboriginal nursing students' experiences. *Nurse Education in Practice, 6*(6), 380–388. doi:10.1016/j.nepr.2006.07.009.

McCloughen, A., O' Brien, L., & Jackson, D. (2011). Nurse leader mentor as a mode of being: Findings from an Australian hermeneutic phenomenological study. *Journal of Nursing Scholarship, 43*(1), 97–104. doi:10.1111/j.1547-5069.2010.01377.x

Osmond, M. W. (1987). Radical-critical theories. In M. B. Sussma & S. K. Steinmetz (Eds.), *Handbook of marriage and the family*. New York: Plenum.

Paterson, J. G., & Zderad, L. T. (1988). *Humanistic nursing* (2nd ed.). New York: National League for Nursing.

Perry, J. A. (2012). Barely legal: Racism and migrant farm labour in the context of Canadian multiculturalism. *Citizenship Studies, 16*(2), 189–201. doi:10.1080/13621025.2012.667611

Potthast-Jutkeit, B. (1997). The history of the family and colonialism. *History of the Family, 2*(2), 115–121.

Puzan, E. (2003). The unbearable whiteness of being (in nursing). *Nursing Inquiry, 10*(3), 193. doi:10.1046/j.1440-1800.2003.00180.x

Pysklywec, M., McLaughlin, J., Tew, M., & Haines, T. (2011). Doctors within borders: Meeting the health care needs of migrant farm workers in Canada. *CMAJ: Canadian Medical Association Journal = Journal De L'association Medicale Canadienne, 183*(9), 1039–1043. doi:10.1503/cmaj.091404

Quayson, A. (2000). *Postcolonialism: Theory, practice or process?* Cornwall, United Kingdom: Polity Press.

Ramirez, S. M., & Villarejo, D. (2012). Poverty, housing, and the rural slum. *American Journal of Public Health, 102*(9), 1664-1675. doi:10.2105/ajph.2011.300864

Raphael, D. (2007). Poverty and the modern welfare state. In D. Raphael (Ed.), *Poverty and policy in Canada: Implications for health and quality of life* (pp. 5–26). Toronto, Ontario, Canada: Canadian Scholar's Press.

Raphael, D. (2010). Social determinants of health: An overview of concepts and issues. In D. Raphael, T. Bryant, & M. Rioux (Eds.), *Staying alive: Critical perspectives on health, illness, and health care* (pp. 145–180). Toronto, Ontario, Canada: Canadian Scholar's Press.

Robbins, P., & Aydede, M. (2009). A short primer on situated cognition. *The Cambridge Handbook of Situated Cognition* (pp. 3–10). New York: Cambridge University Press.

Rodríguez, M. A., & Vega, W. A. (2009). Confronting inequities in Latino health care. *Journal of General Internal Medicine, 24*(Suppl. 3), 505–507. doi:10.1007/s11606-009-1128-0

Russell, H. (2012). *An uneasy subjection: The emergency room encounters of health professionals and women with cardiac symptoms* (Doctoral dissertation). University of Calgary, Canada.

Ryan, L. (2007). Who do you think you are? Irish nurses encountering ethnicity and constructing identity in Britain. *Ethnic & Racial Studies, 30*(3), 416–438. doi:10.1080/01419870701217498

Salvatore, R. D. (2004). Stature, nutrition, and regional convergence. *Social Science History, 28*(2), 297–324.

Scammell, J. M. E., & Olumide, G. (2012). Racism and the mentor-student relationship: Nurse education through a white lens. *Nurse Education Today, 32*(5), 545–550. doi:10.1016/j.nedt.2011.06.012

Sherwin, S. (1998). A relational approach to autonomy in health care. In S. Sherwin (Ed.), *The Politics of Women's Health: Exploring Agency and Autonomy* (pp. 19–47). Philadelphia: Temple University Press.

Shields, M. A., & Price, S. W. (2002). Racial harassment, job satisfaction, and intentions to quit: Evidence from the British nursing profession. *Economica, 69*(274), 295–326. doi:10.2307/3549078

Smith, D., Varcoe, C., & Edwards, N. (2005). Turning around the intergenerational impact of residential schools on Aboriginal people: Implications for health policy and practice. *Canadian Journal of Nursing Research, 37*(4), 38–60.

Smye, V. L., & Browne, A. J. (2002). 'Cultural safety' and the analysis of health policy affecting Aboriginal people. *Nurse Researcher, 9*(3), 42.

Smye, V. L., Browne, A. J., Varcoe, C., & Josewski, V. (2011). Harm reduction, methadone maintenance treatment and the root causes of health and social inequities: An intersectional lens in the Canadian context. *Harm Reduction Journal*, 8–17. doi:10.1186/1477-7517-8-17

Stajduhar, K. (2001). *The idealization of dying at home: The social context of home-based palliative caregiving* (Doctoral dissertation). University of British Columbia, Vancouver, Canada.

Stajduhar, K. (2003). Examining the perspectives of family members involved in the delivery of palliative care at home. *Journal of Palliative Care, 19*(1), 27–35.

Stajduhar, K., Funk, L., Jakobsson, E., & Ohlén, J. (2010). A critical analysis of health promotion and 'empowerment' in the context of palliative family care-giving. *Nursing Inquiry, 17*(3), 221–230.

Stajduhar, K., Funk, L., Roberts, D., McLeod, B., Cloutier-Fisher, D., Wilkinson, C., et al. (2011). Home care nurses' decisions about the need for and amount of service at the end of life. *Journal of Advanced Nursing, 67*(2), 276–286. doi:10.1111/j.1365 -2648.2010.05491.x

Stephenson, P. (1999). Expanding notions of culture for cross-cultural ethics in health and medicine. In H. Coward & P. Ratanakul (Eds.), *A cross-cultural dialogue on health care ethics* (pp. 68–91). Waterloo, Ontario, Canada: Wilfried Laurier University Press.

Turrittin, J., Hagey, R., Guruge, S., Collins, E., & Mitchell, M. (2002). The experiences of professional nurses who have migrated to Canada: cosmopolitan citizenship or democratic racism? *International Journal of Nursing Studies,* p. 655. Retrieved July 16, 2013, from http://search.ebscohost.com /login.aspx?direct=true&db=a9h&AN=7 833520&login.asp&site=ehost-live

Ulrich, C., O'Donnell, P., Taylor, C., Farrar, A., Danis, M., & Grady, C. (2007). Ethical climate, ethics stress, and the job satisfaction of nurses and social workers in the United States. *Social Science & Medicine, 65*(8), 1708–1719. doi:10.1016/j.socscimed.2007.05.050

van Riemsdijk, M. (2010). Variegated privileges of whiteness: Lived experiences of Polish nurses in Norway. *Social & Cultural Geography, 11*(2), 117–137. doi:10.1080/14649360903514376

Varcoe, C. (2001). Abuse obscured: An ethnographic account of emergency nursing in relation to violence against women. *The Canadian Journal Of Nursing Research/Revue Canadienne De Recherche En Sciences Infirmières, 32*(4), 95–115.

Varcoe, C., Brown, H., Calam, B., Harvey, T., & Tallio, M. (2013). Help bring back the celebration of life: A community-based participatory study of rural Aboriginal women's maternity experiences and outcomes. *BMC Pregnancy and Childbirth, 13,* 26.

Varcoe, C., Browne, A. J., Wong, S., & Smye, V. L. (2009). Harms and benefits: Collecting ethnicity data in a clinical context. *Social Science & Medicine,* (68), 1659–1666. doi:10.1016 /j.socscimed.2009.02.034

Varcoe, C., & Hartrick Doane, G. A. (2007). Mothering and women's health. In O. Hankivsky, M. Morrow & C. Varcoe (Eds.), *Women's health in Canada: Critical perspectives on theory and policy* (pp. 297–323). Toronto, Ontario, Canada: University of Toronto.

Vega, W. A., Rodriguez, M. A., & Gruskin, E. (2009). Health disparities in the Latino population. *Epidemiologic Reviews, 31*(1), 99–112.

Walia, H. (2010). Transient servitude: Migrant labour in Canada and the apartheid of citizenship. *Race & Class, 52*(1), 71–84.

Weedon, C. (1981). Principles of poststructuralism. *Feminist practice and poststructuralist theory* (pp. 12–42). New York: Basil Blackwell.

Weedon, C. (1987). *Feminist practice and poststructuralist theory*. New York: Basil Blackwell.

Weedon, C. (1997). *Feminist practice and poststructuralist theory* (2nd ed.). Cambridge, NJ: Blackwell.

Whitehead, M., & Dahlgren, G. (2006). Levelling up (part 1): A discussion paper on concepts and principles for tackling social inequities in health. *Studies on Social and Economic Determinants of Population Health, No. 2*: WHO Collaborating Centre for Policy Research on Social Determinants of Health, University of Liverpool.

Wilby, M. L. (2009). When the world is white. *International Journal for Human Caring, 13*(4), 57–61.

Williams, A. M., Eby, J. A., Crooks, V. A., Stajduhar, K., Giesbrecht, M., Vuksan, M., et al. (2011). Canada's compassionate care benefit: Is it an adequate public health response to addressing the issue of caregiver burden in end-of-life care? *BMC Public Health, 11,* 335–335.

Wuest, J. (1997). Illuminating environmental influences on women's caring. *Journal of Advanced Nursing, 26,* 49–58.

Wuest, J. (2001). Precarious ordering: Toward a formal theory of women's caring. *Health Care for Women International, 22*(1/2), 167–194.

3 Nursing Obligations and Ontologic Capacities: The Five Cs Supporting Relational Inquiry

LEARNING OBJECTIVES

By engaging with the material in this chapter, you will be able to:

1. Understand how nursing obligations are relationally determined.

2. Identify the ontologic capacities that support relational inquiry practice.

3. Explore and develop your own ontologic capacities.

In this chapter, we discuss how relational inquiry can enable you to clearly discern your nursing obligations in complex nursing situations and outline the particular ways of being (ontologic capacities) that support relational inquiry and responsive, health-promoting nursing practice.

HOW DO YOU DETERMINE YOUR NURSING OBLIGATIONS?

As nurses, we are obligated to ensure that our nursing actions promote health and healing, are ethical, and are safe. But how does a nurse determine what actually constitutes "ethical," "safe," and "healing/health promoting" practice in particular situations? Over the past several years, we have repeatedly heard nurses describe the challenges they face in upholding the values of the nursing profession and ensuring competent, effective health care to patients and families. Concerned for patient/family well-being, nurses constantly work *between* their own values and the values of others, *between* competing interests and obligations, and *between* their nursing ideals and health care realities as they strive to ensure quality nursing care (Hartrick Doane, Stajduhar, Bidgood, Causton, & Cox, 2012; Reimer Kirkham et al., 2012; Varcoe et al., 2004; Varcoe, Pauly, Storch, Newton, & Makaroff, 2012; Varcoe, Pauly, Webster, & Storch, 2012).

Clearly discerning your nursing obligations within those complexities can be challenging. Yet clarity of obligation and purpose is necessary to confidently mediate the forces that are pressing in upon you. Such clarity enables you to articulate your nursing concerns to yourself and to others in the health care team and choose the most effective actions.

Challenges in Determining Nursing Obligations

Most often, nursing values and obligations are articulated in the form of ethical codes or principles such as the obligations of beneficence, nonmaleficence, autonomy, and justice. These codes are expected to reinforce professional and societal values and give coherence to professional behavior by disclosing the profession's values and duties (Armstrong, 2006; Thompson, 2002). The norms included in codes are determined by the nursing philosophy of a particular country and at the same time are influenced by the moral problems nurses face in their everyday work (Dobrowolska, Wrońska, Fidecki, & Wysokiński, 2007).

While ethical codes identify what values and principles nurses are obligated to uphold, they do not necessarily delineate *how* to act in specific nursing situations. Specifically, there are three limitations of most codes of ethics that affect nurses at point-of-care. First, the way nursing obligations have been articulated in ethical codes and standards is not necessarily aligned with the complexities of nursing practice (Carnevale, 2005; Hartrick Doane & Varcoe, 2013; McCarthy, 2006). For example, often obligation-based ethics focus on right and wrong action and theoretically assume that there is a definitive "right" response to a situation. Given the complexities of current health care settings, this does not reflect most nursing situations (Thompson, 2002). Second, ethical codes do not offer practical direction for *how* nurses might actually enact their ethical obligations in their day-to-day practice (Armstrong, 2006; MacDonald, 2006; Pattison, 2001; Thompson, 2002). Codes are usually confined to ideals and outline *what* obligations are important but do not provide guidance for *how* a particular nurse in a particular complex situation might proceed (Thompson, 2002). Finally, the way obligations have been conceptualized as an external and universal entity fails to address important features that shape ethical practice, including context, historical changes, culture, character, and relationship (Thompson, 2002). For example, given the dominance of liberalist ideology (remember Chapter 2), codes of ethics tend to promote the values of individualism. In the US and Canadian contexts respectively, Bekemeier and Butterfield (2005) and Kirkham and Browne (2006) argue that codes of ethics encourage us to presume that Western societies are essentially egalitarian, and while we are directed to be aware of broader social issues, we are not committed by professional values as articulated in such codes to act on those broader issues or even to act on issues beyond our assigned patients.

As a result of these three limitations, determining our nursing obligations in particular situations can be challenging. For example, the codes do not necessarily address questions that arise as nurses work within competing obligations. Similarly, codes do not give direction when there is lack of agreement about values—when different values are at play in a particular nursing situation (Thompson, 2002). For example, Provis and Stack (2004) describe how caring work is ripe with conflicting obligations and how personal and organizational obligations might run counter to each other. They offer the example of a caregiver who, interpreting her use of bath towels through the values and norms of the organization, worried that she was being "extravagant." "You're always told how much it costs for linen and that sort of thing . . . I like to put an extra towel over their shoulders to keep them warm while I dry them with the other towel, so that may not be cost-conscious" (p. 6). Even in the smallest moments, various obligations pull us in different directions. Thus, we need a way of determining our nursing obligations when we are obligated in conflicting ways, when our obligations to different patients are in tension, when our obligations to a patient conflict with obligations to a family member (think of knowing that a patient is going to harm a family member), and/ or when our obligations to our organization are at odds with our obligations to patients.

Nursing Obligations Are Relationally Determined

Somewhat in contrast to the dominant understanding that obligations are determined through a rational process of objective reasoning devoid of personal involvement, philosopher John Caputo (1987) contends that obligations are local events; they are matters of flesh and blood. According to Caputo, obligation is the feeling that comes over us in binding ways when others need our help or support and we feel compelled to respond. "When I feel obliged, something demands my response. It is not [simply] a matter of working through a set of principles to conclude whether one is obliged" (p. 22). Caputo asks "Does one really 'conclude' that one is obliged, or does one not just find oneself obliged, without so much as having been consulted or asked for one's consent?" (p. 22). Caputo's description echoes the experience of the majority of nurses with whom we have worked. For example, remember back to the opening story in Chapter 1 of the situation with the dying man who was transferred from the ER. The nurse felt obligated to provide high-quality end-of-life care to the man and his wife, and her inability to do so resulted in her going home in tears.

Relational Inquiry Helps You Discern Your Nursing Obligations

Bergum (2013) contends that it is in the relational spaces of health care where our nursing obligations become evident. While values and ideals such as those articulated in ethical codes can give direction, our nursing obligations become evident through the relational interplay of patients, families, nurses, and the health care situation. For example, what constitutes "preserving dignity" or "promoting justice" (which are ethical obligations outlined in most nursing codes) is dependent on the specific situation, the particular people within that situation, and the system in which care is occurring. As such, the first step toward meeting our nursing obligations is to *be in* those situations as a relational inquirer to develop an in-depth understanding of those elements and an effective response to them (Hartrick Doane & Varcoe, 2007).

TO ILLUSTRATE
Being in Complex Nursing Situations

A few years ago, I (Gweneth) participated in a study with a team of researchers to examine public health nurses' (PHNs) practice with "high-priority" families living in rural and remote areas (Macleod et al., 2004). Using risk assessment tools based on epidemiologic research, the label "high-risk families" is frequently used in public health nursing to identify families with multiple intersecting risk factors (such as poverty, low socioeconomic resources, low social supports, comorbidities, etc.). In response to concerns about the terminology "high-risk" and the labelling of families in that way (remember our discussion in Chapter 2 about labelling), the term "high-priority" has come into use. The label identifies families who might need to be prioritized for public health nurse (PHN) intervention based on their risk indicators. That term was used in the health region in which the PHNs in our study practiced, thus the use of the term in our study.

The study we conducted focused on examining the working relationships between "high-priority" families and the PHNs. The PHNs were interested to know whether the families for whom they cared were benefiting from their current approach. As we gathered and analyzed the data in the study, one of the striking features was the purposeful approach the PHNs took when determining their nursing obligations within what were incredibly complex situations. While on the surface, the PHN mandate offered a clear direction for practice (e.g., they were mandated to immunize a high percentage of the population, assess risk factors, and do subsequent follow-up risk management home visits to new mothers); within the complex family situations, deciding on priorities and determining the most pressing obligations among many competing ones was highly challenging. Below, we briefly highlight some of the elements that were central to the PHNs' effectiveness in determining and meeting their nursing obligations. (For a fuller description, see the published findings in Hartrick Doane, Browne, Reimer, Macleod & Mclellan, 2009; and Browne, Hartrick Doane, Reimer, Macleod, & Mclellan, 2010).

Working effectively with families required that the PHNs worked in concert with the contextual realities of families' lives. This meant understanding the difficulties of the families' lives and the many elements that were shaping their experiences. For example, working with a mother living in challenging social circumstances and hearing her exclaim, "I can't handle my kids" could signal a risk of potential harm, to which the nurses were mandated to assess and alert child protection services (Hartrick Doane et al., 2009). However, the PHNs assessed each situation of potential risk not as an isolated event but within the context of the family's life. Knowing the complexities of a particular family situation, the PHNs mediated between risk and family capacity to discern their obligations. For example, they would weigh the potential harm of removing children from their mother against the possible harm that might come from leaving them in the home. The way the nurses mediated these intricate situations and their competing obligations was through a process of inquiry. What constituted risk and harm became a

continued on page 101

TO ILLUSTRATE *continued*

Being in Complex Nursing Situations

question they considered within the specific situation and time. For example, in one situation, the PHN decided to mediate risk by arranging childcare so the mother could have a break. Her decision arose through a combination of clinical judgment, a sense of obligation to help keep the family together if possible, her empathic understanding of the mother's frustrating circumstances, and the capacity she had witnessed in the mother. Although it would have been within her purview to initiate a call to a child protection social worker to initiate surveillance interventions, she determined her nursing obligations by using her knowledge of the woman's unique needs and vulnerabilities and the particularities of the woman's life situation at that time. Experience had taught the PHNs that to most effectively meet their nursing obligations to families, they had to intentionally focus on the family's context (and its complexities and difficulties) and determine the best action based on who the families were, what they were experiencing, and what they most needed at a particular moment (Hartrick Doane et al., 2009).

Taking a Proximal–Distal View

The PHN example highlights the importance of taking a proximal *and* distal view when determining obligations. Peter and Liaschenko (2004) highlight that proximity to others is one way that nurses understand what their obligations are. "Proximity beckons moral agents to act and therefore has an impact on moral responsiveness" (p. 219). This proximal "relational"

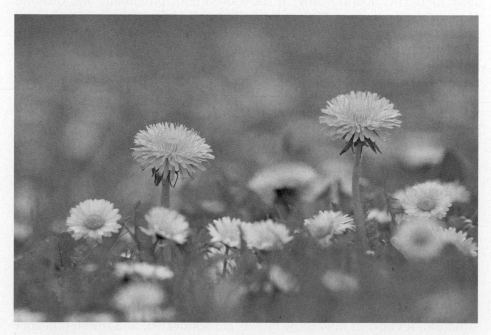

Distal view.

nature of nursing obligations is also evidenced in the way that the nurse in the Chapter 1 story responded within the situation. Her proximity to the wife who was "standing there with her mouth gaping open" compelled the nurse to walk her to her car and ensure that she would not have to go home to an empty house.

However, when taking a relational inquiry approach to discern your nursing obligations, we think it is most effective to consciously take a proximal *and* distal view. For example, while the PHNs had to ensure immediate safety to decide how best to intervene, they also needed to look forward; what would be the immediate *and* long-term effects of any intervention (such as removing a child from the home)? Similarly, to determine obligations, you need to extend your view beyond whomever or whatever is immediately within your sight. Does the pain, suffering, or acuity of the person in front of you obscure someone in greater need? I (Colleen) recall seeing a car accident and running to the first person I saw lying on the road. His throat had been torn open, and he was bleeding profusely and choking. I opened his airway and turned him on his side just as another nurse arrived. We stayed with the man until an ambulance attendant took over. However, neither of us realized that another person was still in one of the cars, in full cardiac arrest.

A relational understanding of nursing obligations and the relational inquiry process enables you to take a proximal–distal view to inquire into and discern best action within the complexities of a particular situation. Returning to the Chapter 1 story, can you think of how the nurse might have enlisted the HP and critical lenses we described in Chapter 2 to help her take a proximal–distal view? For example, while the nurse felt obligated to the man and his wife (who were in her proximal view), what about future patients who might also be affected by the ER transfer policy (distal view)? How might her action change if she looked both proximally and distally? How might looking at the situation intrapersonally, interpersonally, and contextually have expanded her perspective and helped her move beyond an individualist view (where she as a lone nurse is left responsible to provide good care)? Might a relational understanding of nursing obligation help her see how her feelings of inadequacy are not just about her—or how her own actions and response-ability is being hindered by contextual factors that need questioning? Moreover, rather than feeling distressed and powerless, might such a view help her identify a larger range of options for action?

Why a Relational Understanding of Nursing Obligations Is Important

Bringing a relational understanding of nursing obligations to your work both expands your view and the possibilities for action. As you enlist the HP and critical lenses and inquire at the intrapersonal, interpersonal, and contextual levels, you are able to simultaneously (a) move beyond the individualist assumption that you as an individual nurse have the sole responsibility and/or can be a lone moral agent; (b) see and name the intrapersonal, interpersonal, and contextual factors that are shaping the situation; (c) discern how those factors are connected; and the significance of that relational interplay for patient/family, nurse, and system well-being, and (d) extend the range of options for action. There is a range of knowledge and strategies that can support you in that process, and we will be discussing those in the chapters to come. At this point, it is important to first turn attention to the essential ontologic capacities (ways-of-being) you need to develop.

BEING COMPASSIONATE, THE FOUNDATION OF RELATIONAL INQUIRY

While you need to be clear in your nursing obligations to practice effectively as a nurse, we believe that you also need to develop five particular ways of being (what we term the five Cs of relational inquiry). These five Cs include *being* compassionate, curious, committed, competent, and corresponding. We begin with compassion since it is arguably the most fundamental capacity nurses require.

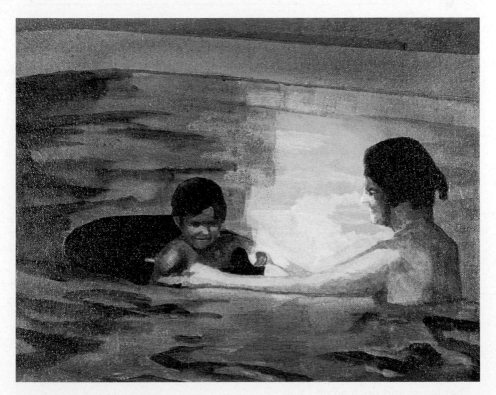

Compassion. (Acrylic painting by Alex Grewal.)

What Is Compassion?

The word *compassion* means "to share suffering." To be compassionate means to be able to relate human being to human being—to share something of ourselves and of what it is to be human. While all nurses would probably say they are compassionate, to act compassionately requires very conscious intent and a particular way of being.

While I (Gweneth) have always sought to be a compassionate nurse, my nursing program and my clinical experiences taught me to see my role as "fixing" my patients' discomfort; I was obligated to somehow alleviate their pain and suffering. In my early career, I worked in critical care units where the importance of biomedical knowledge and technology was foremost. The people and families for whom I cared were experiencing life-threatening illnesses and incredible pain of all forms. While technologies for addressing physiologic issues, including pain, were certainly available, other aspects of my patients' experiences challenged my "fix-it" ability. The following story describes a situation in which, despite being armed with critical care knowledge and skills, I found myself feeling completely unable to offer compassionate care to my patient. I simply did not know *how* to meet the obligation I felt compelled to address.

TO ILLUSTRATE
Unable to Make It Better in the Intensive Care Unit

The intensive care unit (ICU) is quiet, but the hospital is overflowing. As I come on duty, I am told that one of my patients today is in our unit temporarily because she needs a private room. A woman in her late 20s has just been told she has terminal cancer. As I listen to the report, a number of thoughts and feelings flood through me. She's only a few years older than I am! What must she be going through? I have never cared for anyone who is dying. Sure, lots of people die in our unit, but they are in our unit because we are trying to stop them from dying. What do I do for someone who is here because she is dying?

I head out of report and into the young woman's room. I say hello and introduce myself. She just turns around and looks at me. I find myself asking how she is. Inside I am berating myself. "How can you ask such an inadequate question?" She just turns over in her bed. I check her intravenous and flee; I tell myself that my other patient might need me.

A little while later I go back in to check on her. As I enter the room, I hear her crying. I stand there feeling totally inadequate. What should I say? What if I say the wrong thing? I do my check. I don't acknowledge her tears, and once again I flee.

Caputo (1987) describes suffering as something that "humbles us, brings us up short, stops us in our tracks, something surpassing which inspires a mix of fear and awe and admiration, something which both strikes us down and draws us near" (p. 275). I can still remember that feeling of being stopped in my tracks at my inability to influence this situation in a positive way. Although I could leave the room (and flee from my patient's suffering), my own suffering and inability to change the situation went with me. My response was to seek out a colleague who I knew was "really good at talking with people." Interpreting the situation as being a matter of me lacking some knowledge and skill that was outside of my critical care skill set, I asked my colleague if she would go in to see my patient while I looked after hers. I could not ignore or leave my patient's pain uncared for, yet I felt completely inadequate in terms of *being with* her in her situation.

As nurses, we are continuously caring for people who are going through such extraordinary experiences—situations in which illness, trauma, the death of a loved one, or some other form of change has interrupted everyday life. Many of these changes involve pain, fear, anguish, confusion, uncertainty, and so forth. Given this wide range of experiences and the differing responses people and families may have to those experiences, the question becomes: How might we effectively care for them? How does compassion figure into that effective nursing care? And what knowledge or skills do we need to *be* compassionate?

TO ILLUSTRATE

A 4-Year-Old Teaches His Mother about Compassion

My (Gweneth's) son Adrian helped answer those questions for *me*; he demonstrated to me true compassion and also helped me see the vital place compassion has in my nursing practice.

Adrian was 4 years old when my brother died suddenly from an undiagnosed heart condition. One day, after a conversation with a friend who had phoned to offer her condolences, a wave of grief swept over me. Taking a box of tissues, I sat down on the couch to cry. Suddenly, I became aware of Adrian standing in front of me. On his face was an expression of great concern as he asked me what was wrong. "I'm feeling very sad about Uncle Gary so I'm just letting the sadness come out for a while," I replied. With that he nodded and walked off into the family room. I assumed he was leaving me with my grief. A minute or so later, he returned carrying his most precious teddy bear. Without saying a word, he handed me his teddy, crawled up on my lap, and just sat with his arms wrapped around me.

I vividly remember how revelatory this experience was, of having someone be with me *without trying to ease my pain*. Although the storm of grief continued to rush through me, I was aware of something subtly shifting. What was making such a profound difference? Simply put, it was where Adrian was putting his focus and energy. It was *how* he was relating *within* the situation. He had wrapped his arms around me and focused his attention on just *joining me where I was*. He in no way attempted to lessen the force of the pain. He did not try to help me out of the storm or look for

continued on page 106

> **TO ILLUSTRATE** *continued*
>
> ## A 4-Year-Old Teaches His Mother about Compassion
>
> ways to shelter me or himself. He did not try to change anything. *He just related to what was happening.* Consequently, I realized that my own focus of attention gradually began to shift. Mixed in with my grief was the awareness of being cared about and held. That awareness served to change my actual experience. The pain of the grief moved to the background, and the relational connection that my son and I were experiencing *in the grief* moved to the foreground.

That experience changed me forever as a person and a nurse. Before it, although I had understood the idea of compassion, I had most often focused my relational attention and energy on trying to alleviate suffering, to "make it better" in some way. It had never crossed my mind to just be and *endure with* someone. Yet, as I thought back over the various areas in which I had practiced (neonatal and adult ICU, emergency, medicine, psychiatry), it was apparent that most often, there was no way to make the immediate situation better. Patients and families are most often going through extraordinary life situations that have no quick fix. Thus, what patients and families really need is a nurse who joins them in that extraordinary experience. However, the ability to be compassionate and endure their suffering with them, which is such an essential part of competent care, is often sorely lacking.

The experience with Adrian showed me that we all have the capacity to be compassionate; if a 4-year-old can be compassionate in that highly sophisticated and yet profoundly simple way, then surely adult nurses can. Following Adrian's lead, I realized that the secret to compassionate nursing is simply to be the caring human beings that we are right there in the midst of the human experience—to be with people in their uncertainty, anguish, and suffering as it is in any moment.

Perhaps the biggest thing that limits compassionate action is the way we typically relate to and within nursing situations (Hartrick Doane, in press). Focused on controlling and "handling" illness, we fail to fully relate to the people living those human experiences; we fail to *be* compassionate in the true sense of "sharing humanness." Feeling responsible to "fix" suffering is an example of how we relate in ineffective ways and how we can be culturally conditioned *out of* compassionate action. For example, Adrian had not yet experienced the adult-to-adult practice of having a "stiff upper lip" and "being in control." Seeing me upset, he responded to me by merely mirroring the actions he had experienced. When he was upset, I would get his teddy and hug him as he cried.

Importantly, what distinguishes compassionate action is *how* one relates. Compassion is *not* about being an angel of mercy who takes care of those weaker or less fortunate. "Compassion is not a relationship between the healer and the wounded. It's a relationship between equals. . . . Compassion becomes real when we recognize our shared humanity" (Chodron, 2002, p. 50). Thus, compassion is not merely about the emotional realm of nursing, and it is not paternalistic or about doing for or doing to another. Rather it is about being in solidarity and *doing with* another. In their in-depth examination of compassion in nursing, von Dietze and Orb (2000) emphasize that compassion is both rational and action-oriented. Compassionate care is what we do together; it brings reason, emotion, and sentiment together and simultaneously demands that we act (von Dietze & Orb, 2000).

Compassion Requires Us to Be in the Difficulty

How have you learned to "do" compassion? Do you feel responsible to fix people or situations? Do you have the capacity to *be with* people and situations as they are in a particular moment in time? While it is fine to say that compassion requires us to be in the difficulty, it's not easy to be in close proximity with pain and suffering when we experience a heartfelt desire to help. How do we reconcile these competing elements within ourselves—the nursing obligation to *be with* people in their experiences and our own need and mandate to respond in some helpful way?

As my son Adrian demonstrated so well, being compassionate involves joining people in their human vulnerability and frailty *as well as* in their strength and conviction; it involves relating to and experiencing life in that moment "together." To be compassionate requires that we have the strength and fortitude to open to human frailty (including our own) and be physically present with it. "Compassion asks us to go where it hurts, to enter into places of pain, to share in brokenness, fear, confusion, and anguish . . . to mourn with those who are lonely, to weep with those in tears. . . . Compassion means full immersion into the condition of being human" (Nouwen, McNeill, & Morrison, 1982). However, as Nouwen and colleagues (1982) emphasize, the purpose is not to immerse ourselves in suffering, but instead to share the person's burden (and joy). Being compassionate therefore means being in solidarity with patients and families while enabling them to retain their independence and dignity (von Dietze & Orb, 2000). It is this sense of solidarity and the willingness to enter into living experience that distinguishes compassionate nursing action.

Some researchers have argued that being exposed to suffering and difficulty over time may lead to "compassion fatigue" or, in the case of nurses who work with victims of violence, vicarious trauma (Goldblatt, 2009; Sabo, 2011; Sinclair & Hamill, 2007). However, Mitchell and Bunkers (2003) argue that the danger to nurses is not in witnessing such suffering, but rather in turning away when suffering appears. Similar to Naef (2006), who emphasizes the healing power of bearing witness to suffering, these authors share Caputo's (1987, 1993) assertion that it is not suffering itself but rather *how one relates to suffering* that determines the impact.

Currently, I (Colleen) am involved in a practice setting which would be unbearable if I did not actively turn toward suffering. I am working on a health intervention for Aboriginal[1] women who have experienced

---

[1] In Canada, "Aboriginal peoples" refers to indigenous peoples and encompasses first nations, Métis, and Inuit peoples. These three groups reflect "organic political and cultural entities that stem historically from the original peoples of North America, rather than collections of individuals united by so-called 'racial' characteristics" (Royal Commission on Aboriginal Peoples, 1996, p. xii).

violence. Colonization of Aboriginal lands, policy-enforced poverty, and racism have exposed Aboriginal women in Canada, like indigenous women worldwide (Cheers et al., 2006; Stephens, Porter, Nettleton, & Willis, 2009; Weaver, 2009), to far more violence than any other group of Canadian women (Brownridge, 2008; Daoud et al., 2012; Varcoe & Dick, 2008). Indeed, the women who are participating in the intervention have related the most horrendous histories of multiple forms of violence that I have ever heard. Rather than protecting myself or flinching from the inhumanity they have suffered, I try to be with the women and to listen fully to bear witness to their sorrow, suffering, and strength, and to affirm their humanity and deepen my own understanding of their lives. In short, I don't try to stop their tears or my own. My colleagues and I find that such an approach builds trust and promotes healing in ways that any attempt to "fix" could not.

How do *you* see yourself and your nursing role within situations of suffering? Entering into nursing situations feeling obligated to fix the suffering can set us up to feel inadequate as nurses, because we are giving ourselves an impossible responsibility. A complex interplay of multiple factors contributes to the experience of illness and suffering. Expecting ourselves to "make it better" is comparable to expecting ourselves to suddenly shift from Clark Kent to Superman. We do not have super powers; we are merely human. And it is in just being human that our power to help lies.

For example, the more I (Gweneth) felt responsible to ease the young woman's tears in the ICU, the more my own suffering grew. Moreover, the more that I focused on my inability to help, the less I was able to *be with* her. When I fled her hospital room, I was not really fleeing from her, but from myself and the overwhelming angst I felt at not being able to "do" something. In contrast, Adrian's compassionate presence was so powerful and healing because it allowed me to be as I was, to feel what I was feeling. *His human caring presence was his action—that is what he "did."* And that action enabled me to not get lost in my sorrow. The loss of my brother was incredibly painful, but the pain was not a bad thing that needed fixing. It was a deeply felt human experience of grief that needed to be expressed. I liken it to a physical wound that begins to fester if it is covered over and never exposed to the air. Taking the bandage off and cleaning the wound fosters healing. Adrian's presence allowed a clearing of the pain I was feeling in that moment. If a well-meaning nurse had come along and tried to make me feel better, that action might have felt like a denial of the significance of my loss and might have interrupted my grieving process. And therein lies an important paradox at the heart of compassionate nursing practice. In many situations, the most powerful way to help is to relate fully to what is without asking it to be something different and without feeling responsible to fix it.

Compassion involves both joining people in their suffering and responding in ways that are effective. Although we may well engage in interventions to ease pain, treat disease, increase safety, and so forth, most importantly, we need to ensure that our actions are truly compassionate.

TO ILLUSTRATE
Compassion on the Night Shift

The following is a story told to me by a former nursing student who had previously been enrolled in a relational practice course that I (Gweneth) taught. The story depicts how, as nurses, we are with patients and families in their most vulnerable moments—moments of intense sorrow, fear, joy, and uncertainty. Yet, we often fear those moments and feel inadequate, not knowing what to say or do. We share the story because it is one in which the nurse was able to transcend the difficulty of being in her own fears and make a profound difference in the life of a family:

I came on night shift, and the charge nurse asked me if I would special a baby boy who had been born that day with a number of congenital anomalies. The parents had been told that their baby would likely die sometime during the night. I experienced a moment of panic. "Could I actually do this? How would I do it? What would I say? I don't have the skill to do this!" The charge nurse told me that there was no one else, and the parents really needed some support. I began to think back on the relational practice course I had taken. "What did I learn that would help me with this?" I remembered our class discussions about the importance of joining in-relation and that there was never a "right" thing to say or do. I reminded myself that what was important was my desire to connect and to care and my willingness to bring myself to that caring relationship. Those thoughts served as my guide throughout the night I spent with the family.

I went into the room and introduced myself to the parents. I explained that I would be with them during the night. In a very quiet voice, the father told me the doctor had said their son would likely die soon and they wanted to have as much time with him as they could so they would have memories of him after he was gone. As he spoke, his wife began to cry. Without really being aware of what I was doing, I bent down next to the mother and baby and reached out to stroke the baby's face. Through a cracking voice and watering eyes I asked what they had already come to know about their son through their time together. They began to describe the little movements and gestures they had noticed, the family likenesses they could see, and other important things about their son. Throughout the night, we cried, laughed, talked, and were silent together as we watched and came to know their baby. At about 5 in the morning, their son died in his mother's arms.

Weeks later I received a thank you card from the parents. In the card the parents told me that, although I had been with them in their son's death, their memories of that night were more about the short life I had helped them to have and to share with their son. They thanked me for my caring and for my compassion and wrote it was one of the treasured memories from that night they would always carry with them (Hartrick, 1997).[2]

---

[2] This story has been previously published in Hartrick, G. A. (1997). Relational capacity: The foundation for interpersonal nursing practice. *Journal of Advanced Nursing, 26*, 523–528 and is reprinted with permission from Blackwell.

Perhaps the thing that stood out most for me (Gweneth) when the nurse in the story phoned to tell me of her experience was how she had opened up to and honored the family's experience. She did not "do" anything with their tears. Rather she intentionally chose to *be with* the family as they lived the joy as well as the sorrow they were experiencing being with their son. In joining the family, the nurse did not try to "make it better." Rather, what she "did" was simply follow the family's lead. They had told her that the most *significant* and *meaningful* thing to them was their desire to know and experience their son's short life. The nurse *listened* and *honored that meaningful health and healing experience* by joining in with it. In order to do this, she needed to move beyond her own fears and angst—for example, her angst about what *she* as the nurse should say or do for parents of a dying child—to attend to the family's experience. Once she shifted her attention to the family (and away from what was concerning her), she spontaneously and intuitively knew how to join the family and *be-in-relation-with* them.

In recounting the story to me, the nurse said that the experience had also served to transform her own vision of herself as a nurse. She learned from the family that she did "know" how to be-in-relation—that deep within her, she had that innate human capacity and knowledge. This highlights an important aspect of compassion. While the feeling of compassion is spontaneous, to practice compassionately requires cultivation of particular attitudes, values, and actions. For example, the nurse had to prioritize the living experience of the family (as opposed to the alleviation of pain and suffering) and also bring a particular attitude and way-of-being to the situation. Moreover, she had to cultivate a form of compassionate practice that enabled her to *look beyond her own fears and concerns, learn to trust herself, and believe in the strength and capacities of patients and families (and in herself) to be in and live through difficulty.*

Being Compassionate with Ourselves

In addition to having compassion for others, we need to develop the capacity to be compassionate with ourselves. As the example above illustrates, our experience of a particular patient or situation is not separate from who and how we are as people. That is, when we encounter someone who is suffering, we bring our own interpretive frames and the interpretive frames that dominate the larger social world in which we live and practice (Doane, 2003). Thus, paying attention and inquiring into the meaning we are making of any situation is a vital part of compassionate practice. The nurse in the above example had to acknowledge and look beyond her own fears and concerns to join the family where *they were*. They made it clear that although they were living through the death of their son, what *they* wanted to focus on at that moment was his life. Being compassionate in that situation meant joining and responding to that focus on life. In another situation with another family, the nurse might have been called to respond differently.

To be compassionate with others requires that we be compassionate with ourselves when we experience our own suffering. In short, we need to keep current with ourselves moment to moment as we are. Typically, we think of keeping current in nursing as being about staying up to date with knowledge and research. But Nepo (2005) describes another form of keeping current that is central to compassion. Using the metaphor of pipes, Nepo points out that we can get "clogged" as we absorb the vast array of experiences and contextual "debris" within which we work. When we stay current with ourselves and our experiences, we keep our inner pipes clean and keep the current of our own energy flowing.

We keep current with ourselves by giving ourselves the same kind of attention we strive to give to others. "In the course of a single day, we can be momentarily cast down by myriad tiny disappointments, rejections, frustrations, and failures. We are subject to minor physical distress, anxiety . . . fatigue . . . pain, grief, despair" (Armstrong, 2011, p. 83). Attending to our own experience doesn't lead us to become self-absorbed (it is not to clog the pipes with debris). Rather, it leads us to be compassionate with ourselves. The old adage, "Before you can care for someone else, you need to care for yourself," is relevant here. By experiencing our strengths and sorrows, we have the chance to heal the wounds within us and curb any harmful impulses that might arise from them. Keeping current involves acknowledging and moving through any pain we may feel so it does not get stuck within us.

Nepo (2005) explains that the word *sincere* comes from the Latin meaning "without wax." During the Italian Renaissance, it was common for stone sellers to fill cracks in flawed stones with wax and pass them off as flawless. Subsequently, an honest stone seller became known as someone who showed his stone without wax—he was *sincere*, showing the cracks and all (Nepo, 2005). Self-compassion enables us to become more sincere with ourselves and with others—to acknowledge ourselves as imperfect beings who are always in process, always learning and becoming. The places where we have been bruised or struggled can serve as windows of possibility. By consciously looking inward, we see what is constraining our experience and our action and can more intentionally practice and integrate the qualities and attitudes that we wish to cultivate.

How do you relate to yourself as you go about your nursing work? Do you ever inquire into the feelings and thoughts that arise in you as you care for patients and families and/or interact with colleagues? Are you sincere in terms of not covering over your imperfections? Are you compassionate with yourself? For example, when you make an error, what do you do? How do you think about yourself, and how do you act? Do you judge or chastise yourself when you don't adhere to certain standards and values? When you don't know something, what do you think or feel about yourself? One way to keep current with yourself is to pay attention to your emotions.

Keeping Current with Your Emotions

In the Western world, dominant understandings separate the mind from the heart. You just have to think of sayings like "Don't let your heart rule your head" to see the privileging of the rational mind. Yet Nepo (2005) describes how in many Eastern languages and traditions, heart and mind are joined; heart–mind is considered to be one perceptual organ and involves seeing/relating with both detachment and involvement. In heart–mind, one is part of what one is observing.

Consciously noticing the emotions we are experiencing and being as authentic and compassionate with ourselves as we require ourselves to be with others is important. Holecek (2009) describes how we often have four basic strategies in terms of relating with and to emotions. One strategy is to relate to emotions by resisting them (e.g., pushing the feelings away in ourselves and/or dismissing them in others). A second strategy is to try and control them by containing them—for example, weaving a narrative around them ("she must need a holiday to overreact in such a way," or "he is being overly dramatic") or perhaps pushing them down and then distracting our attention elsewhere so we do not have to actually feel them (get busy doing something). A third strategy is to overindulge the emotions and act them out without ever really experiencing them (e.g., indulging our anger by yelling at someone else). The fourth strategy is that of trying to fix or cure feelings, such as talking ourselves or others out of them.

In essence, each of those strategies is a way of avoiding emotions— of trying to *not relate* to them. Yet, as I (Gweneth) experienced when caring for the young woman in the ICU, we can run but we can't hide. Our emotions go where we go. Thus, the most effective way of relating to emotions is to simply let them be (similar to the way Adrian let my emotions be). As Holecek (2009) contends, when one really thinks about it, emotion is not really a problem. However, we add things on to the emotions that are problematic. That is, the interpretations and meanings we associate with situations and emotions create our inner turmoil. Watts (1991) describes the way in which fever was once considered a disease instead of a natural healing process. In a similar way, "we still think of negative feelings as disorders of the mind which need to be cured. But what needs to be cured is the inner resistance to those feelings. . . . To resist the feeling is to be unable to contain it long enough for it to work itself out" (Watts, 1991, p. 92).

By engaging intrapersonally in a compassionate way, you can create the space and openness for emotions to be received and experienced and to work themselves out. Viewing emotion as simply a momentary shift in energy, as a feeling passing through, allows it to do just that (Singer, 2007). Singer uses the analogy of not turning water to ice. Rather than solidifying the feeling by adding a story to the emotion, you simply let it flow through. For example, when feeling anxious in a new clinical setting, rather than solidifying the emotion by narrating yourself as incompetent or inadequate, you recognize the emotion simply as a feeling that has been triggered within the situation. By directly relating to what is (to the emotions that arise) and letting the emotions be, unobstructed feelings can offer a natural and necessary dimension of discriminating intelligence and clear thinking (Wilbur, Patten, Leonard, & Morelli, 2008). For example, our anxiety can point us toward the knowledge we need to develop or the questions we need to ask within an unfamiliar setting. As Donaldson (1991) explains, emotions are our value feelings. They mark what matters to us: "We experience emotion only in regard to that which matters" (p. 2). Thus, Holecek (2009) suggests "The key . . . is to relate to the emotion itself, not the trigger" (p. 205) to see emotions and suffering as signposts that something important is afoot, something that we need to relate to *more* open-heartedly rather than finding ways to avoid feeling the emotion.

As you cultivate the practice of self-compassion, it is important to understand that it does not merely involve paying attention to one's feelings and thoughts and responding based on those feelings and thoughts. Rather, being self-compassionate involves learning to pay attention to the thoughts and emotions and bodily responses one is having at any moment and *reflexively considering those responses in light of what is going on around you and your nursing goals. Most importantly, it involves consciously and intentionally choosing how to act and respond to yourself, others, and the situation to promote well-being at all levels* (Doane, 2003, 2004).Thus, compassionate inquiry involves critically inquiring into the meanings, concerns, emotions, and values that are shaping your experience.

Self-Compassion Supports Choice

Consciously noticing one's experience and scrutinizing the knowledge gleaned through compassionate inquiry at the intrapersonal level can enhance our power and choice in practice in three ways. First, it allows us to more thoughtfully bring ourselves to our work and make conscious choices about how to focus, respond, and use the capacities we have at our disposal. Second, because our bodily sensations, emotions, and thoughts are often sparked in response to what is happening externally, self-experience offers a window to the world and directs our attention to certain aspects of that world. For example, we may value equitable care and "treating all people with dignity" yet also have absorbed values and automatized practices that distinguish between people in terms of their worth and value based on a range of factors such as appearance, demeanor, language, and so on. Thus, when we look at ourselves and our actions more carefully, we can see contradictions in ourselves; we can see the contextual values we have absorbed and taken up that are not really of our choosing. We also may see that we are working between competing values that are pulling us in different directions. As we tune into our conflicted feelings, we become aware of the cost this might be having on ourselves and the patients and families for whom we provide care. Thus, paying attention to and compassionately reflecting on our bodily and emotional experiences can inform us about institutional practices and structures that might be problematic and/or in need of revision and the choices that might be open to us to better promote the well-being of patients, families, ourselves, and the systems in which we work.

Finally, attending to our own experiences is a very direct way of caring for our own well-being. Doing so implies and is based on a belief that what we experience and feel as nurses matters, that *we* matter and are of worth, and it enables us to be as compassionate with ourselves as we hopefully are with others.

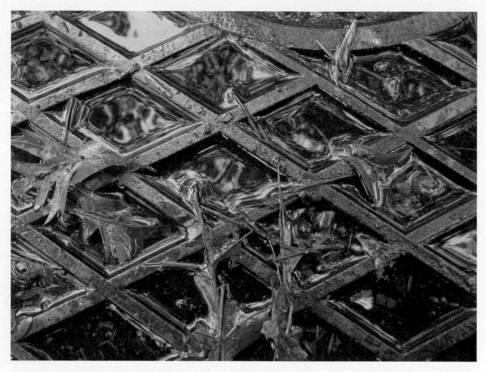

Cleansing the debris. (Photograph by Gweneth Doane.)

TRY IT OUT 3.1

Looking through the Cracks and Cleansing the Debris

A number of years ago during an ethics research project (Rodney, Storch, Varcoe, & Hartrick Doane, 2002–2005), a nurse described to us days when, as she left the unit, she just wanted to go home, take a shower to purge her system, and wash away the residue of the day. Since that time, we have heard countless nurses say similar things. Part of being compassionate is finding ways to help ourselves "keep current" and cleanse any toxic residue we may have absorbed or that may have been laid on us during the day. As you cultivate the capacity of self-compassion, you may find it feels somewhat cumbersome at first, especially if you try to enact it in the moment of your experience.

A good way to start is to bring compassion to yourself retrospectively. For example, think of your last clinical day. Close your eyes and imagine yourself back there.

- What are you feeling (unsure, confident, confused, not knowing, etc.)?
- Of what bodily sensations are you aware?
- What are you thinking to yourself?

continued on page 115

TRY IT OUT 3.1 *continued*

Looking through the Cracks and Cleansing the Debris

- Consider the aspirations and concerns you have. How are they shaping the way you are relating within the situation? What does all of this tell you about yourself?

- What is significant about *your own* experience here? Can you identify any particular values or obligations that are shaping how you are experiencing this situation?

- Do you see any "windows" or cracks you might look through to learn more about yourself and/or to care for yourself more fully? Can you see how these cracks might need some special attention and compassion? Is there anything you are trying to "wax over?"

- How might you clear the debris? For example, the nurse we described earlier would have a shower and visualize washing away the disturbing things that had been said, the concerns with which she was left, and so forth. Other nurses might clear the debris with vigorous exercise, a quiet walk in nature, working in the garden, meditation, playing music, or engaging in some other form of expression and release.

Next, take these ideas with you wherever you are in the next 24 hours. Throughout the next full day, try to note and let flow any emotions you experience. If you are nervous being observed in a clinical lab or practice setting, annoyed at your partner, dog, children, or frustrated with yourself, try to just pay attention to what you feel, and let it flow through you. What happens?

OTHER CAPACITIES SUPPORTING RELATIONAL INQUIRY

Although compassion is perhaps the primary capacity of the relational inquiry approach, four other ontologic capacities are also essential: being curious, competent, committed, and corresponding. We explore these next. Although we discuss the remaining capacities separately ahead, it is important to keep in mind that they are intricately connected. In day-to-day nursing practice, the five Cs show up, shape, and inform one another continually. Each capacity is dependent on the other. For example, as Roach (1987) notes, competence without compassion can result in inhumane action, while compassion without competence "may be no more than a meaningless, if not harmful, intrusion into the life of a person or persons needing help" (p. 61).

Capacity 2: Being Curious

In Chapter 1, we described how being curious is an attitude that is integral to relational inquiry. Being curious is about being interested, inquisitive, and open to the uncertainty that is part of disease and illness experiences. It is the capacity to work *in between* knowing and not knowing. It requires that we see "not knowing" as the pathway to knowledgeable, compassionate care. Being curious means everything can be called into question—your knowledge, values, thoughts, emotions, actions, inaction, habits, inconsistencies, personhood, the truths governing the clinical context in which you work, and so forth.

TO ILLUSTRATE
Cuddling a Neonate

One of my (Gweneth's) early positions in nursing was in a neonatal intensive care unit. At the time, it was "known" that too much stimulation was harmful to babies; for example, experts said that respiratory distress was exacerbated upon touch. Therefore, it was common practice to limit the amount of touching the premature babies received. This limited touching practice continued even after the babies were considered stable. Parents were not allowed to hold their babies until they were completely off oxygen and other treatments. As a new nurse in the unit, I attempted to plead the case for parents' right to hold their babies even briefly when the babies were out of the incubators for tube feedings or other treatments. However, the current "truth" that governed practice in the unit did not support that action.

One of my most vivid memories from that time is of holding a baby I was tube feeding as his mother (who had never held her own child) sat next to me with tears in her eyes. Her longing to hold her baby after weeks of standing by watching him struggle to live was palpable. All through the tube feeding, I sat there feeling in my heart that this practice was wrong. The way that expert knowledge was being used did not seem consistent with responsive practice. That is, it just didn't make sense that a nurse could hold the baby without harm but his own mother could not.

Today, it would be considered ludicrous for parents to not have contact with their babies; expert knowledge now tells us how vitally important that connection is to both mother's and baby's health and healing. Current research shows that skin-to-skin contact in particular improves neonate temperature control, heart rate, oxygen saturation levels, breastfeeding success, parent–child interaction, and child development in both preterm and term neonates, (Blomqvist, Rubertsson, Kylberg, Jöreskog, & Nyqvist, 2012; Cong et al., 2012; Jackson, 2010; Mori, Khanna, Pledge, & Nakayama, 2010; Weber, Harrison, & Steward, 2012). This is an example of the changeability of expert knowledge. What we consider best practice today may well be considered harmful in the future.

The "truth" is knowledge is uncertain as is our ability to know fully (Flanagan, 1996). Thus, having watched as expert truths have changed and evolved, we have come to believe that "good" practice involves shifting some of the confidence we currently place in our "knowing." This does not mean that we do not bring our expert knowledge to our work with people and families or act as if we don't know anything. It requires that we be curious and willing to extend our knowledge and also be uncertain.

The Value of Uncertainty

Uncertainty is an inherent part of most health care experiences. Given the "reality" that health and illness by its very nature is an uncertain experience, how is it that health practitioners approach their work in such a way as to avoid uncertainty?

Nepo (2005) describes how during the "medical gauntlet" of his cancer experience "no one, including the doctors, knew where my life was leading. Yet everyone, in their discomfort with not knowing, offered scenario after scenario of ways that I could die" (p. 219). He describes how, as a patient, he realized that what he really needed to do was wait and "not turn the waiting into something else" (p. 219). That is, he needed to have the capacity to be in uncertainty, to be in that relational space between knowing and not knowing.

There are countless research studies that document how uncertainty is an inherent aspect of the illness experience (Hansen et al., 2012; Neville, 2003). Most of the people/families for whom nurses care are in the midst of some kind of uncertainty and/or in limbo between knowing and not knowing their future, and the actual outcomes of their health/healing situation. There can be complications with even straightforward minor surgeries or seemingly innocuous health conditions. Similarly, it is possible for people with life-threatening illnesses who have been given months to live to survive another decade; conversely, many die sooner than predicted.

While uncertainty (especially as a health practitioner) can be disconcerting, it can also offer a valuable stance from which to practice nursing. Uncertainty is not prevaricating or being timid. *Uncertainty is an opening that can be used to enhance clarity*. As Whyte (2009) describes, "Not knowing what to do, we start to pay real attention. Just as people lost in the wilderness, on a cliff face, or in a blizzard pay attention with a kind of acuity that they would not have if they thought they knew where they were . . . if you think you know where you are you stop looking" (p. 144).

Yet, Mullavey-O'Byrne and West (2001) contend that the "quest for certainty, or at least the deep-seated desire for such a state, is a silent partner in almost every encounter between a health care practitioner and a client" (p. 55). Patients and families expect that their practitioners know and will be able to provide solutions to their health/illness situations. "Similarly, the majority of practitioners desire, even expect, either consciously or unconsciously, that they will be able to provide the answer for the client from the armature of professional knowledge and skill that underpins their practice" (p. 56). As such patients and practitioners often enter into "an unspoken conspiracy to maintain the illusion of certainty in the uncertain world of health care (and this quest or certainty is further strengthened) . . . by the interplay of external pressures" (p. 56).

This quest for certainty is played out in numerous ways in health care; for example, in the growing movement toward evidence-based practice. While supporting clinical decision making with the best available research evidence is vital, Bucknall (2007) argues that much of the knowledge translation research has shown that certainty is an illusion. Rather, personal perceptions and preferences, interpersonal processes, and contexts shape how any research evidence is used in practice. As Bucknall explains, all research findings are contestable and only become evidence (usable knowledge) when a practitioner decides that the information is relevant to a particular circumstance. In short, knowledge is never certain (Dopson, 2007, p. S73).

Cultivating the Capacity for Curiosity

In thinking about illness experiences and patient outcomes, it seems obviously that health care is an uncertain practice. Yet in most settings, to meet the creed of competent, knowledgeable nurse, we are expected to practice with certainty. In contrast, relational inquiry assumes that uncertainty is an inherent and normal aspect of nursing practice. Thus, *it is crucial to learn how to relate within and to uncertainty and how to know and make clinical decisions and act in light of uncertainty.* Being curious is an essential capacity to support that. Being curious gives us the humility and clarity to work in the space between knowing and not knowing, to critically question the knowledge that is guiding us. Being curious leads us to thoughtfully consider what we know and don't know and to ask ourselves in each situation how best to proceed (Dyche & Epstein, 2011). Inherent to curiosity is an eagerness to learn, to explore further.

The ultimate concern guiding our practice should not be ensuring certain practice but rather ensuring we are being as knowledgeable and as sensitive and responsive within health care situations as we can be. Being curious means working the edges of knowledge and developing the capacity to traverse between knowing and not knowing and between certainty and uncertainty.

Capacity 3: Being Committed

To commit means to entrust for safekeeping, to pledge or bind with an obligation, or to promise. Commitment involves a quality of investment of oneself in a conscious course of action.

Being committed means to actively and consciously identify the values and concerns that orient your work as a nurse and continually monitor how your actions are aligning with those commitments.

TO ILLUSTRATE
Commitment through the Screen Door

The following story was told to me (Gweneth) by a PHN during a workshop I was conducting on health-promoting practice with families. As we discussed the intricacies of working with families in ways that were respectful and responsive, a senior PHN shared one of her values, that of honoring the family's right to decide when and how we enter their lives. She offered a story as an example of her deep commitment to this value and the implications that had for her practice.

The nurse told us about a family she was working with that included a teenage mother and her children. The family met all of the criteria for a "high-risk" family; therefore, on discharge, the hospital had requested follow-up

continued on page 119

TO ILLUSTRATE *continued*

Commitment through the Screen Door

from the public health nursing service. The family had not requested a visit from a PHN, and in fact, the young mother had indirectly but clearly communicated her discomfort with the suggestion. However, because the family was deemed high-risk, a PHN was required to visit.

The nurse described how, as she first approached the home, the mother watched her from behind a screen door. When she climbed the stairs outside, the mother did not open the screen door and did not invite her in. The nurse, paying close attention to the unspoken information that was being communicated by the mother and to her own feeling of "what was right," introduced herself through the screen door and explained that she had been asked to visit the family over the next several months to assist them in any way she could. Following this brief exchange, she departed.

The visits had continued in this way for several months. The nurse would contact the mother by telephone to schedule her visit, which would then be conducted through the screen door. Although she made frequent visits to the family, she was never allowed into the house. However, over the next few months, they began to develop a fairly good relationship. The young mother even phoned the nurse occasionally to ask a question or to find out when she would be coming again. One day when the nurse arrived, the woman opened the screen door and invited the nurse in for tea.

As I listened to the PHN tell her story, I was struck by the clarity of her commitment and the way in which it had guided her choices. *Being clear in her commitment* had enabled the PHN to traverse differing needs and expectations, simultaneously honoring both the young mother's choices and her own nursing values and concerns. It was the clarity she had about her nursing values and her living commitment to those values that gave direction to her action and resulted in effective nursing care.

The Question of Commitment

As nurses, we are continually brought face-to-face with the question of commitment. This question is a question about how you will invest yourself, your time, and your energy as a nurse and for what purpose. The questions we regularly face include What is a priority here? What actions am I obligated to take? What authority will I follow? Thus, perhaps more than anything else, *being committed is about power, choice, and investment.*

As I (Gweneth) teach and talk with nurses, I continually hear how powerless they feel in their practice. Citing the numerous realities of their health care settings and what stops them from practicing in the ways they would like, they describe feeling adrift in their work. While they know the nursing ideals they are "supposed" to work toward, the gap between the realities of nursing and those ideals can seem too wide to traverse.

Through my experiences as both a teacher and researcher, I have often observed that nurses wanting to affect their practice in positive ways are missing some key ingredients. The analogy I have used is of a boat that has no navigational system, power source, or anchor (Hartrick Doane, in press). That is, they know who they are (caring, compassionate nurses), and they have an array of workable parts (nursing ideals, knowledge, clinical expertise), but they are not sure *how* to assemble the navigational system, connect to the power source, or anchor themselves, especially in stormy weather (Hartrick Doane, in press).

Commitment can be a nurse's anchor and power source. That is, it can ground and power the navigational system of relational inquiry practice. Within the complex realities and competing obligations that swirl around us as we go about our work, commitment is what ignites our action and what we need to come back to over and over again throughout our day. When we stop and check in with our commitments, if only long enough to take one deep breath, we remember what we are working toward. Being committed does not mean that nurses should overcome the challenges of practice by working harder or being more self-sacrificing. Instead, it means we pay attention to the choices we're making within the very real constraints limiting our practice and note whether or not we are acting in alignment with our values. Again, being committed is *not* about aligning to some romantic vision of nursing, but rather aligning to our commitment to our patients and families and to ourselves as nurses and discovering ways to be the responsive nurses we wish to be.

TRY IT OUT 3.2

Take a Snapshot of Yourself in Practice

The next time you begin your work day, pay attention throughout the first hour to each action you perform and the constraints in which you worked. Make little notes as you go if you can so that later you can reconstruct a chart. If you are not going to be in practice for a while, remember back to the first hour of the last day you were actively in practice. Your chart might look like this:

Time	Action	Analysis

continued on page 121

TRY IT OUT 3.2 *continued*

Take a Snapshot of Yourself in Practice

Fill in the chart with as much detail as possible regarding what you did in each minute. Then, analyze your snapshot, using some of these questions:

- What drove each action (e.g., routine, policies, patient need, someone else's priorities)?
- What part of the hour was planned, routine, expected, or unplanned and unexpected?
- Whose interests are being served by each action?
- What values and goals are implied by each action?
- How much of the time was spent doing what you thought was important, and why?
- What portion of time was spent contributing to patient/family well-being?
- What competing interests, obligations, values, concerns, and constraints can you identify?
- Do you see any room for better aligning your actions with your values and goals?
- How did your actions align with what you are committed to or what you say you value as a nurse?

Difference as a Site for Practicing Commitment

Often, we narrate difference as something unusual or difficult to deal with—as one of the hard spots of nursing. However, if you really think about it, difference is an essential feature of any nursing situation. People come with different backgrounds; each has a different socioeconomic status, a different physiologic status, different resources, and so forth. Thus, working across difference is something that is part and parcel of responsive nursing care. Framing difference as an inherent feature of nursing paves the way, not only for more compassionate nursing practice but also for more effective and responsive nursing practice. It also enables you to consciously enlist difference to support your development as a nurse. Difference offers a window into ourselves; it is where we bump up against ourselves most strongly and can see our own views, assumptions, values, and habits of mind and action at play. Moreover, it is where we find out what matters to us, what we have trouble tolerating, and to what we are committed and not committed. Difference is a site where, as the old saying goes, the rubber hits the road.

The actor Jim Carrey says that his life's motto is, "Always keep your wheels turned toward the skid." (I, Colleen, read that in a glossy magazine!) Living and driving in Canada, I know what this means when driving on ice and snow. When you turn toward difficulty and difference and face it head on, you begin to deal with it. Rather than continuing to skid away, letting difficulty drive you, you drive yourself.

Purposefully enlisting difference begins by seeing it as an opportunity for inquiry. Rather than simply feeling frustrated or powerless with that "difficult patient," "arrogant doctor," or "annoying colleague," purposefully connecting with our power source (our commitments) enables us to respond more effectively to people and practices that might be having a negative impact on well-being. It also offers the opportunity to see the limitations of our commitments—how we might need to extend our proximal–distal view in order to more effectively meet our nursing obligations.

Our sensitivities to the actions of others can become a source of knowledge and fuel for our own practice. For example, let's say we see another nurse acting in a way that is contrary to our own commitments. Rather than labelling this difference as a problem, we can ask ourselves what it might be revealing about our own commitments as a nurse. It can even cue us to more consciously act in accordance with those commitments. That is, rather than letting the difference expand the gulf between us and our colleague by reacting to it, we can use it as a reminder to act in accordance with our values.

TO ILLUSTRATE

Committing to Work across Difference

Situations in which patients harm themselves—for example, through smoking, substance use, or attempted suicide—are often particularly challenging for nurses. A few years ago, I (Colleen) was working with a student who was caring for a patient who "pushed all my buttons" (meaning raised all my personal sensitivities). The patient was a man who was in prison for the murder of his girlfriend. With my concern about violence against women, I found it difficult to support the student nurse, who was herself struggling over how to provide care to this man. Despite the fact that he was under guard on the medical unit, I was concerned for the student's physical safety, and when she began to speak empathically about him, I found myself concerned for her emotional safety. I immediately assumed the man was manipulative and could not entertain any positive ideas about him. I knew that I had to confront my biases against him and came to see that because he challenged my values of nonviolence and gender equality, I was associating him with all male violence and failing to consider how he might have come to be a violent person. Basically, I had to name my discrimination.

After actively reflecting on my biases, I concluded that viewing this man through anger and hostility and letting this view shape my suggestions to the student about how to approach his care would contradict other values I hold (such as unconditional positive regard) and would not be health-promoting for anyone. I was not entirely successful in adjusting my attitude, but I tried to encourage the student to convey positive regard for him as a person without condoning violence. Ironically, in the face of the student's acceptance of him, the man became quite upset and confided remorse that the student was convinced was genuine.

Although the challenge in this situation could appear to have arisen from the man himself, I contributed to the challenge of difference (and extended it to the student). Anticipating your own biases and hot spots allows you to think ahead to how you want to be with particular people, families, and communities—what commitments are central to your nursing practice—rather than simply reacting based on habit. As you read through the rest of this chapter, try and imagine situations that you might find challenging, and try to think through how you would like to act.

TRY IT OUT 3.3
Explore Your Nursing Commitments

Step 1: Have a conversation with another nurse about a particular nursing situation. It might be with a classmate, a nurse on a unit where you are doing your current clinical rotation, or someone in your circle of acquaintances who is or was a nurse. As you discuss the situation, while there may be many shared understandings, pay particular attention to the differences between you. Try to clarify what each of you sees differently and how those differences shape what you see as your nursing commitments. That is, do not try to reach agreement or consensus. Instead, try to illuminate the differences between you.

Your conversation might explore some or all of the following ideas:
■ What is the primary concern in the situation?
■ What are the primary nursing commitments?
■ What are the important factors to consider in identifying those concerns and commitments?
■ What do you feel obligated to address?
■ What is challenging for you in this situation?

Step 2: Analyze the conversation. Answer these questions:
■ What was it like to focus on illuminating the differences between you rather than working to find areas of agreement?
■ What surprised you?
■ What similarities and differences did you experience?
■ What factors influenced those differences?
■ What understandings of nursing and nursing obligations can you identify in the other person's thinking? What understandings can you identify in yourself?
■ What different commitments do you hold in contrast to the person you talked to?
■ If the other nurse was a colleague with whom you were working closely, what would you find particularly challenging about the differences between you?

Committing to Developing a Proximal–Distal View

Earlier, in Chapter 2, we described the importance of developing a proximal–distal view to determine one's nursing obligations. Committing yourself to cultivating a proximal–distal view is central to relational inquiry practice. Discussing violence, Žižek (2008) illustrates the relevance of a proximal–distal view. When pain and suffering is witnessed directly, we have the ethical illusion of attending sympathetically, yet we tolerate less visible forms of suffering. He uses the example of how social abhorrence of local acts of violence against single individuals co-occurs with tolerance for widespread war against thousands of people. So, we may find ourselves touched or disturbed by an article in the newspaper about someone who was shot and killed in our hometown or about a local family whose home and possessions have been lost in a fire. Yet, reading the same newspaper, we skim over an article about thousands of people being killed or displaced by civil war in another country or refugee families trying to get into countries such as the United States or Canada after having to leave their homes, jobs, and communities to survive.

TO ILLUSTRATE

Expanding Our Proximal-Relational View

My (Gweneth's) son Taylor found his proximal-relational view widened and extended when he attended an international school. Returning home at the end of his first year after having lived and studied with 200 people from 85 different countries, Taylor noticed some changes in himself. One such change became evident while reading the newspaper at the kitchen table one morning. Sitting in his comfortable home, leisurely enjoying his breakfast, he suddenly looked up at me with great concern on his face. He had just read about an atrocity that had occurred in a distant country. As he took in the story, he began telling me about one of his classmates who was from that county and what he had learned about the contextual elements that had shaped and led up to this situation. As he talked, I could see that he was with some urgency trying to figure out what this might mean for his friend and his friend's family and community as well as what it meant for himself in terms of how he, Taylor, might respond.

It became clear that what had in the past been just distant pieces of information in a newspaper were now being read and *related to* as living experiences. As he exclaimed, "I will never read a newspaper in the same way again," I could see how Taylor himself was changed—how his proximal view had been widened and extended. Diverse people and issues were now proximal. It was not just having friends from Kazakhstan, Iraq, or Rwanda that broadened his understanding of those contexts. Rather, as his view of the world and how it is shaped was widened, his view of himself

continued on page 125

> **TO ILLUSTRATE** *continued*
>
> ## Expanding Our Proximal-Relational View
>
> *in* the world and his obligations and commitments were also widened. He now experienced himself and the world relationally. It was not just a widening of "what and who" were within his scope of concern, but why and how it was relevant to him and to his own actions. Relational inquiry provides a set of practices and tools to help you purposefully consider what and who should be brought into your view and why, and to consider your commitments more thoughtfully.

Capacity 4: Competence

Being competent is most often associated with possessing knowledge and skills and having the ability to integrate that knowledge and skill set into practice (Smith, 2012). Analyzing the varying definitions and perspectives offered in the nursing literature, Smith points out that overall, *competence* refers to two main elements: (a) nurses' ability to perform their work without harm to patients and (b) the evaluation of nurses' knowledge and skills. In addition, while possessing and integrating knowledge into practice is an essential element of competence, other elements such as critical thinking, the ability to communicate well, proficiency in clinical skills, caring, and professionalism are also considered features of a competent nurse (Smith, 2012).

Roach (1987) defined competence as "the state of having the knowledge, judgment, skills, energy, experience, and motivation required to respond adequately to the demands of one's professional responsibilities" (p. 61). In essence, *being competent* translates into being a confident and safe practitioner who is able to provide holistic care (Smith, 2012). However, when one examines discussions of competence in the nursing literature and strategies used to measure competence, one begins to see that an individualist understanding of competence dominates. That is, underpinning the descriptions and evaluative strategies is the assumption that competence is located within the individual nurse. It is about the knowledge and skill set of an individual and how that individual uses his or her knowledge and skills. Given that nursing is always done in concert with others (patients, families, interprofessional colleagues, etc.) and is thus by its essence a relational practice, this individualist orientation raises a question—how does individual competence translate into safe nursing practice?

Although it is possible to distinguish competence at the individual level, when considered as a relational phenomenon, competence becomes broader and more robust. Practically speaking, from a relational perspective, *being competent* is not just about you and the knowledge and skills you possess. Rather, it is person/context-dependent and is determined in and by what transpires in particular relational situations.

TO ILLUSTRATE
Competence Is Relationally Determined

During research on ethical practice, I (Colleen) was following a nurse working at the triage desk in the emergency department of a large urban hospital serving a diverse population. The waiting room was full of "difference" (e.g., people with different illness conditions, of different ages, ethnicities, skin color, people speaking different languages, etc.). Children were crying, people who appeared to be in pain were standing because there was nowhere to sit, and there was a long line at the triage desk. I could see that the nurse was tired and frustrated at having to tell patients that the wait to be seen would be hours long. She saw about 18 patients within the first hour I observed her working, but the line did not get any shorter.

Then a young woman with a little girl of about 2 came next in line. Both were blond and blue-eyed. Like many of the children we had seen, the little girl looked feverish. The nurse took the history from the mother, took the child's temperature (it was 38.1 °C), and suddenly stood up. "Follow me," she said and led the mother through the doors to the pediatric stretchers. When the nurse returned, I asked her what I had missed, saying that I could not see how the child was any more acute than many who were waiting. She said that I had not missed anything, clearly understanding that I was implying she had allowed the woman and her child to jump the line. I asked, "So, why did you take her through?" The nurse replied, "Because I can."

This is not a story about a nurse enacting her nursing obligations according to her own value system or in a way that was inequitable or unjust. It is a story about a nurse who was practicing in circumstances in which she felt overwhelmed and (she told me) powerless to change the situation. She only had room for one child in the pediatric area, and thus only one opportunity to feel that she could do something positive. She acted, because she could, within immediate proximity.

As you think about this situation, how would *you* evaluate the nurse's competence? What indicators would you use? For example, as the nurse triaged patients, I observed that she enlisted sophisticated clinical knowledge and demonstrated sound analytic and clinical decision-making skills. Yet, I could see that the decision to take the little girl into the stretcher area was not solely based on clinical considerations. The child was of a similar ethnicity as the nurse, in contrast to the majority of other people in the waiting room. Both spoke English as a first language, also in contrast with the majority of people waiting. Did these or other influences factor into her decision? If another family who had been waiting for an hour with a child who also had a high fever were to evaluate the nurse's competence, what do you think they would say? In some ways, the nurse's response was in line with Caputo's (1987) assertion that obligation arises in the moment.

The nurse felt obligated to care for the patients, and her action of taking the little girl into the stretcher area was her way of exercising her power to respond to that obligation in the moment. However, while she may have been well-intentioned in her action, from a relational perspective, what is called into question is how she actually responded and what sparked that response.

Discerning Competence

What constitutes competence or "best" practice? The evaluation of competence can vary depending on contexts, values, and normative practices. How one nurse in a particular context uses clinical knowledge and expertise to be competent may, in another context, be questionable. For example, competence might be highly dependent on power and the interests and concerns that dominate a situation. Kelley Doucette, an ER nurse who recently told me (Gweneth) of changes she had made to nursing approach as a result of the relational inquiry course she had taken, offers a good example of this. Kelley decided to more consciously live her nursing values and exercise the power she had to "do good" in the ER. One particular change she made was to presence with each person who came to the triage desk. She figured out that while the context was what it was, she could choose how she related within and to that context. Thus, she decided that in the 1 or 2 minutes she had with each person, she would ensure that she communicated that they and their health concern mattered and that someone (she) was going to do what was possible to have them attended to.

Since the triage was in a high traffic area and people either walked directly through or stood behind the presenting patient as they waited in the queue, she changed her practice considerably just by asking each patient to close the pocket door between the triage area and the waiting room. This created a physical barrier for their privacy and a relational space for them to connect with each other.

These seemingly minor adjustments had a significant impact on her "competent" practice. Previously, she had always been focused on wait times and acuity levels and how many beds were free. However, she now realized that she had been privileging those elements; they were taking attention from the people who needed care, and she was able to consciously refocus her attention on the person who was sitting in front of her.

We believe that to determine competence, one must look to the relational realities and identify indicators that are relevant to the particular situation. Discerning competent practice is highly dependent upon and strongly linked to the nursing commitment and obligations within a particular situation.

While competence is sometimes evaluated by how nurses align their practice with proscribed protocols, there are also times when being competent requires challenging the status quo. As Higgs and Titchen (2001) point out, "best practice is frequently interpreted as merely the best of what currently exists." The fact that those practices are often grounded in existing and/or normative frameworks "guarantees neither the most ideal practice experience, process, or outcomes for the individual client, nor the best practice that can be imagined and created" (p. 13). Subsequently, being competent is intricately interwoven with being compassionate, being curious, and being committed. Manifesting these capacities together enables you to scrutinize what is being held up as best practice. They focus you on nursing situations, orient you to the living experience of the people and families in those situations, and bring your nursing commitments to life. And as Higgs and Titchen (2001) suggest, at times, this may mean stepping beyond the normative practices that dominate a particular health care setting.

TO ILLUSTRATE
A Crazy Day

A fourth-year nursing student shared this story during an ethics research project (Varcoe et al., 2004). The story exemplifies the process of discernment we are describing. It also depicts how different capacities work in concert to affect competent, safe nursing care.

It was a crazy day on the ward. My preceptor was busy with other things going on . . . this woman was going for ECT due to psychotic depression. And she did not want that at all. She was in severe pain, and she was upset that they weren't looking into what the pain was due to. They were telling her it was in her head. And I was looking at the situation . . . there was something going on . . . it was not just pain, she did need psychiatric help. But the way they were planning on going about it, I didn't like. So I just tried to make a change for her . . . I was feeling powerless because I didn't know, like that was my own constraint on myself, because I'm thinking, "I'm just a student, really, what can I do?" But I just kept phoning the doctor. . .

Within the story, it is possible to hear the student's compassion, curiosity, commitment, and competence. Although she understood the need for psychiatric treatment, she could also see what was amiss in the way the woman's report of pain was being ignored. By listening to her own response ("I didn't like [it]," "I was feeling powerless"), the student nurse was able to identify what really mattered to her (her nursing commitments), step beyond her feeling of powerlessness, and live her obligation of responsive ethical nursing care. She was able to work within the contextual realities and normative practices and at the same time assert her own nursing commitments and effect change for her patient.

Capacity 5: Corresponding to What Is

Nepo (2005) describes that in its origins, the word "relate" actually has an interesting twin root. The Latin root means "to bear or endure," and its Indo-European root means "to lift or support." These two aspects capture the essence of corresponding in relational inquiry practice.

Nepo's (2005) description of the difference between two nurses illustrates the importance of relational corresponding. He describes how, while "barely awake," the "burly nurse" pulled back his covers wanting him to walk. "'I just looked at her,' (and) she swung my legs to the edge of the bed" (Nepo, 2005, p. 130). In contrast, the second nurse "appeared with a washcloth for my forehead. She looked at me with compassion, took my hand and said in a firm whisper, 'The rest of your life starts here.' I started to weep. The rib that was removed the day before was now cooling in a jar in the lab while I, sore in every way, was straining to get out of bed . . . But she was right, and so, with much help, I put my feet to the floor and began" (Nepo, 2005, p. 131).

In Nepo's (2005) description, you can see how the second nurse acted in correspondence with what he was experiencing. While the two nurses shared the concern of getting their patient ambulated postoperatively, what made the qualitative difference in terms of compassionate, competent care was corresponding to the man who was the patient. Given his postanalgesic drowsiness, his pain, and his emotional anguish, getting out of bed was not a priority for him. He needed something to make getting out of bed meaningful (which was not a lecture on why postoperative mobilization is important). To correspond means "to be in harmony," "to be in sync with," and "to co-respond to." It also means to communicate, to relate to. Within Nepo's story, it is possible to see how the second nurse corresponded in both ways. Yet, how often does our best-intended care fail to correspond? How many times have you heard nurses cajoling patients to get out of bed or lecturing them on why they should do something the nurse wants them to do? Have you heard nurses speaking about that "noncompliant" patient or the patient with a poor pain tolerance who wouldn't get moving for his or her own good?

Corresponding is about striking up a correspondence—relating to and with people in a way that is meaningful to *them*. It involves paying attention to the meaning, concerns, and life situations of people and families. As one PHN in the study we described earlier stated about her relational approach with families, *"You [have to be and convey that you're] sincerely interested in them as a family, and that each of them are striving to be the best that they can be. And that 'bar' may be different for some families than others but it's not an arbitrary bar that I set . . . Because we all have strengths"* (Browne et al., 2010, p. 32).

Relational inquiry also involves paying attention to how you are corresponding energetically. For example, as a community nurse, walking into the home of a busy family with young children, it is probably out of sync to expect to sit quietly for half an hour and discuss their situation. Engaging with the children as they come and go or engaging as the parent wipes a nose, settles a squabble, or changes diapers would be more energetically "in sync." Similarly, rushing into a hospital room where an elderly man is lying in bed quietly talking with his partner and his spiritual advisor and hurriedly checking an IV before rushing out of the room would be out of sync energetically. To slow one's movements would probably add only a matter of seconds to the action yet would be far less disruptive and more in correspondence to the situation and experience.

Stop for a minute and think about how you correspond with people/ families. Think back to that hour of your clinical day that you analyzed. Do you enter lightly and respectfully? Do you sometimes trample in with your busy nursing gait? Do you enter in a way that enables you to see the texture and richness of the person or family, or do you come armed with nurse-driven assessment tools, treatments, and interventions? Think of other nurses with whom you have worked. How do they appear to correspond?

How we correspond also shapes our own experiences as nurses. An analogy that speaks to this that I (Gweneth) once heard someone use was that of going on a walk in the forest (Mitha, 2000). Depending on how we enter the forest and upon what we are focused, we experience the forest in different ways. For example, if we set out to walk our two large dogs that have not had a run in a few days, it is likely we will be entering the forest with a flurry of force and energy. The dogs will be noisily running through the trees, and we will be walking at a clip to keep up with them. Entering in such a way, we will most definitely disturb the quietness of the forest and the chirping of birds that may quickly flee upon our arrival. Entering through this storm of activity, we are unlikely to notice the multitude of sensations the forest has to offer us. We may fail to feel the moisture in the trees, smell the freshness of new rain, or feel the peacefulness of being amongst the trees that are centuries old. Our activity distracts us and limits our ability to experience the forest in its fullness. On another day if we feel we would like to escape from the noise and activity of the day and set off to have a quiet walk in the forest by ourselves, we are likely to experience the forest quite differently than we did previously. We may find ourselves surprised at the wildflowers we hadn't notice before, at the many shades of green that previously seemed to blend together, and if we pay attention to ourselves, we will likely notice how different we feel as we step into the forest and join in relation with nature.

This forest analogy offers a way of thinking about *how* we relate and correspond in our nursing work. It highlights how our own way of corresponding shapes what we see, experience, and take away. It also highlights how corresponding can profoundly affect the people and families with whom we are. The analogy reminds us that people, as the forest, have a life and harmony all of their own and that it is important for visitors (such as nurses) to tread lightly and respectfully as they enter people's life spaces.

DEVELOPING THE FIVE CS: BEING COMPASSIONATE, CURIOUS, COMMITTED, COMPETENT, AND CORRESPONDING

> One cannot learn to drive by reading a car manual; you have to get into the vehicle and practice manipulating it until the skills you acquire so laboriously become second nature. You cannot learn to swim by sitting on the edge of the pool watching others cavort in the water; you have to take the plunge. (Armstrong, 2011, p. 25)

The five ontologic capacities we have described are integral to relational inquiry practice. As ways-of-being, these capacities can be thought of as the ingredients that bring form to your nursing way-of-being. For example, using the metaphor of a cake, the five Cs are the key ingredients; they are like the sugar, butter, flour, vanilla, baking soda, and salt that combine and give form to the cake. Each ingredient is needed and affects the other, and how you combine the different ingredients affects the nature of the cake you end up with, whether it is large or small, whether it will rise in the oven, and so forth.

In a similar way, the five Cs set the parameters for the kinds of knowledge you will enlist and how you will enlist it, the types of observations and analyses you will engage in, how you will go about making clinical judgments, the nature of those judgments, and ultimately how you will act as a nurse.

Developing these capacities is a lifelong practice. It is not a simple matter of reading about them and understanding them conceptually. As Armstrong (2011) describes in the quote above, to "know" them, you have to live them; you have to take the plunge into the deep waters of nursing and slowly but deliberately practice. While most people understand that competence requires development, it is also important to understand that commitment, compassion, curiosity, and corresponding are not simply "natural" characteristics; they are also cultivated ontologic capacities that you can deliberately enhance. It is our hope that you will develop the capacities in a way that enhances your own nursing practice. Consequently, we expect that even though all nurses who read this book might be striving toward the ways-of-being we have described, if we were to observe you in practice, each reader would "look" different. In common would be the response-ability to nursing situations that you manifest.

THIS WEEK IN PRACTICE
Scrutinizing Nursing Obligations and the Five Cs

The five Cs are foundational to your relational inquiry tool kit. This week in practice, choose one nursing situation to critically analyze. First, consider the situation in terms of nursing obligations. How did you determine your nursing obligations? How were the nursing obligations similar and/or different from that of the doctors, the physiotherapists, or other health practitioners who might have been part of the health care team? Next, reread the descriptions of each of the five Cs and consider your way of being—*how* were you in the situation? Were you compassionate, curious, competent, committed, and corresponding?

YOUR RELATIONAL INQUIRY TOOLBOX

Add the following tools to your relational inquiry toolbox:
- Assess your obligations "relationally" (inquiring intrapersonally, interpersonally, and contextually).
- Take both a proximal view (of those in front of you in the immediate moment) and a distal view (those people, situations, and organizations beyond your view and in the future).

continued on page 132

YOUR RELATIONAL INQUIRY TOOLBOX *continued*

- Consciously discern priorities within competing obligations.
- Be compassionate with others, with yourself, and your own "flaws."
- Relate to emotions rather than trying to avoid or fix them.
- Be curious, identifying what you know and don't know.
- Check in with your nursing commitments.
- Be competent by enlisting uncertainty and difference.
- Intentionally correspond by getting in sync with people and situations.

REFERENCES

Armstrong, A. E. (2006). Towards a strong virtue ethics for nursing practice. *Nursing Philosophy, 7*(3), 110–124.

Armstrong, K. (2011). *Twelve steps to a compassionate life.* Toronto, Ontario, Canada: Vintage Canada.

Bekemeier, B., & Butterfield, P. (2005). Unreconciled inconsistencies: A critical review of the concept of social justice in 3 national nursing documents. *Advances in Nursing Science, 28*(2), 152–162.

Bergum, V. (2013). Relational ethics for health care. In J. Storch, P. Rodney, & R. Starzomski (Eds.), *Toward a moral horizon: Nursing ethics for leadership and practice* (2nd ed., pp. 127–142). Toronto, Ontario, Canada: Pearson.

Blomqvist, Y. T., Rubertsson, C., Kylberg, E., Jöreskog, K., & Nyqvist, K. H. (2012). Kangaroo mother care helps fathers of preterm infants gain confidence in the paternal role. *Journal of Advanced Nursing, 68*(9), 1988–1996.

Browne, A. J., Hartrick Doane, G. A., Reimer, J., Macleod, M., & Mclellan, E. (2010). Public health nursing practice with 'high priority' families: The significance of contextualizing 'risk.' *Nursing Inquiry, 17*(1), 27–38.

Brownridge, D. A. (2008). Understanding the elevated risk of partner violence against Aboriginal women: A comparison of two nationally representative surveys of Canada. *Journal of Family Violence, 23*(5), 353–367.

Bucknall, T. (2007). A gaze through the lens of decision theory toward knowledge translation science. *Nursing Research, 56*(4S), S60–S66.

Caputo, J. (1987). *Radical hermeneutics: Repetition, deconstruction and the hermeneutic project.* Bloomington, IN: Indiana University Press.

Caputo, J. (1993). *Against ethics.* Bloomington, IN: Indiana University Press.

Carnevale, F. A. (2005). Ethical care of the critically ill child: A conception of a 'thick' bioethics. *Nursing Ethics, 12*(3), 239–252.

Cheers, B., Binell, M., Coleman, H., Gentle, I., Miller, G., Taylor, J., et al. (2006). Family violence: An Australian Indigenous community tells its story. *International Social Work, 49*(1), 51–63.

Chodron, P. (2002*). The places that scare you. A guide to fearlessness in difficult times.* Boston: Shambhala Press.

Cong, X., Cusson, R. M., Walsh, S., Hussain, N., Ludington-Hoe, S. M., & Zhang, D. (2012). Effects of skin-to-skin contact on autonomic pain responses in preterm infants. *Journal of Pain, 13*(7), 636–645.

Daoud, N., Urquia, M. L., O'Campo, P., Heaman, M., Janssen, P. A., Smylie, J., et al. (2012). Prevalence of abuse and violence before, during, and after pregnancy in a national sample of Canadian women. *American Journal of Public Health, 102*(10), 1893–1901.

Doane, G. H. (2003). Reflexivity as presence: A journey of self-inquiry. In L. Finlay & B. Gough (Eds.), *Reflexivity. A practical guide for researchers in health and social sciences.* Oxford, United Kingdom: Blackwell.

Doane, G. H. (2004). Being an ethical practitioner: The embodiment of mind, emotion and action. In J. Storch,

P. Rodney, & R. Starzomski (Eds.), *Toward a moral horizon: Nursing ethics for leadership and practice* (pp. 433–446). Toronto, Ontario, Canada: Pearson.

Dobrowolska, B., Wrońska, I., Fidecki, W., & Wysokiński, M. (2007). Moral obligations of nurses based on the ICN, UK, Irish and Polish Codes of Ethics for nurses. *Nursing Ethics, 14*, 171–180.

Donaldson, M. (1991). *Human minds: An exploration.* London: Penguin.

Dopson, S. (2007). A view from organizational studies. *Nursing Research, 56*(4S), S72–S77.

Dyche, L., & Epstein, R. M. (2011). Curiosity and medical education. *Medical Education, 45*(7), 663–668.

Flanagan, O. (1996). *Self expressions: Mind, morals, and the meaning of life.* New York: Oxford University Press.

Goldblatt, H. (2009). Caring for abused women: Impact on nurses' professional and personal life experiences. *Journal of Advanced Nursing, 65*(8), 1645–1654.

Hansen, B. S., Rørtveit, K., Leiknes, I., Morken, I., Testad, I., Joa, I., et al. (2012). Patient experiences of uncertainty—A synthesis to guide nursing practice and research. *Journal of Nursing Management, 20*(2), 266–277.

Hartrick, G. A. (1997). Relational capacity: The foundation for interpersonal nursing practice. *Journal of Advanced Nursing, 26*, 523–528.

Hartrick Doane, G. A. (in press). Cultivating relational consciousness in social justice practice. In P. Kagan, M. Smith, & P. Chinn (Eds.), *Philosophies and practices of emancipatory nursing: Social justice as praxis.* New York: Routledge.

Hartrick Doane, G. A., Browne, A. J., Reimer, J., Macleod, M., & Mclellan, E. (2009). Enacting nursing obligations: Public health nurses' theorizing in practice. *Research and Theory for Nursing Practice, 23*(2), 88–96.

Hartrick Doane, G. A., Stajduhar, K., Bidgood, D., Causton, E., & Cox, A. (2012). End-of-life care and inter-professional practice: Not simply a matter of more. *Health and Interprofessional Practice, 11*(3), EP1028.

Hartrick Doane, G. A., & Varcoe, C. (2007). Relational practice and nursing obligations. *Advances in Nursing Science, 30*(3), 192–205.

Hartrick Doane, G. A., & Varcoe, C. (2013). Relational practice and nursing obligations. In J. Storch, R.

Starzomski, & P. Rodney (Eds.), *Toward a moral horizon: Nursing ethics for leadership and practice* (2nd ed., pp. 143–157). Toronto, Ontario, Canada: Pearson-Prentice Hall.

Higgs, J., & Titchen, A. (2001). Framing professional practice: Knowing and doing in context. In J. Higgs & A. Titchen (Eds.), *Professional practice in health, education and the creative arts* (pp. 3–15). Oxford, United Kingdom: Blackwell Science Ltd.

Holecek, A. (2009). *The power and the pain.* Ithaca, NY: Snow Lion.

Jackson, P. C. (2010). Complementary and alternative methods of increasing breast milk supply for lactating mothers of infants in the NICU. *Neonatal Network, 29*(4), 225–234.

Kirkham, S. R., & Browne, A. J. (2006). Toward a critical theoretical interpretation of social justice discourses in nursing. *Advances in Nursing Science, 29*(4), 324–339.

MacDonald, H. (2006). Relational ethics and advocacy in nursing: Literature review. *Journal of Advanced Nursing, 57*(2), 119–126.

Macleod, M., Browne, A. J., Hartrick Doane, G. A., Cerny, L., Moules, N., Hanlon, N., et al. (2004). *The working relationships of public health nurses and high-priority families in northern communities.* Canadian Institutes of Health Research.

McCarthy, J. (2006). A pluralist view of nursing ethics. *Nursing Philosophy, 7*(3), 157–164.

Mitchell, G. J., & Bunkers, S. S. (2003). Engaging the abyss: A miss-take of opportunity. *Nursing Science Quarterly, 16*(2), 121.

Mitha, F. (2000). *Spirituality in education.* Paper presented at the University of Victoria, British Columbia, Canada.

Mori, R., Khanna, R., Pledge, D., & Nakayama, T. (2010). Meta-analysis of physiological effects of skin-to-skin contact for newborns and mothers. *Pediatrics International, 52*(2), 161–170.

Mullavey-O'Byrne, C., & West, S. (2001). Practising without certainty: Providing health care in an uncertain world. In J. Higgs & A. Titchen (Eds.), *Professional practice in health, education and the creative arts* (pp. 49–61). Oxford, United Kingdom: Blackwell Science Ltd.

Naef, R. (2006). Bearing witness: A moral way of engaging in the nurse-person relationship. *Nursing Philosophy, 7*(3), 146–156.

Nepo, M. (2005). *The book of awakening.* San Francisco: Canari Press.

Neville, K. L. (2003). Uncertainty in illness: An integrative review. *Orthopaedic Nursing, 22*(3), 206–214.

Nouwen, H. J., McNeill, D. P., & Morrison, D. A. (1982). *Compassion: A reflection on the Christian life.* London: Darton, Longman and Todd.

Pattison, S. (2001). Are nursing codes of practice ethical? *Nursing Ethics, 8,* 5–18.

Peter, E., & Liaschenko, J. (2004). Perils of proximity: A spatiotemporal analysis of moral distress and moral ambiguity. *Nursing Inquiry, 11,* 218–225.

Provis, C., & Stack, S. (2004). Caring work, personal obligation, and collective responsibility. *Nursing Ethics, 11*(1), 5–14.

Reimer Kirkham, S., Antifeau, E., Hartrick Doane, G. A., Pesut, B., Porterfield, P., Roberts, D., et al. (2012). *Integrated knowledge translation: Examining a collaborative knowledge translation approach.* Michael Smith Foundation for Health Research.

Roach, M. S. (1987). *The human act of caring: A blueprint for the health professions.* Ottawa, Ontario, Canada: Canadian Hospital.

Rodney, P., Storch, J. L., Varcoe, C., & Hartrick Doane, G. A. (2002–2005). *Ethics in action: Strengthening nurses' enactment of their moral agency within the cultural context of health care delivery.* British Columbia, Canada: Social Sciences and Humanities Research Council, University of Victoria.

Royal Commission on Aboriginal Peoples (1996). *Report of the Royal Commission on Aboriginal Peoples: Volume 3, Gathering Strength.* Ottawa, Ontario, Canada: Author.

Sabo, B. (2011). Reflecting on the concept of compassion fatigue. *Online Journal of Issues in Nursing, 16*(1), 1.

Sinclair, H. A. H., & Hamill, C. (2007). Does vicarious traumatisation affect oncology nurses? A literature review. *European Journal of Oncology Nursing, 11*(4), 348–356.

Singer, M. A. (2007). *The untethered soul.* Oakland, CA: New Harbinger.

Smith, S. (2012). Nurse competence: A concept analysis. *International Journal of Nursing Knowledge, 23*(3), 172–182.

Stephens, C., Porter, J., Nettleton, C., & Willis, R. (2009). Disappearing, displaced, and undervalued: A call to action for Indigenous health worldwide. *The Lancet, 367*(9527), 2019–2028.

Thompson, F. (2002). Moving from codes of ethics to ethical relationships for midwifery practice. *Nursing Ethics, 9*(5), 522–536.

Varcoe, C., & Dick, S. (2008). Intersecting risks of violence and HIV for rural and Aboriginal women in a neocolonial Canadian context. *Journal of Aboriginal Health, 4,* 42–52.

Varcoe, C., Doane, G., Pauly, B., Rodney, P., Storch, J. L., Mahoney, K., et al. (2004). Ethical practice in nursing: Working the in-betweens. *Journal of Advanced Nursing, 45*(3), 316–325.

Varcoe, C., Pauly, B., Storch, J., Newton, L., & Makaroff, K. (2012). Nurses' perceptions of and responses to morally distressing situations. *Nursing Ethics, 19*(4), 488–500.

Varcoe, C., Pauly, B., Webster, G., & Storch, J. (2012). Moral distress: Tensions as springboards for action. *HEC forum: An interdisciplinary journal on hospitals' ethical and legal issues, 24*(1), 51–62.

von Dietze, E., & Orb, A. (2000). Compassionate care: A moral dimension of nursing. *Nursing Inquiry, 7,* 166–174.

Watts, A. W. (1991). *Nature, man, and woman.* New York: Vintage Books.

Weaver, H. N. (2009). The colonial context of violence: Reflections on violence in the lives of Native American women. *Journal of Interpersonal Violence, 24*(9), 1552–1563.

Weber, A. M., Harrison, T. M., & Steward, D. K. (2012). Schore's regulation theory: Maternal–infant interaction in the NICU as a mechanism for reducing the effects of allostatic load on neurodevelopment in premature infants. *Biological Research for Nursing, 14*(4), 375–386.

Whyte, D. (2009). *The three marriages. Reimagining work, self and relationship.* New York: Riverhead Books.

Wilbur, K., Patten, T., Leonard, A., & Morelli, M. (2008). *Integral life practice.* Boston: Integral Books.

Žižek, S. (2008). *Violence.* New York: Picador.

4 All Nursing Is Cultural and Contextual

LEARNING OBJECTIVES

By engaging with the material in this chapter, you will be able to:

1. Define context and culture relationally and explain the benefits of seeing culture contextually.

2. Identify multiple contexts that shape and are shaped by people.

3. Explain the ways in which health is socially determined and how contexts can produce inequities.

4. Identify and discuss several strategies for practicing based on a relational understanding of culture and context.

This chapter explores the relevance of context and culture within day-to-day nursing practice. Although the terms *context* and *culture* are not synonymous, the concepts are inseparable in lived experience. People and their health are socially produced as they live in and embody their contexts and cultures. This understanding provides a foundation for inquiry into how health is socially determined and the implications of that for nursing practice. The chapter closes with strategies that can help nurses negotiate effectively across differences in people's experiences and to understand and honor what is of meaning and significance to them.

RELATIONAL DEFINITIONS OF CONTEXT AND CULTURE

A relational understanding of context and culture is important to nursing because it provides a basis for nurses to: (a) practice based on knowledge of how people, their health, nursing, and health care are all being shaped by their multiple contexts and cultures; (b) intervene to produce situations in which health and well-being can be optimized; and (c) work across differences. That understanding begins with relational definitions of the terms themselves.

Context: Beyond the Container

What comes to mind when you think of the word *context*? If you pay attention to how context is written and talked about, you may notice that it is primarily discussed as a container, an inert backdrop to life. Certainly, contexts can be seen as containers; after all, there are real physical places, such as homes, communities, and health care settings in which lives and health care are conducted. A relational perspective helps nurses look beyond the container. We define contexts as the structures and living processes that shape and are shaped by people's lives. Multiple dynamic interacting historical, economic, sociopolitical, physical, and linguistic structures and processes shape people's health experiences and nursing practice. Different people experience and embody different contexts. Therefore, how people influence and are influenced by any given context has implications for health and nursing care.

For example, think about intensive care units (ICUs). They are physical places with technology, certain layouts, nursing protocols, and so forth. While these contextual elements could be thought of in a static sense—as containers—if one looks relationally, it is possible to see how the physical context of the ICU is shaping people, their experiences, and their interactions. Within the ICU are health care practitioners with certain skills, organized to achieve certain goals, with a certain relationship to other aspects of health care systems. Because they are settings for people with acute illnesses and injuries, ICUs have a characteristic physical appearance, language, access to resources, power structure, level of urgency, and so on compared to long-term care units, maternity care units, emergency departments, and mental health, community, or primary health care settings. However, far from being merely an inert container, the ICU is also shaping and being shaped by every person that is in any way related to it. When you enter an ICU as a nurse for the first time, you immediately notice and begin to learn the language, activities, and usual ways of acting toward patients and colleagues. As you become oriented in the ICU, you are shaped as a nurse. You have a changed sense of what constitutes an emergency, a different emphasis on physiologic parameters, and a different comfort level with technology. You also shape the culture of the ICU, influencing its evolution. At the same time, no two nurses experience or shape the ICU in the same way. Some have a heightened sense of anxiety about this setting, some less. Some strive for proficiency with technical skills, whereas others strive to find ways to "humanize" the technology, and so on.

Moreover, as a result of practicing in the context of the ICU, you are shaped as a nurse. For example, I (Gweneth) found it very challenging when I temporarily worked on a medical unit after spending a few years in ICU. I had become so used to knowing and being able to monitor my patients from head to toe that I found it incredibly stressful to give less intensive care to a greater number of patients who I did not feel I knew well. I (Colleen) had a similar experience moving from ICU to work in emergency, where I felt disoriented by continuously having to leave work with patients incomplete in order to care for new patients.

Similarly, patients and families are shaped by and shape health care settings. As soon as a person is sent to emergency, palliative care, a discharge planning unit, or an ICU, there is a shift in how that person's health situation is understood by the person, family, and care providers. In some cases, when a person is transferred to ICU, the gravity of the situation becomes clearer to everyone; in other cases, it may feel as though a situation considered grave to some is now being taken more seriously by others; in yet other cases, admission to the ICU engenders despair while in others, hope. Although different for each person, the experience has an effect to which people respond. People's responses in turn shape their contexts. For example, because of the influence of various people over time, ICUs have become more "family friendly." Some have integrated a palliative approach for the many people likely to die. Rehabilitation principles have increasingly informed practice early in the ICU trajectory.

This ICU example illustrates how when you take a relational view, your attention is extended to the dynamic interplay of people and contexts. As we explain shortly, you begin to notice how context is embodied and experienced. As a result, your choices expand and your effectiveness as a nurse increases. This happens in at least three specific ways.

First, when you consciously pay attention to the interplay between your own assumptions, values, and beliefs and the contexts of your practice, you can make better decisions. For example, when a nurse in an ICU is conscious of the multiple influences that draw attention to technology (including the pressure to convey competence, the need to stay on top of alarms, or the dominance of the physiologic concerns being monitored, etc.), he or she can more deliberately decide how much attention to devote to technology versus other aspects of care—the person receiving care, family members, and so on. Similarly, rather than accepting the normative organizational practices as given, a nurse who focuses on the interplay among a variety of contexts can work to orient organizational practices to the well-being of individuals/families. So, for example, instead of insisting that families cooperate with the rules regarding who can visit and when, a nurse can work to develop rules that best foster all forms of well-being (e.g., rules that balance physiologic well-being with psychosocial needs).

Second, when you attend to the interplay between people and the contexts of health and health care experiences, you can better understand and respond to the differences among people. For example, Helen Brown's research in neonatal intensive care units (NICUs) explored the importance of context in mothers' responses to the nurses providing their babies' care (Brown, 2008). Depending on the circumstances of their lives (e.g., varied levels of familiarity with technology or fluency in English), mothers felt varying levels of competence. Some compared themselves unfavorably to expert NICU nurses, becoming reluctant to provide care to their premature neonates or even to visit. If nurses understood how the contexts shaping these women's lives influenced their confidence, the nurses could have chosen ways of practicing that would build the women's confidence, engage them, and prepare them for parenting at home.

Third, when you are able to analyze the interplay among contexts, the individuals and families receiving care, and your practice, you are able to intervene at the contextual level. For example, nurses have been instrumental in changing visiting policies (including and beyond ICUs and NICUs) to be more responsive to the well-being of individuals and families. In doing so, they have shaped the contexts of their practice, including how resources are used. For example, in one unit, nurses persuaded administrators to prioritize the building of a family and visitor lounge over purchasing new blood gas monitors.

TRY IT OUT 4.1

Examine a Context of Practice

Find someone to interview (or to have a purposeful conversation with) to learn about a particular health care context. Find someone who has experience with a particular setting—either as a health care provider or as a patient or family member of a patient. If you are in a practice setting now, you might interview a nurse who works there about that context of practice or about another setting with which that person has experience. If you are not in a practice setting, find someone who has had experience with a health care context—it might be emergency, palliative care, long-term care, or a surgical unit. Perhaps pick someone from an area in which you are interested in working.

Your goal is to learn about the features of that practice context, how those features influence people's experiences of health care and how people try to influence that context. Also, listen for how the context aligns with what that person values and finds meaningful and significant. I (Colleen) just did this with a woman whose mother has dementia and is in a long-term care unit. Her description of the institutional-looking context, unrelieved by "failed attempts to make the place look home-like," and of staff behavior, which seemed more appropriate to "custodians than nurses," helped me more fully understand the woman's distress over her mother's care. When she told me all that she does to make her mother's surroundings "more human," such as putting up photos of her mom's prior life, bringing a range of visitors regularly, making the surroundings as home-like as possible, displaying her mother's paintings and so on, I understood how she experienced "dehumanizing care" more fully.

Try asking questions such as:

- What is (LTC, maternity, surgery, diagnostic imaging, etc.) like?
- How is the context different from other practice settings (ask about history, resources, politics)?
- What is unique about the language used in (hemodialysis, the chemo unit, the diabetic clinic, etc.)?
- How do the characteristics of (the burn unit, emergency, the outpatient department, etc.) affect the people working there? The patients?
- How do staff try to influence what happens in the unit? What role do patients and families have in influencing what happens? What is one thing you have tried to change?

After your conversation, compare what you learned with someone else who has done the same exercise. Do you see how these contexts of practice are constantly exerting influence and being changed? Do you see how people's own values and experiences shape their interpretations and the way they respond? Can you articulate several ways in which each practice context is unique and ways in which it is similar to other health care contexts?

Culture: Beyond Population Groups

What comes to mind when you think of the word *culture*? The term is used in diverse ways, including as a reference to sophisticated forms of art, music, and literature. However, culture is perhaps most commonly defined as the values, beliefs, attitudes, and practices of particular groups. We find this definition narrow and misleading for a number of reasons.

First, the fact that these dimensions of culture (values, behaviors, etc.) arise from multiple contexts is rarely specified. For example, dietary preferences are often seen as cultural, yet such preferences usually arise from what is available and affordable. People living in areas conducive to rice cultivation tend to eat rice. As global trade and transportation allow people to consume rice in areas where it can't be grown, new cultures incorporate rice as a common food.

Second, when the notion of culture is applied to individual people, the fact that people belong to multiple groups simultaneously and that their allegiance to any given group is always partial and changing is also commonly overlooked. So, for example, it's commonly assumed that someone who has descended from inhabitants of Japan (perhaps someone who identifies as Japanese American) eats rice, whether that person likes rice or not. Yet, a person who identifies as American never embraces all things deemed American, a person who identifies as Muslim never embraces all things Muslim, and so on. Group membership is not a useful indicator of individual values, beliefs, or practices because individual participation in a culture is a dynamic process mediated by multiple contexts.

For these reasons, we define *culture* as a dynamic relational process of selectively responding to and integrating particular historical, social, political, economic, physical, and linguistic structures and processes. That is, culture is relationally determined and contextual. These responses are expressed in multiple ways, including values, beliefs, attitudes, and practices. In the words of Stephenson (1999, p. 85), "culture is a process that happens between people"; culture is a relational process.

Why do nurses need this new definition of culture? Traditionally, health care providers have focused on categorizing people/groups by ethnicity, race, and/or nationality, using single categories to identify the relevant values, beliefs, attitudes, and practices that should be considered when providing care. So, for example, nursing textbooks often draw attention to the values, beliefs, and practices associated with groups defined by ethnicity, race, or nation (e.g., Italian, Hmong, Chinese, Salvadorian). Our definition avoids the limitations of such practices. Rather than setting nurses up to make erroneous assumptions, draw on stereotypes, and overlook other important influences, a relational definition of culture encourages you to dispense with the idea that categories based on race, ethnicity, or nationality will be useful in understanding individuals or families in any full way and to inquire about the range of contextually mediated influences shaping people's lives and health.

Understanding culture from a relational perspective also provides a more effective basis for nursing practice. A relational view enables you to take the influence of multiple contexts into account and draws your attention to the interplay among different people's values, beliefs, attitudes, and practices as well as to the interplay between these and the multiple contexts that shape them. In short, cultural difference is not limited to difference based on membership in an ethnic or racial group, but rather it encompasses differences in experience, meanings, and what is significant to particular individuals and families.

Specifically, seeing culture relationally offers at least five advantages. It helps you:

- See culture contextually.
- Avoid confusing and conflating culture with race, ethnicity, or nationality.
- See how group membership, beliefs, and values do not necessarily dictate the culture of individuals.
- See how culture is infused with power.
- See culture as dynamic and always changing.

Seeing Culture Contextually

Razack (1998) says that the most common view of culture is a decontextualized view in which "culture is taken to mean values, beliefs, knowledge, and customs that exist outside of patriarchy, racism, imperialism, and colonialism" (p. 58). In this view, people's values, beliefs, and customs are identified as "cultural" and separate from their life circumstances. This habit of seeing some aspects of people's lives as cultural and separate from life circumstances is important because it has major implications for how you practice as a nurse. For example, if you brought this decontextualized understanding of culture to your work, you might focus on looking for cultural practices such as the wearing of certain clothing or symbols of faith for certain groups. While these practices are important, there is far more to culture that needs to be brought into view if you are to nurse effectively—namely the larger contextual circumstances that are inseparable from culture. Overlooking these contextual circumstances serves to (a) trivialize culture, (b) confine attention to traditions that differ from the dominant norm, and (c) overlook the webs of social and political influences that shape cultures.

In health care practice, culture is often understood in this decontextualized way. Stephenson's (1999) description of a news report of a 5-year-old girl who dies from chicken pox offers a prime example. Attributing the child's death to "Mexican culture" obscured the dynamics of colonialism and overlooked the family's poverty, unfamiliarity with services, immigration status, and the language barriers they faced and instead blamed her parents for not seeking care.

These dynamics echo the experience that I (Colleen) have had doing research on violence against women. Many people ask me, "What is it about their [referring to any culture that they see as different] culture that leads the women to stay with abusive men?" Understanding culture as being people's values and beliefs disconnected from their wider life circumstances overlooks broader contextual issues. In the case of women with abusive male partners, such a view overlooks gendered role expectations, power differences, wage differences, and so on. At the same time, problems that arise from those broader contexts (e.g., poverty, unemployment) are seen as linked with culture thought of narrowly in association with groups often defined by ethnicity or race. For example, although the chances of entering or leaving an abusive relationship are influenced by economic independence for all women (and people of other genders), this influence is only labeled as "cultural" for racialized groups. As described in Chapter 2, by racialized we mean the assigning of racial categories to people so that their apparent race becomes a salient feature, a process experienced more often by nondominant groups.

Another way that a decontextualized view of culture can be seen is when health care practitioners treat culture as though it determines health or health practices. For example, assuming that a person's culture leads them to live, eat, and behave in certain ways and/or that people are unhealthy (or smoke or stay with abusive partners) because of their cultural beliefs obscures the influences of economic, sociopolitical, historical, and linguistic contexts. For example, saying that women from a particular ethnic group stay with abusive partners because of their beliefs overlooks the role of power dynamics in shaping their beliefs and how economics, social expectations, and language shape and limit the possibilities of doing otherwise.

In order to understand people's practices, the circumstances of their lives must be understood. A relational understanding "contextualizes" culture and extends your view beyond shared beliefs or group membership to consider these larger contextual circumstances. Specifically, contextualizing culture draws your attention to how differences between people are shaped by patriarchy, racism, imperialism, and colonialism and these factors' economic, political, and social effects. For example, people travelling in Mexico from other parts of North America often comment on garbage on the roadside as cultural, overlooking how it is actually the product of tax policies within the global economy that do not support social services such as recycling programs, garbage pickup, and clean up. A relational view helps you see in this example how cultures of consumerism and environmentalism intersect with economic contexts. People's practices, such as how much garbage they produce and how they dispose of it, are never simply the product of beliefs. Even without a strong commitment to environmental protection, a person may recycle garbage because policies requiring such practice are becoming embedded in Western culture. People will present themselves in certain ways with regard to environmental practices in relation to what is acceptable in their local setting. A person may reject consumerism or not have any material resources, but they still have a relationship to and are shaped by consumerism. These multiple influences converge and influence us all.

Not Confusing Culture with Race, Ethnicity, or Nationality

Culture is often only seen as relevant to people who differ from the dominant group. For example, in North America if you speak English with an accent that is different from the dominant norm or have a skin color other than white, people have probably asked you questions about your race, ethnicity, or nationality. If you are white and speak English with an accent close to the dominant norm, it is likely that you have not been asked such questions.

This understanding of culture as a thing determined by race and/or ethnicity is highly limiting. As David Allen (1999) argues, culture is not an object: "There is no such 'thing' as culture" (p. 227). Yet often we treat culture as a thing that is located in people or groups. In many Western countries, the dominant culture is unremarkable as the norm, while non-Western cultures (e.g., Indian, Chinese, Thai, Vietnamese, etc.) are made visible and often associated with "other than." Whether defining a culture by location (e.g., urban culture), ethnicity (e.g., Irish culture), identity (e.g., queer culture), or something else, this static view of culture invites making assumptions and taking a stance of knowing, increasing the risk of erroneously applying stereotypical ideas to particular people. For instance, if you link culture to nationality and you know something about Irish culture, you may be tempted to assume those characteristics apply to all individuals who identify as Irish.

Associating culture with race, ethnicity, or nationality is inadequate for at least four reasons:

- It supports a tendency to associate individuals with groups and make incorrect assumptions that individuals share presumed group values or practices.
- It supports a tendency to ascribe salience to culture only with certain groups (those defined as different from the dominant group).
- It promotes a static view and overlooks tensions within and among groups.
- It often overlooks what is of meaning and significance to particular individuals and families.

Defining culture relationally helps you avoid conflating people's cultures with their ethnicity, race, or nationality, and it widens your understanding of the multiple influences that shape culture and people. When you don't confuse culture with ethnicity, race, or nationality, you will inquire with individuals about what is of meaning and significance to them without making assumptions, drawing on stereotypes, or confining your inquiry to values, beliefs, or practices that are associated with a single group and that may or may not be relevant.

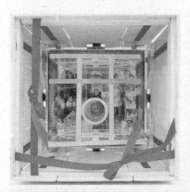
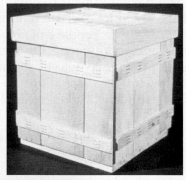

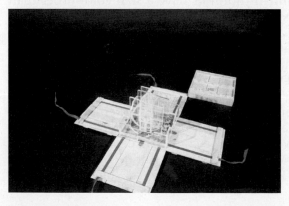

Cultural baggage. (Mixed media by Connie Sabo.)

Defining culture relationally can also enable you to better recognize the problematic effects of using the idea of culture in a way that conflates it with ethnicity, race, or nationality. This kind of culture talk can operate in two different ways. It can be used to signal difference from the dominant norm and imply inferiority or aberrance to certain groups of people (often disguised as fascination with the exotic) and to justify unfair treatment. For example, changes to employment policies that facilitate access for new immigrants to Western countries have been blocked by ideas expressed like, "Those people [any racialized ethnic group] are lazy and just came to this country for a free ride. Why should they get our jobs?" It can also be used to create solidarity and to counter oppression. Razack (1998) says that "culture talk is a double-edged sword" in that it "packages difference as inferiority . . . yet is important for contextualizing oppressed groups' claims for justice, improving their access to services and for requiring dominant groups to examine the invisible cultural advantages they enjoy" (p. 58). It is crucial for nurses to understand that while a nurse should work against applying single, ethnic-based identities to people, the same people may claim those identities. So, for example, in my (Colleen's) work, I am very careful not to racialize violence against women; yet, at the same time, my South Asian colleagues find it politically useful to marshal activism in their communities by talking about violence against women in the South Asian community.

Defining culture relationally enables you to be discerning around culture talk and identify the effects of how it is being used. Sometimes, naming culture in the sense of ethnicity serves to illuminate discriminatory practices. At other times, naming culture as ethnicity functions to obscure salient underlying issues, such as poverty or discriminatory policies, to shift responsibility, or to obscure diversity.

Seeing Culture as More than Single-Group Membership

From a relational view, a person's culture is not limited to the values, beliefs, and preferences associated with membership in any single group, whether that group is defined by race, ethnicity, nationality, or any other characteristic, including gender, age, socioeconomic bracket, and so forth. Stop for a minute and think about this idea in terms of yourself. For example, can you think of how you share certain values, beliefs, and preferences with a particular group and at the same time have other "different" values and practices? Similarly, you live within a particular country, but you probably only align with certain values that are ascribed to that country. Moreover, because you are from a particular country, would assuming you are the same as everyone else in that country obscure ways that you are unique and/or different from those who share your ethnicity or citizenship? Similarly, you are also part of the nursing profession, but to which nursing values do you fully subscribe? You share some values with your family of origin, and others you question. You share some and reject other values that are associated with your ethnic group(s), however you define them. Your values are shifting as you evolve as a nurse and hopefully as you read this book.

Seeing culture as more than beliefs, values, and practices associated with a particular group enables you to move beyond stereotyping people. It prompts you to ask individuals and families what they actually value, rather than making assumptions based on what you perceive to be their group membership. Similarly, you can look to see how culture is being lived and meaningfully experienced between groups and people.

Seeing Culture as Infused with Power

The fourth feature of a relational perspective of culture is that it helps you see how power dynamics shape culture. When culture is intentionally looked at as more than ethnicity, more than a collection of shared beliefs, and inseparable from social, political, and economic circumstances, the importance of power relations comes into view. For example, when we examine the experiences of people who immigrate to the United States (or Canada, Britain, etc.) and are racialized in their new country, the salience of the power dynamics of migration processes and racialization become more evident. In contrast, when structural issues, such as poverty, unemployment, access to health care, and so on are labeled cultural issues, and when unwanted life circumstances are labeled personal choices, then individuals and families can unjustly be held responsible for them.

Defining culture relationally will help you see when culture is being problematically used to explain and deal with "others" in ways that sustain economic exclusion (Swendson & Windsor, 1996). For example, the phrase "the culture of poverty" implies that poverty is a matter of choice that arises from beliefs or that poverty gives rise to a self-sustaining culture. When you hear groups of people being labeled as lazy or unmotivated and blamed for their experiences of poverty rather than poverty being understood as arising from their life circumstances, you will be better able to challenge these ideas for yourself and others. I (Colleen) often try to respond to discourses about people on social assistance (the dole, welfare) by pointing out the high percentage of women on social assistance who have left abusive partners.

TO ILLUSTRATE
Looking White People in the Eye

Have you ever heard about certain groups who don't make eye contact? Has anyone told you that for certain people, avoidance of eye contact is a "cultural norm?" Razack (1998) points out that eye contact is a common topic when discussing cultural difference, "a perennial favorite as a marker of the perils associated with cross-cultural encounters" (p. 57). Razack shows how perceiving eye contact as "cultural" overlooks the effects of power, racism, and colonialism. It also overlooks the fact that eye contact is often being judged within a context of white supremacy, usually by members of dominant groups. She asks to what extent is avoidance of eye contact with white people by racialized groups a safety strategy? To what extent is it an aversion to what racialized people might expect to see in the eyes of white people (such as aversion, fear, or disregard)? Referring to the criminal justice system, Razack also shows how a focus on behaviors as cultural (such as avoidance of eye contact, which those in power often consider indicative of guilt) draws attention away from systemic oppression. Thus, in her example, discriminatory justice system practices (such as disproportionately high arrest and incarceration rates of people of color and indigenous people) are explained as cultural problems rather than as

continued on page 145

> **TO ILLUSTRATE** *continued*
> ## Looking White People in the Eye
>
> consequences of institutionalized racism. Eye contact is a complex behavior influenced by power and meaning, gender norms, religious proscriptions, and many other factors and must be understood in its complexity rather than as a simple group-related behavior.

Seeing Culture as Dynamic and Changing

Because culture is a process that is experienced in and between people, it is dynamic and always in the process of being made. Therefore, to engage relationally in nursing is also to engage culturally. It is to practice from the assumption that culture is created, culture is lived, and culture is always in process. The values, beliefs, and practices of individuals and families come together in dynamic interplay with those of the nurse, all within the values and priorities of the health care context.

Understanding that culture is always changing and in process and that multiple influences intersect in dynamic ways supports inquiry as the best approach to culture and difference. It draws your attention to the tensions within and between various groups and individuals.

>
> ## TO ILLUSTRATE
> ### Food Practices as "Cultural"
>
> Interviewing diverse people about food, eating, and its meaning, Brenda Beagan, Gwen Chapman, and their colleagues (Beagan et al., in press) show the complexity of culture. For example, in families who emigrated from non-Western to Western countries, adolescents often wanted to eat Western foods in a Western style rather than following and maintaining their families' traditional practices, creating tension between parents and children. Food and practices were not just sources of nutrition with social meaning. Rather, they were also performances through which people expressed a sense of superiority in relation to others. People conveyed their moral superiority by contrasting their own superior eating habits to what they saw as the inferior habits of others (e.g., "healthy eating" versus junk or fast food; fresh, local, organic food versus processed packaged food; adventurous, cosmopolitan food versus bland meat and potatoes). Often, these symbolic boundaries marked social class differences.

Taking up a relational view of culture requires attention to the dynamic interplay of values, beliefs, and practices at all levels. It highlights how people can never stand outside of their own experiences, values, beliefs, and attitudes to view others and to understand differences. Thus, when engaging across any difference, it is important to begin with interrogating our own perspectives, our cultures, and the views to which they might give rise.

TRY IT OUT 4.2

Map Your Own Cultures

List the multiple cultures to which you belong. Figure 4.1 shows a few of the cultures to which I (Colleen) belong at present. What are the key cultures to which you belong? Western culture? The culture of health care? Student culture? How does membership in these cultures influence your life? What about your ethnic background? Does it dominate? What are the tensions among these cultures? What is the interplay between your intrapersonal values and beliefs and those that dominate the context?

Identify one key value, belief, or attitude each of your cultures contributes to your world view. How does each complement the others within your overall world view? What are the tensions? From being embedded in Western culture with a well-paying job, I (Colleen) value and take for granted a certain level of material affluence. At the same time, having grown up in a rural setting in a low-income family, I bring a critique of my current class privilege. I am an Anglophone, but being embedded within Canadian culture (as well as Francophone culture

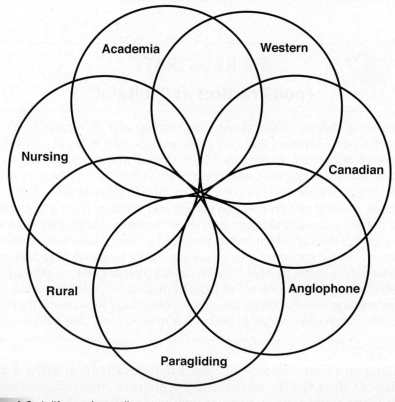

Fig. 4.1 A "few cultures."

continued on page 147

> ### TRY IT OUT 4.2 *continued*
>
> ## Map Your Own Cultures
>
> and indigenous activism about language rights) has heightened my awareness of my unearned privilege that flows from speaking English as I travel the world.
>
> Compare yourself to others you know. Do you share the same culture with your parents as you do with your friends or with any children you know? Do you enact your culture differently depending on whom you are with? For example, with nursing versus non-nursing friends, or with older versus younger people? Can you see your own culture as a relational process, something changing and dynamic that you influence and shape?

The Benefits of Seeing Context and Culture Relationally in Nursing Practice

Holding relational definitions of context and culture enables you to purposefully examine context and culture as you interpret people and situations and act in response to them. It does this in three key ways.

First, a relational view enables you to understand that context and culture are inseparable. Not only is culture always contextual, it is always "perspectival" (Allen, 1999), meaning that people are always viewing from their own perspectives and being viewed within and from particular contexts. For instance, a colleague who is originally from Pakistan described how she is seen differently depending on where she is. In Canada, she is seen as being from Pakistani culture in that she originates from Pakistan, speaks English with a certain accent, at times dresses in clothing from Pakistan, and so forth. Yet, when she returns to Pakistan, she is seen as a "white Westerner" because people there see her as having Western ways and a Western accent. This underscores the fluid nature of culture and cultural identity and the limitations of categories and generalizations. As you examine how your own values, beliefs, and attitudes arise from the contexts of your life, you can better identify the stereotypes to which you have been exposed and thus better avoid reductionist ways of understanding and approaching people. At the same time, you can appreciate your differences from others as arising from differences in experiences and contexts and as more than mere clashes of values or beliefs.

Second, contextualizing culture helps you remember that given how people are situated and constituted within multiple contexts, no two people who share an ethnic, religious, or national background can be lumped together and seen as having the same culture. Two people who emigrate from Pakistan to New Zealand will differ on at least some dimensions of experience, perhaps including their education, income, religion, language, age, and gender; all of these shape values, beliefs, and practices. What those two people eat, for example, may be partially due to ethnic influences but is also shaped by what each can afford, what is available, what they enjoy, and what is acceptable in their varied environments.

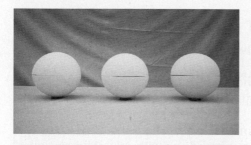
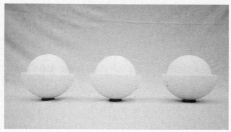
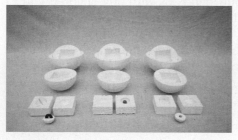

The life within. (Mixed media by Connie Sabo.)

Third, intertwining context and culture helps you consider how multiple influences (e.g., historical, economic, geographical, etc.) may be intersecting at any one time and what the implications of those intersections may be for individual and family well-being. To take a simple example, by seeing context and culture as inseparable, you are better able to help people improve their diets. If one works from the assumption that different people will have different food preferences and those preferences are shaped contextually/culturally, you will see food preferences as more than "ethnic" practices and also more than simple health choices. Rather than making any assumption about ethnic preferences based on people's appearances, you are automatically triggered to extend your view and inquire. into what is shaping their preferences and decisions. What can they afford? What is available? How have their economic and geographic circumstances shaped their exposure to certain foods and not others? You are also guided to consider your own food biases (e.g., what you consider to be a healthy, "normal" diet, your ethics in relation to food), anticipate how your preferences and nursing concerns might be different from those of others, and lessen negative judgment on your part when those differences arise. By intertwining context/culture as you inquire, you are better positioned to determine people's food preferences/choices and to understand the source of those differences. Understanding the basis of preferences and differences lessens conflict and judgment. It also provides a basis for negotiation.

CONTEXTS AND THE PEOPLE WHO LIVE THEM

As you explore how contexts give rise to cultures and cultures shape contexts, your knowledge and understanding of people and families increases and you are able to make more informed decisions about how to intervene and provide care. As part of that process of exploration, let's look at precisely how people shape and are shaped by their multiple contexts.

People Shape and Are Shaped by Their Multiple Contexts

The old adage "children are products of their environments" seems self-evident. Children are produced physically by what they eat (or don't eat), the level of safety in their environments, and so on; they are produced socially by what they are exposed to and taught, including language and behaviors. These dynamics, easy to see with children, are less easy to keep in mind with adults. However, all adults, families, and nurses are also produced in an ongoing way by their environments. This is because people are embedded in and embody their contexts in an ongoing process throughout their lifespans.

In thinking about how contexts are embodied in people, it is helpful to think about how we understand the body and what the idea of "embodiment" means. The dominant Western way of thinking about the body aligns with the world in which the mind and body are treated as distinct and separate entities. This view is often termed the "Cartesian view" because the ideas of René Descartes, a French philosopher and mathematician, have been so influential. Within the dualism that characterizes this perspective, not only are the body and mind separate, but as Davis and Walker (2010) explain, "the body cannot be a 'knower' within this schema, and the body and its experiences are always subordinate to the objective reason of the mind. Within this polarization, the mind is associated with the masculine, and the body is associated with the feminine. Women are closely connected to the body, emotion, and irrationality while men are connected with the mind, control, and reason" (p. 458). This effectively diminishes the body as a source of knowledge and women as knowers. Cartesian dualism works with and reinforces other binaries such as male/female and emotional/rational.

How nurses understand the body matters. Nurses continually have opportunities to help people pay attention to and trust their bodies as well as to understand how they are embodying their contexts. If nurses uncritically take up a dualist view of the body as separate from the mind and uncritically separate reason and emotion, associating them with the mind and body, male and female respectively, then they will be less effective in supporting people's health and will be more likely to accept gender stereotypes, particularly those related to reason and emotion.

The Cartesian understanding leads us to approach people as separate from their worlds and as composed of discrete parts. For example, we separate mental illness from physical illness. We privilege physical comfort that we can verify through something we can either see or know from information other than the person's perspective. For example, nurses are much more likely to believe patient's pain assessments when a verifiable cause can be known, such as a wound, fracture, tumor, and so on. We are constantly influenced to think in this way. For example, think of the sayings "It's all in your head" or "Think with your head, not your heart." In our practices, we can reinforce this view. For example, in my research in primary health care settings for people who are highly marginalized by poverty and racism, I (Colleen) have observed that in order to decide which patients can be prescribed narcotics, nurses and physicians continuously try to determine who has "legitimate pain" and who does not. These dynamics are predicated on physical pain with a known etiology as more legitimate than other forms of pain (e.g., undiagnosed problems, diffuse chronic pain, mental and emotional trauma, etc.). Further, nurses often judge women differently from men, such as devaluing more "emotional" responses to pain by women in contrast to men.

In contrast to a Cartesian view, a relational view highlights the inseparability of mind and body and people and their worlds. A relational view takes into account how bodies simultaneously are both material and biologic entities. In this view, the body is knowledgeable and also a source of knowledge. For example, think about how your body knows when you are tired, hungry, anxious, happy, and so on. Bergum (2013) described embodiment as the incorporation of the body as a material object with the lived body in a way "so that scientific knowledge and human compassion are given equal weight: emotions and feeling are understood to be as important to human life as physical signs and symptoms" (p. 132). For example, nurses can be effective in assisting people with enduring suffering and pain, and that effectiveness is greatly enhanced when you attend to the whole person and the inseparability of the physical, mental, emotional, and spiritual dimensions of people. Think about what happens physiologically when you ask a person to take a deep breath and exhale slowly and relax. Are the effects only physical?

It is crucial that nurses understand the inseparability of the body and mind and the inseparability of the body and its multiple contexts. Each time a nurse interacts with a person, he or she is engaging with the whole person and their lived experiences as they are embodied in that person. For example, think about how powerfully certain sounds, smells, and sights can evoke memories and even physical reactions. For myself (Colleen), I can feel myself relaxing when I smell lavender—at least in part because of numerous positive memories with which I associate the smell. Similarly, when I (Gweneth) worked with people who had experienced severe trauma, bodily sensation and memory were integral to the healing process. Often, the therapeutic process focused more explicitly on accessing and healing the connections between the contextual elements (i.e., the sounds and sights of a frightening car accident) to the person's physical symptoms and current health challenges.

Understanding the inseparability of the body, mind, and context highlights the importance of your own actions as a nurse. Each time you interact with a person, you, as part of that person's social context, are influencing the person's responses physically, mentally, and emotionally. Whether you are intentional or not, your level of energy, your attitude, your mood, your patience (or impatience), and your confidence (or lack of confidence) are conveyed and have influence. Ignoring your "contextual" impact simply limits your ability to have a more purposeful and intentionally positive effect. At the same time, systematically considering the multiple contexts that shape people and how people embody their different contexts will provide you with a stronger basis from which to understand particular people, differences among people, how you are responding, and what is shaping your responses.

TRY IT OUT 4.3

An Influence Experiment

Next time you are about to enter a social situation—a family dinner, classroom, coffee shop to meet friends—consciously choose a mode of interaction. Try to "get in sync" with the way people are being, or try to change the energy of the context. Try being a calming influence, a wild enthusiast, or a thought provocateur. Watch what happens to other people around you. Who do you shut down or draw closer? Who do you engage or disengage? How do people look at you, and do they lean toward you or away from you? Can you bring the whole energy of the context up or down with your presence? Can you influence people *physically* with your mode of interaction? Can you carry that over to a patient situation? For example, through your approach (not just with words), can you influence a person to whom you are providing care to relax more fully?

Multiple interrelated environments shape and are shaped by people and are always influencing their health experiences. People simultaneously shape their contexts both purposefully and simply by existing. For example, even when people are unconscious, their inert bodies still produce effects. As nurses, we respond in particular ways to people when they are unconscious, depending on the practice context. An inert body in ICU has a different meaning than in a community mental health setting. However, each response is a complex interplay among nurses, people, and contexts. The inert body of a child on a street will evoke different responses than an older person who is dressed in poor and dirty clothing in the same setting.

TO ILLUSTRATE

Two Strokes

Consider two people who have the same medical diagnoses. Both Mrs. Zhang, a 68-year-old woman, and Mr. Stephen, a 56-year-old man, have had strokes, are mildly aphasic, and have some right-sided paralysis. Mrs. Zhang immigrated to the United States to live with her son about 10 years ago when her husband died in an accident in a shipbuilding yard. She recently lost her job at a garment factory when it moved from the United States to Bangladesh, and she now cares for her three young grandchildren while her son and daughter-in-law run a small import business. She speaks Shanghainese and understands some Mandarin. Mr. Stephen was born in England and is a British citizen. He is a well-known news writer and public personality. He speaks only English. Both are receiving care in a Western-style, acute care, English-speaking hospital.

continued on page 152

TO ILLUSTRATE *continued*

Two Strokes

Although both people have the same medical diagnosis, and the same clinical pathways (also referred to as care pathways or care maps) might be used to guide their care related to the physiologic effects of stroke and medical treatment, their health and thus nursing practice requires more. As you can already imagine, their contexts, experiences, and what is of meaning and significance to each differs in important ways.

Multiple Contexts Are Always at Work

There are multiple types of interrelated and overlapping contexts that are important to pay attention to as a nurse. While there are many more possibilities, for the purpose of this book, we have chosen to draw your attention to historical, sociopolitical, material-economic, physical, and linguistic-discursive environments or contexts (see Figure 4.2). We have chosen these contexts because we think that they capture some of the greatest influences on health and health care.

Historical Contexts

First, consider historical contexts. History is always present and shaping the future of people to whom you provide care as well as of nursing and health care practice. Each patient you encounter has a history that is not confined to his or her immediate life but rather stretches back many generations,

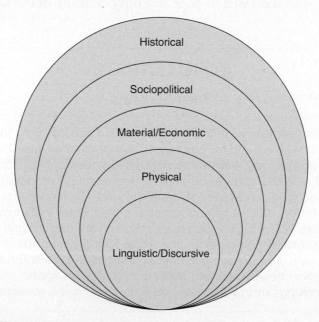

Fig. 4.2 One typology of interrelated health contexts.

shaping his or her social life, material conditions, language, and physical form, even at the level of genetics. For example, think of Mrs. Zhang and Mr. Stephen prior to their stroke experiences. How might their social, political, and economic histories be contributing to their risk of stroke and stroke experiences?

The histories of both nurses and the individuals and families to whom they provide care come together in each health care encounter. Emphasizing the connectedness between one's past, present, and future, Paterson and Zderad argue that humanistic nursing is always inclusive of both nurses' and patients' histories (O'Connor, 1993). This is important to nursing because your own history shapes your perceptions and knowledge and, consequently, how you relate. For example, if you have a parent who has had a stroke, you will be influenced by this history in various ways. If you encountered Mr. Stephen, how would his history likely differ from yours, and how would it be similar? Then consider Mrs. Zhang. Even based on age and country of birth alone, you likely would have experienced and embodied different contexts than each person.

The histories of the individuals and families to whom you provide care are clearly important because they shape health and health care. In health care influenced by individualist and biomedical view, histories are often narrowly focused on an individual's immediate health history and/or a family's genetic history, overlooking the broader social determinants of health and often overlooking key features of a person's life. However, nursing requires a broader understanding of the circumstances of individual and families' lives.

History is always exerting influence for individuals and families. Similarly, history is always exerting influence over groups, communities, and organizations. But how much history do you need? How far back do you go? Integrating understanding of historical contexts in nursing practice does not mean taking a detailed history of each person you encounter following a proscribed guide. Rather, from a relational inquiry perspective it means:

- Practicing with an awareness of history
- Following the lead of the individual and family to learn what is relevant
- Continuous inquiry at all levels regarding the history influencing the immediate situation

For example, when the nurse caring for Mrs. Zhang was able to work through an interpreter, she learned that Mrs. Zhang was able to communicate more than the physicians and other nurses had thought; her dysphasia was not as pronounced as previously thought, or it was improving. The nurse also learned that Mrs. Zhang was very distressed about what might happen if she is unable to care for her grandchildren as the family cannot afford to run the business and pay for childcare. Finally, the nurse also learned that Mrs. Zhang is diabetic, something in her personal health history that had somehow been overlooked, illustrating how a relational inquiry approach simultaneously widens beyond and complements a biomedical approach.

BOX 4.1

Integrating Awareness of Historical Contexts

Ask yourself and others:
- What do you think led to this [situation, problem, illness]?
- Is there anything from the past that I should know about?
- How did you/your family deal with this [situation, problem, illness] previously?

The more deliberately conscious you are about your inquiry into history, the better able you will be to learn what is of meaning and significance to people, how situations have been produced, and how they might be further influenced. Again, knowing your own history, inquiring about the histories of others with as few preconceptions as possible, and taking contexts actively into account in your thinking attunes you to differences that are important.

Sociopolitical Contexts

We refer to social environments as "sociopolitical" to draw attention to how power is an inherent aspect of our social world. Power operates in every context and social process and influences what transpires and is experienced by and among people within any given context. For example, can you think of social situations or environments that bring out the best in you? Do you recognize how you behave differently across different contexts? Can you identify contextual aspects that influence your experiences? For example, I (Gweneth) have found within the context of a hierarchical health care culture I experience power differently depending on whether I am professionally identified as a psychologist or a nurse. Across contexts, I am seen and experienced as having more or less power in relation to other colleagues, the organization assigns me a particular position in the hierarchy, colleagues respond somewhat differently, and so forth. Have you found yourself being treated according to your student designation?

Understanding how you influence and are influenced by context is crucial to nursing practice. You are exerting influence and creating context in every moment of practice whether you are conscious of doing so or not. More conscious attention allows you to be more purposeful in your effort to influence the sociopolitical context of care to be health-promoting for others and to contribute to a healthy work environment.

One of the most important ways nurses promote health through sociopolitical contexts is by reducing barriers and enhancing access to health care. Health care access is often thought about only at the level of social or organizational policy. Of course, cost, insurance coverage, availability of services, distance to services, and transportation affordability and availability are critical elements to access to health care. Nurses can intervene at the contextual level to influence these. However, nurses also have a role influencing the sociopolitical context at the intra- and interpersonal levels and at contextual levels more locally to reduce barriers and enhance access.

People do not come for care, fail to return for care, leave care, and do not listen to health care advice for a wide range of reasons, including fear of being judged, demeaned, dismissed or disrespected, and real experiences of being treated poorly. Nurses have the opportunity on a daily basis to anticipate such fears and provide care to prevent such fears from becoming realities. Repeatedly, our research has shown that people and families can be supported or discouraged from accessing the health care they need by how nurses practice in particular contexts. For example, each health care context has particular forms of judgment, stigma, and discrimination that people fear, which in turn can deter access. Thus, any effort a nurse can make to reduce people's fear, anticipation, and experiences of judgment, stigma, and discriminatory treatment can improve access. If the normative practice of nurses in a renal unit is to meet patients in renal failure with a scolding regarding their water and salt intake, patients may be more likely to miss appointments or skip lab tests. Conversely, by creating a culture of unconditional positive regard (Rogers, 1961) in the renal unit that shapes nurses to convey a nonjudgmental attitude and cultivate a compassionate practice recognizing the difficulties of living with dietary restrictions, feelings of deprivation and loss, and so on, nurses are more likely to create a helpful, supportive space that the person will feel more comfortable accessing.

To integrate attention to sociopolitical contexts, including your own, those of people and families to whom you provide care, and those of health care contexts, it is useful to analyze how power is playing out in each situation, how those dynamics are influencing care, and how they might be further influenced.

For example, ask yourself the questions from Box 4.2 in relation to what you know of Mr. Stephen and Mrs. Zhang. There are obvious ways in which access to care can be enhanced, such as getting an interpreter to facilitate communication between Mrs. Zhang and her caregivers. Read Mr. Stephen's account of his stroke, and see if you can identify various influences that are enhancing and deterring his access to health care. Focus on the interplay between his experience and his sociopolitical context.

> My stroke happened at 10:28 p.m. on a Wednesday in 2005. I was 56. A conference I was attending was winding down, and I had gone to the bar to order a drink for an old friend who had been abroad and who I had not seen for several years.

BOX 4.2

Integrating Awareness of Sociopolitical Contexts

Ask yourself and others:
- How is power playing out in this situation?
- What are the barriers to health and health care in this situation?
- How is access to optimal health care being deterred, and how can it be better facilitated?

I glanced up at the bar clock, for the last time in the physical state into which I had been born. My next glance was down at the bar to see my left hand sweeping the drink I had ordered into the lap of the gaping and embarrassed barman.

What then happened was pure hell. One by one, I lost the ability to order my hands, my feet, my mouth, my eyes to do what I asked them to do. I didn't have a clue what was happening to me. Out of nowhere, someone was switching off all the lights in my head. I was helped back to my hotel room by well-meaning people who clearly thought I was drunk—I'd been on Diet Coke—and could just about manage to sit upright on my bed while an intense ambulance driver sought to persuade me to allow him to take me to [the] hospital.

I remember a blur of lights, voices, movement, and being left on a trolley in a darkened A&E [accident and emergency] unit, still fouled by my own vomit. Someone was screaming and moaning, and for several minutes I thought it was me. The transfer to a ward was no better; my lump of an unresponsive body flung into a hastily made bed and left there. No one explained what was happening to me.

The horror was knowing that inside my skull the same person was still there, but he had lost all ability to communicate, except with rolling eyes, slurred speech, and a part-paralyzed face, so that I could see in the eyes of those around me that they thought my mental capacities had gone forever. I was experiencing solitary confinement of the most extreme kind: confinement inside my own skull. (Stephen, 2013)

How is power playing out? How are his social position, social expectations, and the social environment of the health care settings contributing to this man's horror and solitary confinement? What role might fear of judgment, stigma, or unfair treatment be playing? How could his health have been promoted better? If you were his nurse, what might you have done? As a nurse, how could you have influenced the conditions he was experiencing?

Material/Economic Contexts

Material and economic contexts are interrelated with historical and sociopolitical contexts. At the level of countries, global resources are distributed according to historical enactments of power—war, colonization, displacement of people, appropriation of land, forced migration, and so on. Think of the history of your own country. For example, how have wars influenced the economy, and how have those wars affected health and health care? For example, what health consequences do war veterans face from exposure to chronic stress, extreme violence, toxins, and direct physical harm? Currently, to what extent does military spending in your country compete with health care spending? Where do the profits from military and health care corporations go? Similarly, at the level of communities, relative wealth is a consequence of history and power and how they play out. For example, most cities and towns in North America have poorer and wealthier communities with those divisions usually going back generations.

Although within Western liberal individualist thinking we are encouraged to think that at the level of individuals, wealth and poverty are

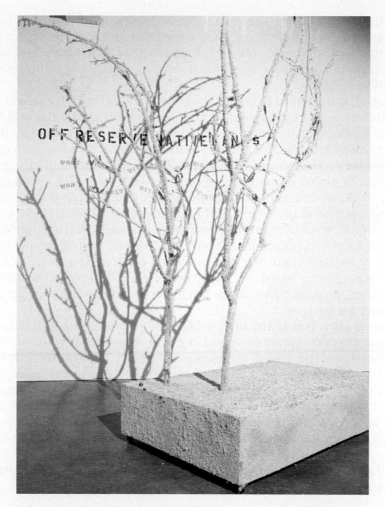

Reserved land. (Wood and sawdust sculpture by Jocelyne Robinson.)

a consequence of individual effort, they are largely accidents of birth. For example, a person who is born poor is more likely to remain poor than his or her more affluent counterpart. Corak (2006) writes that "in the United States, almost half of children born to low-income parents become low-income adults. This is an extreme case, but the fraction is also high in the UK at one in four and in Canada where about one third of low-income children do not escape low income in adulthood" (p. 143). Myths, fairy tales, and cautionary tales convey that hard work almost inevitably leads to economic success, but globally, economic upward mobility is the exception rather than the rule for most people, and it is still not the rule in countries that have enjoyed increasing prosperity overall. People's economic contexts have profound influences on their health, and although they generally have little control over their life chances, they are often held accountable.

Understanding the dynamics of economic and material resources and how they affect health is central to providing health-promoting nursing care. First, nurses must understand how health is affected by material resources at a population level. Such knowledge helps nurses better understand how such dynamics play out for particular individuals and families and help them participate in efforts to improve health at community and population levels.

Second, nurses need to understand how material resources affect health for particular people by drawing on population-level knowledge and inquiring into particular situations. In the absence of such knowledge, nursing practice will be less effective and can even be harmful if nurses convey judgment or blame. For example, both Mrs. Zhang and Mr. Stephen are living the impact of global economics. Labor laws, work safety laws, immigration laws, and global economies affect industries (e.g., shipbuilding, garment and news media industries, etc.) with real effects on people. Understanding something of these dynamics helps nurses evaluate Mrs. Zhang's English skills, stroke risk prevention strategies, or diabetic management within a framework broader than that of "individual choice." If a nurse negatively judged Mrs. Zhang based on the attitude that "people who immigrate should learn English," that nurse might be less diligent about getting an interpreter for her.

It is equally important to consider Mr. Stephen within his material/economic context. While he may have had fewer negative personal consequences from the global economies in which he has lived, his privileges (e.g., relative to Mrs. Zhang) do not protect him from suffering nor from potential economic consequences of poor health. For example, his stroke threatens his livelihood. Understanding the fears and concerns of people and their families helps nurses provide more responsive, supportive, and health-promoting care. Again, continuously striving to test your own assumptions, inquiring nonjudgmentally, and attending to context helps you understand differences in ways that will make nursing care more effective.

BOX 4.3

Integrating Awareness of Material/Economic Contexts

Learn about the communities you serve:

- What are the range of economic situations of individuals and families to whom I am likely to provide care?
- What key historical events have shaped economic realities at the national, regional, and local levels?
- How is health affected by these varied and shifting economic situations?

Inquire about particular individuals and families you serve:

- How is the health and health care of this individual/family affected by their access to material resources?
- How is this individual's/family's health likely to impact their material well-being?

Physical Contexts

Physical environments affect health. In the global environment, pollution, radiation, water, and hazards such as unexploded mines, occupational stressors, and toxins pose risks to health. In local communities, the common forms of work (e.g., mining versus farming versus service industry versus office work) and recreation (e.g., video games versus swimming versus drag racing) shape patterns of health issues. The immediate spaces of health care influence the care provided. A significant proportion of the global burden of disease is attributable to physical environmental risks, and the broad physical environment is contiguous with immediate environments of care. Think, for example, of the differences between a hospital set in a rural setting versus one in an urban setting within the same state or province. The physical resources in a given hospital vary with the economic resources of the community, including the funding structure, the tax base, and the level of philanthropy. This in turn has a direct impact on the care you are able to provide.

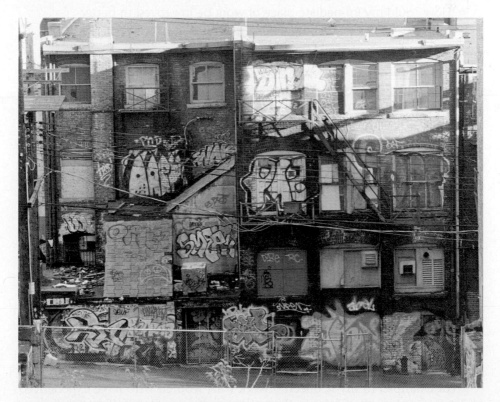

Patterns. (Photograph by Len Budiwski.)

Whether you are providing care in a labor and delivery room, an outpost clinic, a refugee camp, an ICU, an outpatient clinic, a palliative care unit, an acute care hospital room, or any other setting, the environment matters to the health of individual patients and families as well as to your own well-being. Each specific nursing environment poses particular challenges to health. Operating room nurses are often exposed to various chemicals and high levels of radiation; ICU patients are subject to high levels of noise and light that limit rest and sleep; street environments pose a range of health risks to both nurses and those to whom they provide care.

BOX 4.4

Integrating Awareness of Physical Contexts

Ask yourself:

- What are the key environmental influences on health in my immediate community?
- How do these influences affect the patterns of health problems in the community?
- How does this individual or family fit with the usual patterns of health in this community, and what other physical environmental influences might be operating?
- How does my immediate place of work optimize/mitigate against health and well-being?
- How could my immediate place of work be improved to better promote health and safety?

Nurses need to develop a relational consciousness regarding the influence of physical environments both so that they can anticipate effects and so that they can work to create healthier environments.

Linguistic/Discursive Contexts

> The environment can be conceptualized not only as the physical surroundings but the discourses to which one has access. From a poststructuralist methodology that focuses on the creative aspects of language, the . . . question becomes not the discovery of 'truth' but instead asking how truths are created, by whom, and for what purposes. (Hardin, 2001, p. 12)

Pam Hardin (2001) argues that the environment is not just made up of social, historical, and physical surroundings, but also of the language and discourses to which one has access. She shows how thinking about language as an environment makes it possible to bridge between how people talk about their lives and health and the language and ideas that are available to them. That is, it becomes easier to see how our understandings are shaped by the ideas and language to which we are exposed.

For example, in my (Colleen's) work with women who have experienced violence, women often refer to themselves as having "low self-esteem," coming from "dysfunctional families," and being an "abused woman." These ideas are part of discourses that have emerged from psychology and "the battered women's movement" and become integrated in everyday language. These ideas are not necessarily problematic in themselves, but they can come to serve as a short-hand for experience in ways that do not really communicate that experience. For example, often, when I ask women what they mean by "having low self-esteem," some are well able to articulate that they have been told that they are "worthless" so often that they have trouble believing that they are worthy as human beings. Others quickly contradict themselves, saying that they feel fine about themselves but feel that other people (service providers, family members, health care workers) judge them poorly. Ideas such as these can operate as labels that quickly narrow a person's experience. Often, families labeled as "dysfunctional" can have considerable strength and resilience; women who are "abused" are invariably much more than their abuse experiences.

Hardin (2001) also shows how understanding individual experiences as nested within available explanations and discourses helps us see that individuals are neither agents of free choice (because we can't just think "anything" without being influenced by the ideas to which we previously have been exposed) nor mere puppets at the mercy of preexisting ideas. So, for example, a person who is struggling with the stigma of being on social assistance (in our area terms such as "welfare bum" are used) might buffer that stigma by focusing on the circumstances beyond that person's control that led to being on social assistance or challenging the assumption that having money connotes being a worthy person.

It is useful for nurses to conceptualize language as environment because it attunes nurses to the language and discourses they are taking up and using and the effects of doing so, and it allows them to be more conscious in using or countering the available discourses. For example, when nurses think about the stigmatizing effects of terms used to ridicule poverty (e.g., "trailer trash," "welfare bunny"), they can counter such effects by drawing attention to the economic conditions that create poverty and make economic dependence necessary. They can also more consciously look for ways in which the normative discourse and ways of speaking/labeling might be negatively shaping their reactions to people.

Such understanding also helps nurses recognize when and how others are taking up available discourses. For example, in nursing practice, the discourse of "the difficult patient" often plays out in ways that are harmful (Khalil, 2009; Maupin, 1995; Podrasky & Sexton, 1988). Indeed, it is remarkably easy to become the "difficult" patient or the "difficult family" (Cleveland, 2008; Kemp, Ball, Perkins, Hollingsworth, & Lepore, 2009). Nursing research has shown repeatedly that categorizing patients as "difficult" is a common form of labeling or stereotyping in nursing practice (Arnaert, Seller, & Wainwright, 2009; Caveth, 1995; Khalil, 2009; Liaschenko, 1994; Peternelj-Taylor, 2004; Podrasky & Sexton, 1988). In each context, certain people are more likely than others to be labeled. Patients may be labeled as good or bad, difficult or demanding, and/or likeable or unlikeable on the basis of individual characteristics and behaviors or as a result of association with certain social groups (Caveth, 1995; Corley & Goren, 1998; Kelly & May, 1982; Liaschenko, 1994, 1995). When nurses and others care for people who differ from dominant groups in terms of race, class, religion, age, income, or sexual orientation, there is a greater risk of labeling, stereotyping, and negative social judgments (Carveth, 1995; Grief & Elliott, 1994; Johnson & Webb, 1995a, 1995b; Liaschenko, 1994; Malone, 1996; Podrasky & Sexton, 1988; Stevens, 1992, 1994). Women, people who are poor, have substance use problems, or are from ethnic minorities are more likely to experience negative social judgments in their relationships with health care providers. This underscores the importance of nurses anticipating harmful discourses, paying attention to their own values and beliefs, using such understanding to be thoughtful about how they participate, and learning how to intervene to reduce the negative effects of language practices such as labeling.

Each health care setting has particular issues or groups of people that are more likely to be the subject of harmful discourses, and these discourses work with broader social discourses. For example, in emergency nursing practice, the discourse of the patient as a "frequent flyer" works with economic efficiency and the discourse of people overusing or inappropriately using emergency services to discourage certain people from seeking emergency care (such as those with chronic pain or mental health problems). In many settings, the discourse of compliance and noncompliance operates to enforce the power of health care providers and reinforce the social discourse of personal responsibility for health that overlooks life circumstances.

Certain discourses can have harmful effects on nurses as well. For example, in emergency nursing, images and stereotypes of emergency nurses as "tough" can work in some ways to help nurses deal with the harsh realities of the suffering they see, but at the same time can work to prevent them from getting healthy support. For instance, early in my research in emergency, I (Colleen) worked with a nurse who was traumatized by an incident she had experienced years earlier. She had provided care to two preschool children who were beaten by their father with an axe. It was not the trauma of the deaths of the children within hours of their admission that she could not live with; it was the derision of her coworkers who belittled her for "falling apart" and failing to meet stereotypical expectations of emergency nurses as hard and unemotional; she was instead considered a "bleeding heart."

Nurses can work to improve such dynamics by (a) developing greater awareness of the effects of the language being used, (b) not using discourses that are potentially harmful, and (c) helping others develop new understanding. For example, if people with chronic pain are returning repeatedly to emergency, rather than referring to them as a "frequent flyer," a nurse can draw attention to the need to more effectively deal with pain both in terms of particular individuals and in terms of having adequate health care system resources, such as pain management education, specialists, or clinics.

BOX 4.5

Integrating Awareness of Linguistic/Discursive Contexts

In any health care setting, ask:

- What are the stereotypes about people (including nurses) or health problems common in this setting? What are common labeling practices? How do these relate to broader social practices?
- Who or what is usually seen as problematic?
- What language and ideas (discourses) support practices that discourage people from accessing health care?
- What is my relationship to this language (do I use it without thinking, silently resist using it, or actively offer alternatives)?

In reference to any individual/family, ask:

- What labels, stereotypes, or other language practices are likely to be harmful to these people?
- How will I relate to these practices (conform to dominant practices, passively resist, actively offer alternatives)?

TRY IT OUT 4.4
Integrate Awareness of a Context

In the preceding section, we offered questions in the text boxes that can help you integrate awareness of particular aspects of context and culture in your nursing practice. Select the questions in one of these text boxes (perhaps the one that you find the most unfamiliar), and apply those questions to your current or most recent practice setting. If you are not yet in a clinical practice context, then use the context that was the subject of your interview in Try It Out 4.1.

What do you learn by applying these questions? Compare your thinking with that of your colleagues or classmates who are in different practice contexts and of those who used a different set of text box questions. What do you learn from these conversations?

Multiple contexts are interrelated and mutually reinforcing. Therefore, taking contexts into account means seeing how language, physical environments, material, sociopolitical contexts, and history are mutually situating and constituting people. For example, at a global level, the modern welfare state arose and has been undermined through historical and ongoing enactments of power leading to varied effects on physical environments (think of the different environmental laws of different countries or of nuclear accidents in Russia, Japan, and the United States); and varied social arrangements (think of different labor laws in various countries over time), supported by different discourses (think of tree huggers, draft dodgers, and Wall Street "occupiers"). The dynamics are similar at the level of health care units. For example, ICUs were invented in the 1960s as a product of medical and technologic advances in a context of economic prosperity supported by discourses that valued individual well-being. Language use involves enactments of power infused throughout social contexts; material resources are reflected in physical environments, all of which shape social possibilities and all of which have historical antecedents and evolve over time. People and their health have variously been shaped by these shifting environments and in turn have shaped those environments with consequences for health, health care, and nursing.

HEALTH IS SOCIALLY DETERMINED

Health and illness can be understood from a range of perspectives. Because contemporary health care often emphasizes biomedical treatment, our understanding of health and illness often begins with the physiologic and pathophysiologic aspects, then considers risk factors for those and sometimes links those risk factors to contextual factors.

Bringing attention to the way in which people and their experiences are socially produced and the multiple contexts and cultures that are influencing and shaping them highlights the ways in which health is socially determined. That is, a relational view draws attention to the social determinants of health and how they are always operating. For example, in Chapter 3, I (Gweneth) shared an example of extending the view of a woman with breast cancer from the perspective of a cytology slide to a photo of her with her husband. In essence, the photo "contextualized" the physiologic aspect of the disease and drew attention to the woman's meaningful health experience. Each health problem can be similarly understood. Stroke, for example, may have common pathophysiologic and physical etiologic features, which are important for medical treatment aimed at cure or alleviation of symptoms, but understanding people in their immediate and more distant social contexts is required for nursing care aimed at promoting well-being more broadly.

TRY IT OUT 4.5

Examine the Multiple Contexts of a Health Issue

Pick a health issue you know something about. Diabetes? Hypertension? Autism? Depression? Eczema? Place it in the center of a circle surrounded by the various contexts we have been discussing. First, what are the obvious contextual influences? List what you immediately think of when you think about the historical, physical, political, economic, social, and linguistic environments influencing your chosen health issue. For example, contemporary social environments of stress, food supply, and nutritional norms are obvious influences in the development of hypertension. Now, what are less obvious influences? What do you know, for example, about the strong relationship between racism and hypertension? What about the relationship between poverty, stress, and hypertension? Now, where are your "blanks," and can you inquire to fill them in? What language is relevant, and how does it shape our understanding of the health issue? For example, if you have chosen a form of cancer, how does the language of "fighting" cancer shape people's experiences? What are the political aspects to your chosen health issue? At first try, it might be quite difficult for you to see how some of these contexts are relevant. However, as you develop your inquiry skills, you will see more and more connections. What does your inquiry suggest about what would be required to optimize health care?

Health is socially determined for all people, including each individual you meet and yourself. Health care is generally considered one of many determinants of health. Thus, as Figure 4.3 depicts, each nursing encounter brings together the multiple embodied environments of the individuals/families receiving care and the nurse within an influential health care context. Understanding health in this relational, socially mediated way leads to understanding that many of the vast differences in health seen at population and individual levels (inequalities) can be seen as consequences of the

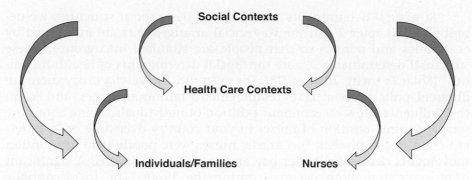

Fig. 4.3 Social and health care contexts shape each nursing encounter.

embodiment of contexts. Thus, while knowledge about physiology, patho-physiology, medical treatment, and risk factors are all essential to good nursing practice, nurses need more than biomedical knowledge. They need to consider the social determinants of health.

Social Determinants of Health

Social determinants of health are those contextual factors that influence health. Solar and Irwin (2010) define the social determinants of health as "access to power, money, and resources and the conditions of daily life—the circumstances in which people are born, grow, live, work, and age" (p. i). The World Health Organization's Commission on Social Determinants of Health Conceptual Framework (see Figure 4.4) differentiates among various elements that determine health. The first element is the socioeconomic and political context. The second element includes structural determinants and socioeconomic position.

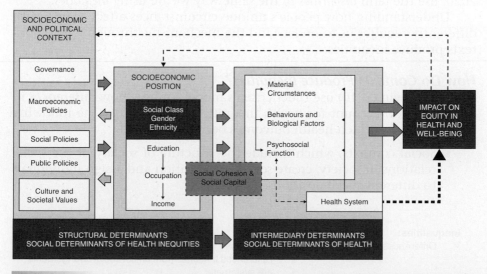

Fig. 4.4 Commission on Social Determinants of Health Conceptual Framework. (From Solar, O., & Irwin, A. (2010). *A conceptual framework for action on the social determinants of health*. Geneva, Switzerland: World Health Organization.)

"Structural determinants" refers to the basic social structures we described in Chapter 2 and the way social arrangements are influenced by economics and politics so that people are stratified into groups. These structural determinants . . . are the "social determinants of health inequities" (Solar & Irwin, 2010, p. 28). For example, in every country there are different policies about taxes, employment, minimum wages, and so on that influence the socioeconomic position of individuals. Think about the socioeconomic position of nurses in your country over time or in different countries at present. In Canada, nurses were poorly paid until union movements demanded better pay and working conditions. A significant improvement in both occurred during the 1960s. The socioeconomic position of any nurse is shaped not only by that nurse's own motivation, quest for education, skills, and work ethic, but also by the larger structural conditions that shape employment opportunities, wages, and working conditions.

Context and Inequities

Because people live in and embody different contexts, they are affected unequally; therefore, considering the social determinants of health—income, education, occupation, social class, gender, and race/ethnicity—always means considering inequities.

Inequities are *avoidable* differences that arise from *social arrangements* that are *unfair* (Whitehead & Dahlgren, 2006). Many things are unequal—that is, inequalities, which may or may not be fair and may or may not be social in origin and thus modifiable. Although in some contexts (e.g., often in Europe), the terms *inequalities* and *inequities* are used interchangeably, we reserve the term *inequities* for differences that are unfair because they arise from social conditions that are modifiable (see Figure 4.5). Some sources, such as the U.S. Department of Health and Human Services' *Healthy People 2020*, use the term *disparities* in the same way we are using *inequities*.

Understanding how people's unique circumstances affect their health differently requires us to understand the mechanisms through which contexts produce inequities.

How Do Contexts Produce Inequities?

Solar and Irwin (2010) use Diderichsen's model to show how differences in social position account for health inequities. They identify the following mechanisms by which health outcomes become stratified:

■ Social contexts, which include the structure of society or the social relations in society, create social stratification and assign individuals to different social positions.

Inequalities:	Inequities:
✓ Differences	✓ Differences that are unfair
	✓ Differences that arise from unjust social arrangements are systematic
	✓ Differences that are modifiable

Fig. 4.5 Inequalities vs. Inequities

- Social stratification in turn engenders differential exposure to health-damaging conditions and differential vulnerability in terms of health conditions and material resource availability.
- Social stratification likewise determines differential consequences of ill health for more and less advantaged groups (including economic and social consequences, as well as differential health outcomes) (Solar & Irwin, 2010, p. 5).

TO ILLUSTRATE

How Does Poverty "Work" on Health?

We all know that poverty is one of the biggest risks to health. However, as we have discussed, poverty is often thought of as avoidable, somehow the product of "bad choices," something people could change if they "worked harder." We are encouraged to hold this view by many contemporary discourses, including novels and movies that repeatedly feature "rags to riches" stories with a happy (wealthy) ending. This view of the world requires people who have access to material wealth to overlook how their own personal contexts have facilitated that access. Further, the effect of poverty on health is often thought about in fairly limited ways as being primarily the direct and most obvious effects of material deprivation (e.g., not enough quality food). Alternatively, Figure 4.6 shows some of the multiple pathways between material resources and health.

Since nurses will encounter people across the spectrum from those who are wealthy to those who are impoverished, having a more

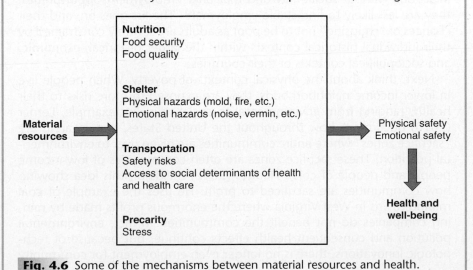

Fig. 4.6 Some of the mechanisms between material resources and health.

continued on page 168

TO ILLUSTRATE *continued*

How Does Poverty "Work" on Health?

comprehensive understanding of poverty and the relationship between access to material resources and health is crucial. Moreover, nurses have to be very careful not to make assumptions about people's access to resources based on the nurses' own experiences. They need to anticipate a wide range of economic circumstances and to understand the effects of those circumstances.

First of all, consider the historical context of poverty. At a population level, as mentioned in Chapter 2, in most countries (with a few exceptions in South America), the gap between the very wealthy and the very poor has been widening over recent decades (Beddoes, 2012; Lustig, Lopez-Calva, & Ortiz-Juarez, 2012; Milanovic, 2012). Such inequities have significant negative effects on populations; the health of the entire population declines, not just the health of the poorest people. Individuals are thus affected by their own historical circumstances. For example, in so called "first-world countries," a high percentage of children live in poverty. In Canada, for example, approximately 10% of children live in poverty (Conference Board of Canada, 2009). Among 29 of the "richest countries" in the world, Canada's child poverty rate is midway between those with the lowest child poverty rates (less than 5% in the Netherlands) and those with the highest, with over 15% in Greece, the United States, Lithuania, Latvia, and Romania (UNICEF Office of Research, 2013). Other estimates put the US rate at 23% (UNICEF Innocenti Research Centre, 2012).

Children who live in poverty often experience food insecurity, housing insecurity, poor access to health care, and lower educational opportunities. Without adequate nutrition, they are unable to focus and learn in school; without social networks that offer employment opportunities, they are less likely to find stable employment. The list goes on, and their chances of "choosing" not to be poor as adults are severely constrained by their individual historical contexts within the larger historical, economic, and sociopolitical contexts of their countries.

Next, think about the physical contexts of poverty. When people live in lower income neighborhoods, they are exposed to more risks to their health, ranging from environmental to social risks. For example, Lerner (2010) documents how throughout the United States, certain areas are "sacrifice zones" where entire communities are given over to environmental pollution. These sacrifice zones are often communities of low-income people and people of color. Hedges (2012) builds on this idea showing how communities are sacrificed to profit. He uses the example of coal mining towns in West Virginia where the enormous profits made by mining companies do not benefit the communities. In fact, environmental pollution and consequent health effects continue, but because of technologic innovations, there is no longer even employment for community

continued on page 169

TO ILLUSTRATE *continued*

How Does Poverty "Work" on Health?

---

residents. The consequence is that the communities are among the poorest and unhealthiest in the United States despite being among the richest in natural resources.

These dynamics show how physical and sociopolitical contexts are deeply interrelated. Of course, sociopolitical contexts are inseparable from these economic and physical contexts in their effects on health; for example, lower income neighborhoods have poorer schools, and a reduced level of education negatively affects health. On a more global level, Bales (2012) shows how within economic globalism, entire populations are rendered disposable. Despite slavery being globally "illegal," at least 27 million people are enslaved, including people displaced from farmland by large corporations using neocolonial processes (e.g., mines, factories) and forced into subsistence living with factory work, sex trade work, drug trade work, and so forth. This matters to nurses because all people to whom they provide care are affected by their socioeconomic positions, which are structurally determined. Poverty has compounding effects on other social determinants of health. For example, take the issue of transportation. In many urban settings, lower priced food is often available at large stores located in suburbs. People who can afford transportation to such stores, can afford to buy in bulk, and can afford to transport bulk supplies can lower their food costs. But very low-income people often do not have such means and thus are forced to buy higher priced food in smaller amounts.

In tandem with direct material deprivation, research has clearly shown that the stress of living under conditions of chronic poverty has physical, mental, and emotional effects (Conroy, Sandel, & Zuckerman, 2010; Evans & Kim, 2007; Santiago, Wadsworth, & Stump, 2011). People embody their stressful conditions, including worries about economic and food security, fear due to greater exposure to a range of physical harms (e.g., vermin, violence, pollutants, fires), and the direct effects of those poverty-induced harms, which in turn makes it more difficult for them to manage their stress (Evans & Kim, 2007; Santiago et al., 2011).

Finally, think how language (discursive contexts) shapes the experience of poverty. What terms are commonly used in your contexts to label people who are impoverished, and what moral judgments are inherent in those labels? Where we (Gweneth and Colleen) live, terms such as "welfare mom" and "welfare bum" are used to describe people on social assistance. Other terms such as "trailer trash" are used to demean people who cannot afford houses or apartments. Discursive practices also function to obscure the relationship between sociopolitical and economic contexts and health and place responsibility on individuals for their circumstances, even when they are beyond individual control. Look at the many websites that make fun of "trailer trash"—

continued on page 170

TO ILLUSTRATE *continued*

How Does Poverty "Work" on Health?

for example, www.missouritrailertrash.com. Look at the photos, and think about them and the discourses they support in relation to structural issues such as changing global economics, interest rates, corporate tax policies, or minimum wage policies that shape employment and educational opportunities, income levels, and so on.

TRY IT OUT 4.6

Map the Mechanisms

Preferably in a group, pick a social determinant of health (other than income or poverty). You might pick education, occupation, social class, social support, gender, or racism. In the same way as we have explored the mechanisms between poverty and health, brainstorm the relationships between your selected "determinant" and health. Use Figure 4.2 to remind yourself to consider the historical, sociopolitical, material-economic, physical, and linguistic-discursive environments.

Next, have each person in your group find a research article (in a peer-reviewed journal) that discusses the relationship between the selected determinant and health with one or more of these contexts in mind. In what ways does the article support your brainstorming? What did you miss?

If you are in a class, compare and contrast your thinking with groups who have chosen the same and different determinants. What are the similarities, overlaps, and differences?

How Do You Relate to Inequities?

Every day, we are surrounded by visual evidence of inequities. We walk by people begging on streets; we see disproportionate numbers of people of certain ethnicities in low-paying jobs; and we see deference paid to some people based on gender, size, age, or how well dressed they are. Each of us relates to this evidence of inequities in some way: sometimes we ignore and turn away from it, sometimes we become defensive about our own privileges, sometimes we blame people for their own circumstances, and sometimes we feel overwhelmed and helpless.

Awareness of inequities is and should be uncomfortable. If you value fairness, then inequities challenge your values. As a result, you may turn to charity, such as by sponsoring a child, making a donation, and so on. Even as you do this, you can't help recognizing that no one person can rectify the injustices of the world. However, when you understand inequities as structural in origin, then you are led to recognize that the solutions are also structural. For example, many countries that depend on foreign aid, particularly in the global south, are maintained in this dependence by loans with exorbitant interest rates through global financial institutions such as the World Bank and the International Monetary Fund. While charity may offer some relief to countries in extreme impoverishment and during times of crisis, sustainable change must be structural.

The dynamics are similar at a local level. People and societies often relate to inequities with solutions that do not address the root causes. For instance, social assistance is an important support that helps women leave abusive partners. In Canada, we know that about one in four women who are on social assistance have experienced intimate partner violence (IPV) in the past year. However, there are few measures that address the underlying gender inequities that make women more vulnerable than men to economic dependence and partner violence. Further, social assistance rates in most countries are such that people on such assistance must live in extreme poverty. Gender, gender-based power and violence, and economics intersect so that structural poverty is continuously reinforced. Gendered employment opportunities and social expectations influence women to prioritize child-rearing over labor force participation; such influences also direct women to deal with IPV by leaving abusive partners. When women with children are unable to support themselves when leaving an abusive partner and require social assistance, they must choose between enduring poverty or further abuse. While charity and public social assistance helps many women, such support is often in the form of an undignified "handout" and comes with contingencies. On the other hand, there is considerable evidence that structural solutions, such as providing people with a guaranteed annual income, allows people to live with dignity and has greatest impact on those who are most disadvantaged, such as those vulnerable to gender-based violence (Hodgson, 2011; Young & Mulvale, 2009).

The dynamics of inequity also play out in similar ways in health care contexts. First, people who have more resources (social, economic, political, linguistic) can access health care more easily. Second, people with more resources can access better health care (e.g., by being able to afford transportation to a "better" clinic, by having a social network that can connect to the "best" physician). Third, even when access is similar, those with more resources receive better treatment.

A relational perspective helps us keep in mind that when we believe we are seeing health inequities at the individual level, we are actually seeing the culmination of multiple, dynamic, contextual elements. Rather than intervening only in relation to the particular individual or family (interpersonally), you need to simultaneously intervene to address structural conditions at the contextual level (taking both the proximal and distal views), as well as intrapersonally—examining your own assumptions and thinking.

Specifically addressing inequities from a relational perspective requires:

- Conscious attention to see decontextualizing as it is happening in your own thinking and that of others
- Integrating knowledge of how health is socially determined in inequitable ways
- Developing skills to infuse your practice with a contextualized view

This requires attention to how language is used and applied to people as well as developing ways of using language and knowledge and inquiring to counter decontextualizing of inequities.

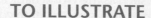

TO ILLUSTRATE

Using the Discourses of Risk, Vulnerability, Marginalization, and Precarity to Address Inequities

The concepts of risk, vulnerability, marginalization, and precarity are useful for understanding how contexts produce people and communities in ways that harm health and produce inequities. Let's take a look at the use of each of these terms.

In contemporary health care, it is fairly common practice to use the terms "high risk" and "at risk" without specifying what the risk *is* or what is producing risk. For example, it is common to talk about "at-risk youth" without specifying that they are at risk of certain problems such as homelessness and without specifying that their risks generally arise from the contexts in which they live—poverty, violence, housing instability, and so on. As mentioned in Chapter 3, the PHNs with whom Gweneth and her colleagues did research shifted the language to "high-priority" to move away from language that located risk in the people rather than in their circumstances.

Vulnerability can also be understood in an individualizing way that moves responsibility toward the people experiencing the inequity and away from the causal conditions. For example, indigenous groups with whom I (Colleen) have worked have expressed outrage at being referred to as vulnerable. One indigenous leader said to me, "We are not vulnerable. We are strong and resilient and have survived the worst conditions imaginable."

The term *marginalization* generally turns attention to conditions and mechanisms and has been used in nursing to understand how health is socially determined (Hall, 1999; Hall, Stevens, & Meleis, 1994; Lynam & Cowley, 2007). The term refers to how some people are pushed to the edges of society; that is, they are more excluded than others from access to power, money, resources, and the conditions of daily life.

Finally, the terms *precariousness* and *precarity* increasingly are used to draw attention to inequities and the uncertainty of people's social circumstances. I (Colleen) recently heard Judith Butler (n.d.) point out how each of us lives amidst uncertainty (think of how both Mr. Stephen's and Mrs. Zhang's livelihoods were similarly threatened despite their different circumstances) and how we are all implicated in the social networks that sustain or fail to sustain ourselves and other beings. She has written that precariousness

characterizes every embodied and finite human being, and non-human beings as well . . . each of us could be subject to deprivation, injury, debilitation or death by virtue of events or processes outside of our control. It is also, importantly, a feature of what we might call the social bond, the various relations that establish our interdependency. In other words, no one person suffers a lack of shelter without a social failure to organize shelter in such a way that it is accessible to each and every person. And no one person suffers unemployment without a system or a political economy that fails to safeguard against that possibility (Butler, n.d.).

BOX 4.6

Countering Individualizing Discourses

When you hear "choice," ask: "What is constraining and enabling choice for particular groups and individuals?"

When you hear "at risk," ask:

- "At risk of what?"
- "What is the source of risk?"

When you hear "vulnerable," ask:

- "Vulnerable to what?"
- "What is creating the vulnerability?

When you hear "marginalized," ask:

- "Marginalized by what?"
- "Marginalized from what?"

Try out alternative language such as:

- Life circumstances
- Precarious conditions
- Marginalizing conditions

Nurses have opportunities to use these various ideas to promote a contextualized view of health and to counter inequities. Box 4.6 offers some suggestions about language and ideas that signal such opportunities, and it poses questions you can ask and answer to do so.

Integrating understanding of health as socially determined in nursing practice means bringing knowledge of contexts and inequities to bear to determine what is salient in particular situations. This in turn means treating every moment of practice as contextual and cultural.

STRATEGIES FOR CULTURALLY AND CONTEXTUALLY RESPONSIVE NURSING PRACTICE

How can you translate what you have just read about context, culture, social determinants, and inequities into your day-to-day nursing practice? How might the understanding that people and their health are being produced by multiple influences—by cultures and contexts—shape your decisions and actions? Throughout the past few decades, various ideas for enacting nursing in more contextually and culturally responsive ways have been explored in nursing to integrate the concept of "environment" (Chopoorian, 1986; Kleffel, 1996; Stevens, 1989) and, to a greater extent, integrate the concept of culture. We explore some of these ideas and consider their usefulness in terms of relational inquiry practice.

Integrate Attention to Context and Culture

As you encounter people as a nurse and purposefully inquire as to how history, economics, language, physical, and social environments are influencing their lives, health, and health care experiences, to integrate attention to

BOX 4.7

Inquiring with Individuals and Families

Inquiring with individuals and families to better understand their contexts does not mean asking a set of proscribed questions. It does mean using a range of information sources, making and testing assumptions, and building your understanding in these areas:

- How has history, including colonization and migration, shaped these people's lives?
- What sociopolitical circumstances are particularly relevant to these people's lives?
- How are economics and access to material resources shaping these people's lives?
- What discourses might be particularly relevant to the well-being of these people?
- How are the particular health issues facing this individual/family shaped by history, physical environments, economics, sociopolitical factors, and language?
- How is this health care context influencing these people's experience?
- How might a better situation be produced?

culture and context, begin with the environmental conditions and consider how they shape people, families and communities, and thus their health (See Box 4.7). Examining the economic, temporal-historical, sociopolitical, and linguistic circumstances of people's lives widens our understanding of the range of influences that might be shaping people's experiences and offers us a broader range of ways to intervene. At the same time, consider how these various contexts shape the health issues the person is facing. For example, if you met Mrs. Zhang and Mr. Stephen during their hospitalization following their strokes, you would inquire as to their particular circumstances and link that to your understanding of stroke.

As you develop your physiologic, pathophysiologic, and treatment-related knowledge of various health issues, consider each health issue as contextual and cultural. For example, consider different forms of cancer. Each form not only has different pathophysiologic characteristics but also has different and changing physical environmental influences, historical, sociopolitical, economic, and linguistic characteristics. Consider breast cancer, for example. What do you know about the links between breast cancer and environmental hazards? What are the risk factors for breast cancer, and how do they link to income and social experiences such as racism? How has the history of breast cancer evolved with effects on fundraising efforts? Is the emphasis in research disproportionately on genetic versus environmental risk factors? And if so, why? What are the discourses related to breast cancer, and how are they related to gender? Students with whom I (Colleen) worked analyzed various forms of cancer from a contextual and cultural perspective and concluded that breast cancer had achieved a level of popularity at least in part due to gender stereotypes about women and the importance of breasts, as well as stigma and blame associated with other forms of cancer (e.g., colorectal cancer and lung cancer). The students asked, "Why think pink? Cancer affects everyone." They argued that the emphasis on breast cancer overshadowed concern and funding for treatment and research for other forms of cancer such as colorectal, uterine, and prostate cancer. They found that gender stereotypes were problematic not only for women with breast cancer but also for people experiencing various forms. Producing better situations in the context of cancer care would include countering stigma, blame, and gender stereotyping.

Practicing with a conscious awareness of how people are socially produced is about understanding the dynamics so you can figure out what is salient in any given situation—salient to what is shaping the person in front of you and your response to that person. Understanding how people are socially produced leads to understanding health as socially determined.

Distinguish Different Approaches to Culture in Nursing

In the past several decades, Western nursing has begun to grapple with the idea of culture and cultural difference as important to practice. Nurses have developed a number of useful concepts and have taken several approaches. These approaches range from those that advocate cultural sensitivity based on understanding culture as ethnicity or race to those that advocate cultural safety based on understanding culture as relational (Browne et al., 2009; Reimer-Kirkham et al., 2009; Varcoe, Browne, & Anderson, 2010; Varcoe & Browne, in press). The term "cultural competence" has been applied across this range of approaches.

Recognize the Limitations of Multiculturalism and Cultural Sensitivity

In recognition of diversity and the need to cross differences, nurses have taken up the ideas of multiculturalism and advocated being "sensitive" to cultural difference. In many former European colonies with diverse populations, including Canada, the United Kingdom (Culley, 1996, 2006) and Australia (Swendson & Windsor, 1996), multiculturalism has become policy, and this policy has been widely disseminated in state organizations, including health care settings.

Multiculturalism is based on understanding culture as shared beliefs, as a thing that belongs to groups of individuals, groups that are primarily identified by race/ethnicity. In nursing, the ideas of multiculturalism, sometimes using the language of "diversity," are used to focus on bringing "culture" into nursing care. Thus, nurses are encouraged to learn about "different" cultures (note the implied norm and the implication that culture is a group "thing") and be more sensitive to differences. In health care and nursing, multiculturalism is an approach that deals with problems of difference as being mismatches between minority and dominant cultures. Dealing with difference is seen as a matter of being more sensitive to others and of reducing the prejudices of individuals. While being sensitive is important, it suggests a passive response that from a relational perspective is not adequate to promote health.

TO ILLUSTRATE
The Multicultural Corner

A few years ago, I (Colleen) picked up a health care organization newsletter that had a "Multicultural Corner" feature "designed to help health service providers become more aware of the cultural sensitivities of patients, clients, and residents." In this edition of the newsletter, "Indo Canadians" were featured. This one-page feature listed the "Countries of Origin" as "Pakistan, India, Sri Lanka, Bangladesh, Nepal, Fiji, East Africa, United Kingdom, and Hong Kong." "Religion and Religious Practices" were identified as "Sikhism, Hinduism, and Islam" with information about practices such as hair cutting and prayer beads, and a list of languages—"English, Hindi, Punjabi, Guharate, and Urdu. Most speak English." The page also had information under the categories of "Family Support," "Hospitalization," "Diet," "Death," and "Child Care." The "Family Support" section read:

■ Extended families are common.

■ Family spokesperson is usually the most established male (i.e., language skills, financially established, seniority in family).

■ Role of women—caregivers, nurturers, generally submissive but respected.

■ Elderly—have authority and are accorded respect, help with child care, arrange marriages, provide advice.

The "Hospitalization" section contained items such as:

■ Lots of support from family and friends.

■ Expectation that friends will visit to show concern and caring (if it's a problem, talk to the family spokesperson).

■ Cleanliness is important.

■ Embarrassment and resistance to have male health care professional look after patient.

The section on "Diet" made points such as "vegetarianism is common" and "fasting may be observed."

The intention of this "Multicultural Corner" was to help nurses and others provide more sensitive care. However, it is likely that the intent was undermined because of the approach taken. First, the document lumped an incredibly diverse group of people into one category. This kind of categorization begs the question of who is doing the categorizing. To what extent can this information possibly apply to millions of diverse people? Second, it offered a stereotypical and overly general view. To what extent could the hospitalization statements, for example, be applied to most people? If one takes a relational view and draws on the hermeneutic phenomenologic (HP) lens and the ideas of people as situated and constituted, it becomes evident that individuals are constituted by the multitude of experiences and locations in which they live. This means that a person who came to Canada from India as an adult will be constituted differently than someone who came as an infant, someone who was born and grew up in Canada, or from someone who grew up in India. For example, my (Gweneth's) son's friend who was born and grew up in Mumbai described how during a flight to Canada she felt very "un-Indian" as she conversed with two Indo-Canadians sitting next to her. Her family in Mumbai had not adhered to many of the traditions that the two Indo-Canadian people practiced. She actually described feeling a bit out of her element as the "cultural divide" between their values, beliefs, and practices and hers became evident. This shows how, although people may share particular sociocultural ethnicities, experiences, and even traditions, there are in most cases significant differences between them; their cultures are therefore different. Thus, how can such standardized information lead to being more sensitive? Might the information lead to unwarranted assumptions about individual people and families?

Finally, whose interests are most served by something like the "Multicultural Corner" feature? For example, one of the worst possibilities is that the brochure could be used to provide a shortcut for nursing practice. Based on having this information, nurses can think they know what is important and not have to inquire into the particularities of the people and families for whom they provide care. Another concerning possibility is that the brochure could promote negative judgments. In the document, "friends visiting to show concern and caring" is identified as a potential problem, pointing to tensions that commonly arise. As we illustrated in Chapter 2, health care providers often complain that people from certain groups have "too many visitors," suggesting that the interests of providers should supersede the interests of the individuals and families.

While multiculturalism has drawn attention to diversity, it uses narrow understandings of culture and thus overlooks social inequities and structural determinants of health. It reduces all practices to culture understood narrowly as synonymous with race/ethnicity/nationality and overlooks other influences, such as gender roles or economics, which might be similar across cultures. With a narrow definition of culture, the historical impact of colonization, immigration, and racism are also overlooked. When trying to bring culture into care as an "add-on," it is easy to confuse culture with ethnicity.

When the problem is defined as mismatches between minority and dominant cultures, political and economic forces are overlooked. For example, in the "Multicultural Corner," immigration policies that disadvantage women and contribute to confining them to caregiving roles do not figure in the description of the role of women; similarly, the many "Indo-Canadian" women who are leaders, professionals, and so on are discounted. Also, when the problem is defined as mismatches between minority and dominant cultures, the "different" culture becomes the problem (e.g., too many friends visiting) and the solutions become bringing "others" into line ("talk to the family spokesperson"). Finally, focusing on "prejudiced individuals," another hallmark of multiculturalism, overlooks how racism is deeply embedded in language, structures, and institutions.

A nurse shooing Indo-Canadian visitors out the door is not just an individual practicing in a discriminatory manner; the nurse is acting in concert with ideas sanctioned by the health care organization that reflect wider dominant social mores.

Cultural sensitivity is one of the central practices of multiculturalism. Being more sensitive to values and beliefs of people who are not members of the dominant group is the primary way that dealing with ethnic/racial difference (under the banner of cultural difference) has been conceptualized in health care and service delivery, and nursing has widely embraced this idea. Based on the narrow understandings of culture that underlie multiculturalism and the confusion of culture, ethnicity, and race, however, cultural sensitivity is highly inadequate in that it overlooks and obscures issues of racial supremacy and inequality and the way that cultural relations are embedded in and shaped by sociopolitical and economic contexts (Culley, 1996, 2006; Swendson & Windsor, 1996).

Cultural sensitivity implies that those operating from the dominant norm and who wield the most power ought to be sensitive to difference. This sensitivity requires no social action. Sensitivity to cultural difference, when culture is seen as values and beliefs associated with ethnic groups, means sensitivity to values and beliefs but does not require sensitivity to context and the structural determinants of health. Our overriding concern with the idea of cultural sensitivity is how it gives rise to a "recipe book" approach to culture as illustrated in the "Multicultural Corner" feature. Nurses are encouraged to learn about "others'" values, beliefs, and practices (e.g., Chinese do this, African Americans do that, Jews think this, Muslims think that, etc.) as recipes to guide practice with others. Naturally, this places the dominant white Eurocentric norm at the center and leaves the culturally sensitive practitioner open to generalizations and stereotypes based on race, class, religion, and so on. Working from the ideas of multiculturalism and sensitivity, it is perhaps not surprising that, as Gray and Thomas (2002) have concluded, nurses often have taken up a limited view of culture and focused upon "difference," particularly racial/ethnic or religious differences without bridging those differences. Clearly, such an approach is not congruent with relational nursing practice or with promoting health.

Integrate Cultural Safety in Your Practice

Over the past two decades, nursing scholars have introduced the idea of "cultural safety" as a tool for practice in diverse contexts. Cultural safety begins with recognition that cultures are dynamic and constantly shifting in relation to power dynamics in our society and historical, economic, political, and local trends (Browne et al., 2009; Reimer-Kirkham et al., 2009; Varcoe & Browne, in press). The idea of safety is predicated on an understanding of "un-safety" as anything that diminishes, demeans, or disempowers the cultural identity and well-being of an individual or group (Wood & Schwass, 1993). Promoting safety requires actions that recognize, respect, and nurture the unique cultural identity of people/families and safely meet their needs, expectations, and rights.

Maori nurse educators initially introduced the idea of cultural safety in Aeotara/New Zealand to facilitate health care interactions between the indigenous Maori people and Pakuha (the nonindigenous, predominantly white immigrants) (Papps & Ramsden, 1996; Wood & Schwass, 1993). The idea has since been explored as a way of promoting ethical practice within ethnically diverse populations (Anderson et al., 2003; Browne & Fiske, 2001; Polashek, 1998; Reimer-Kirkham et al., 2002; Smye & Browne, 2002). Cultural safety involves the "recognition of the social, economic, and political position of certain groups within society . . . and is concerned with fostering an understanding of the relationship between minority status and health status. The intent is to change nurses' attitudes from those which continue to support current dominant practices and systems of health care to those which are more supportive of the health of minority groups" (Smye & Browne, 2002, pp. 46–47). The concept of cultural safety not only turns attention to the attitudes and practices of individuals but also directs attention to examining how dominant organizational, institutional, and structural contexts shape health and social relations and practices and prompts the unmasking of the ways that policies and practices may perpetuate neocolonial approaches to health care (Smye & Browne, 2002).

The central ideas of cultural safety are that:

■ Culture is dynamic and embedded within and changing in response to historical, economic, political, and social contexts.

■ When working to promote safety, it is how a group "is perceived and treated that is relevant rather than the different things its members think or do"(Polashek, 1998, p. 452).

■ The social, economic, and political positions of groups within society influence health and health care.

■ Individual and institutional discrimination in health care creates risks for patients, particularly when people from a specific group perceive they are "demeaned, diminished, or disempowered by actions and delivery systems," including by those who typically hold the power in health care contexts (Ramsden & Spoonley, 1994, p. 164).

■ Health care providers must "reflect on their own personal and cultural history and the values and beliefs they bring in their interaction with clients, rather than an uncritical imposition of their own understandings and beliefs on clients and their families" (Anderson et al., 2003, p. 198). Providers must also consider how their own social locations influence how they see others.

■ Promoting safety requires actions that (a) recognize, respect, and nurture the unique and dynamic cultural identities of all people and families, and (b) safely meet people's needs, expectations, and rights given the unique contexts of their lives.

It is clear that the ideas of cultural safety are harmonious with a relational approach. They are based on understanding context and culture as inseparable, developing a relational consciousness, and inquiring at all levels. Box 4.8 suggests questions to ask yourself to integrate cultural safety in your practice.

BOX 4.8

Using the Ideas of Cultural Safety

Start with the organization to inquire at the level of context:

■ How are organizational practices supporting the health of nondominant groups?

■ What policies or organizational practices diminish, demean, or disempower the cultural identity and well-being of any individual or group? How do such policies or practices support discrimination?

■ What policies or organizational practices would recognize, respect, and nurture the unique cultural identities of people and families and safely meet their needs, expectations, and rights?

Examine nursing practices to inquire interpersonally:

■ What is the unique identity of this person or family? What are this person's or family's needs and expectations?

■ How can I practice to recognize, respect, and nurture that identity and meet those needs and expectations?

Use reflexivity to inquire intrapersonally:

■ How do my own personal and cultural history, values, and beliefs influence my practice?

■ How do my own economic, political, social, and historical location shape my practice?

The ideas of cultural safety are congruent with and parallel to the process of relational inquiry. Rather than directing nurses to learn about "other" cultures (where we can never know enough) and fearing cultural blunders, relational inquiry focuses on understanding the complex dynamics of contexts within which culture is embedded. Relational inquiry rests on the assumption that every moment of practice is cultural and contextual. Enacting nursing practice through relational inquiry directs you to consciously consider:

■ The contextual circumstances and cultures of people's lives that are relevant to the immediate situation

■ How your own values, beliefs, and attitudes are shaping your understanding of people's life circumstances and their different effects

■ How health care contexts are shaping practice and might be optimized toward well-being

What distinguishes relational inquiry from other nursing approaches is (a) the expanded view of context/culture that focuses attention on the relational interplay and (b) how one very intentionally acts in response to that interplay. Relational inquiry is specifically oriented toward the complexities of context/culture with the goal of producing situations that support and foster well-being of people and contexts.

TO ILLUSTRATE

A Drug-Seeking Woman

When I (Colleen) was doing research in emergency settings, because the nurses knew I was studying health care responses to violence against women, they would point out women they thought were experiencing violence. One evening, the nurse I was working with and another nurse noticed a well-dressed woman at triage. "Oh, she's back again," said one nurse, rolling her eyes. "She's a doctor's wife. She comes in for her shot of Demerol, but she won't leave him." In that moment, I recognized that the idea of leaving violence as a simple "choice" was operating, along with stereotypes about women too "weak" to leave a violent relationship. I didn't want to embarrass or alienate the nurses or make them feel defensive. I wanted to engage them in thinking about the woman's context, but I didn't want to lecture them. I said, "You guys must be doing something right, if she keeps coming back." Somehow, that opened up rather than closing down the conversation, and I was able to talk about how women's fears of judgment often deter them from getting help when dealing with abusive partners.

Several days later, one of the two nurses told me that she had realized that she had been assuming that because the woman appeared to have an adequate income that she could easily leave her husband. The nurse said, "We've offered her help before, but maybe what we offered wasn't what she needed." She suggested that next time she saw the woman, she would find out. This was a small moment and may have affected only one nurse's thinking. However, many small moments can add up to a sea of change, for example, in how the contexts of people's lives might be better understood. I was seeking to produce a situation in which the nurses could inquire about their own thinking, the woman's situation, and health care practice. In doing so, I felt positive about my own practice, opened dialogue with the nurses, and possibly contributed to enhancing a culture of responsiveness.

Work across Differences

The example Colleen describes above illustrates how when one takes a relational inquiry approach and begins enacting contextual, culturally safe nursing practice, working across differences becomes a central feature of day-to-day nursing work. It also reveals how thoughtfully intervening at one level can have an impact beyond the immediate situation. For example, by taking the well-being of the patient, the nurses, and the health care system into consideration and specifically targeting her action in a way that would both support the well-being of the people involved and respond to the various cultural elements at play, Colleen was able to have an impact beyond the specific patient and situation.

Below, we describe some concrete habits that can support you to effectively practice in a contextual, culturally safe way—habits of practice that will enable you to work across difference and promote well-being.

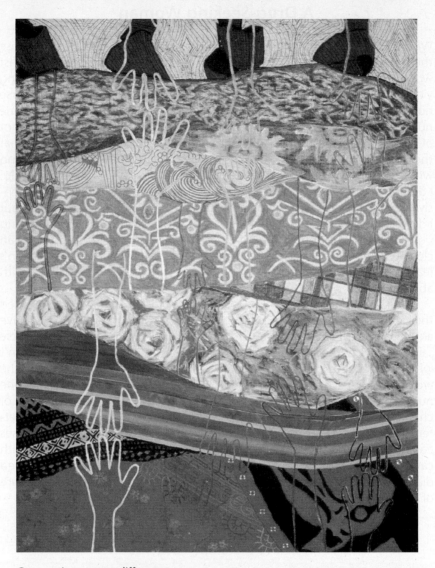

Connecting across difference.

See and Address Systemic Structures

As nurses, we often take systemic structures for granted and/or do not notice how they are shaping our practice. For example, as described in Chapter 2, the nurse in the COPD clinic took the power structure for granted that assigned her the privilege of knowing what was best for patients. She did not question her authority and/or the practice of expecting patients to comply with the authority of expert knowledge. Similarly, given the business model of health care shaping health care reform, structures that organize practices of efficiency can become taken for granted. Yet, for patients and families, they may have an entirely different meaning. To meet our obligations to them, we need to consider that meaning. For example, putting patients in holding areas or on stretchers in hallways while waiting for admission to a bed is normal, everyday practice within many health care institutions. Yet, for someone who is ill, in pain, and has not slept for 2 days due to noise, blinding overhead lighting and the constant chaos of people running by is anything but normal. Think of Mr. Stephen's description of this in the hospital after his stroke. How to meet the obligation to patients within those system constraints is a question that needs to be asked. Seeing yourself as an agent in context and seeing contexts as sites for change supports such questioning as a continuous aspect of practice. It also supports you to take action to improve situations, both for particular people and more generally. While you may not immediately be able to change policy or get a specific patient moved to a bed, enlisting the HP and critical lenses and inquiring intrapersonally (to notice what you are taking for granted, what is concerning you); interpersonally (to notice what is happening and concerning for the patient, what the nursing issues are, what is being taken for granted, what changes might be possible within the interpersonal space); and contextually (what structures, values, powers are at play, how those elements are impeding well-being), you can more strategically consider the available options. Thus, developing the habit of seeing and impacting systemic structures supports your choice and potential effectiveness in terms of promoting well-being.

Avoid Labeling

Another problematic practice in health care is that of decontextualizing by labeling, objectifying, and commodifying people and families. "I have 15 high-risks [families] to see," "We had three codes going on at once," and "The appendectomy in room 5 needs vital signs done" are just a few examples of how we reduce people to the moral status of objects (Buber, 1958), seeing and relating to them as objects to be observed, assessed, labeled, and treated.

As these examples suggest, decontextualizing people often begins with categorizing and labeling. As we discussed in Chapter 2, categorizing and labeling are acts of power. Labeling has significant performative effects (i.e., it performs an influential function). Think of the powerful consequences that the label "terminal" can have, both on a person's health and health care. Think back to the story of the nurse in Chapter 1 caring for the man transferred from the emergency department. When he was determined to be terminal, a whole cascade of events followed. As this example suggests, all labels and categories need to be scrutinized critically for how they are being used and what their effects are, and their harmful effects need to be countered in every moment (see Box 4.9).

Labels are problematic in at least five ways when applied uncritically to people. First, through labels, people are reduced to a small aspect of their experience. In my (Colleen's) area of research, the terms "abused woman" and "battered woman" are used commonly, reducing a woman to only her experience of violence. This is not mere wordplay or semantics. Rather, such labels have practical consequences. By taking up these labels, nurses are influenced to think that violence in a woman's life is the most salient feature, and they overlook other features that may be more significant. For example, women's feelings for and commitment to their partners is often dismissed by well-intentioned helpers who think they know what is

---

BOX 4.9

Useful "Rules" for Countering the Negative Effects of Labels

- Keep the person in the foreground ("person who injects drugs" instead of "IDU").
- Make the causes of risk, marginality, precarity, or vulnerability explicit ("people at risk of homelessness" instead of "the homeless").
- Locate contextual problems contextually ("children living in poverty" instead of "at-risk children").
- Question the salience of labels being used (When is being "white" relevant, and why?).
- Question the effects of labeling (How does the diagnosis "Asperger syndrome" simultaneously stigmatize, gain additional resources for a family, and provide a helpful explanation of behavior that has been difficult to understand?).

---

best. In turn, this deters women from seeking support and help and results in missed opportunities to assist women to assess the danger they might face and plan for their safety and well-being. To counter this labeling, a useful "rule" is always to keep the person in view. The phrase "women who experience violence" requires a few more words, but it can have the profound effect of widening understanding.

Second, labels can be pejorative, judgmental, and stigmatizing, such as the examples we have used: "broken family," "welfare mom," "white trash," and so forth. However, problematic labels can be countered. Think of how powerfully the language of "persons living with AIDS" shifted from "AIDS patients" or "HIV-positives."

Third, because labeling reduces people to less than their full human status, such acts can contribute to treating people as less than fully human. For example, the literature on HIV routinely labels people who use injection drugs as "IDUs" (e.g. German & Latkin, 2012; Maas et al., 2007). This reduces them to their drug use and stigmatizes and paves the way for further "less than" treatment.

Fourth, labels often draw attention to features that may not even be salient to a given situation or may convey attention that is erroneous. For example, labeling families according to risk factors without specifying which risks are significant can misdirect attention; a family may be considered "high-risk" prenatally for genetic, social, or economic reasons. Labeling people by their presumed ethnicity or race implies salience that may not be accurate. Even though it is widespread practice in research to use racial categories to study the social effects of racial categorization, doing so often is misunderstood as implying the study of genetic characteristics. Further, such categorization is almost never relevant in relation to a particular individual in a health care context. A common error in doing so is assuming characteristics that have no relevance. Assuming that "Mr. Singh" is a vegetarian, speaks Punjabi fluently, or has emigrated from India is more likely to be wrong than right. He may well be a third- or fourth-generation American whose ancestry (perhaps from Africa) may be completely irrelevant to his current life and lifestyle. A further helpful rule is to question the salience of any label or category.

Fifth, labeling truncates the experience of individuals to a specific problem and locates that problem in the person. To return to the example of the label of "abused woman," this act of labeling makes abuse a characteristic of the woman, locates the problem in the woman, and leaves the perpetrator of abuse invisible. The phrases "woman abused by her partner" or "woman assaulted by her son" more accurately locates the problem.

Finally, categorizing and labeling people lays the ground for commodification of people. To commodify means to assign economic value to something not usually or previously considered in economic terms. The process of considering people in economic terms aligns with an emphasis on efficiency in health care without attention to effectiveness. That is, when nurses talk about people in economic and numerical terms, it can function to accomplish all of the above effects. When a nurse says, "I have 15 high-risk families," the effect can be to locate the problem in the families, reduce families to problems, dehumanize them, and convey stigma. Declaring a person or family as being "at risk" shifts the location of the problem from the cause to the victim. So a family might be at risk of the effects of poverty, or a youth might be at risk because of the failure of entire social systems, but risk is transferred to become the problem of the people who are bearing the risk. Therefore, another useful rule is to make causes explicit. Saying "children at risk of exploitation," "women at risk of the effects of poverty," or "men at risk of deportation" specifies the nature of the risk and locates the problem more accurately. Better yet, language such as "young women living in stressful and low-income conditions" can locate the problem contextually, another useful rule.

TRY IT OUT 4.7
Listening for and Countering Labels

The next time you are in a practice context, listen actively for how labels are being deployed, and see how far you can go in shifting those practices. The skills of standing your ground and not participating in problematic practices are fundamental to you being able to practice in alignment with values such as fairness. Further, because your practice is always in relation to others, you will need to develop the ability to skillfully and respectfully interrupt problematic practices and support others to be less harmful without provoking defensiveness.

1. Listen for labels. Listen for what labels are commonly deployed in your practice setting. For example, if you are in emergency, you might hear labels such as "frequent flyer" applied to patients or "bleeding heart" applied to nurses.

continued on page 186

TRY IT OUT 4.7 *continued*

Listening for and Countering Labels

2. Practice alternatives. If you hear labels being used, join the conversation with an alternative. For example, if you hear "she's terminal," join the conversation in some way to widen attention to other features of the person who is dying. "How is her family dealing with the idea she is dying?"

3. Practice countering with "I" statements. When I hear "abused woman," I (Colleen) find it useful to say something such as, "I always try to keep the woman in the foreground when women have experienced abuse." Practice this countering in relatively symmetrical power relations. That is, try it out with friends, fellow students, or anyone you feel you can safely challenge without reprisal. If you practice, you will become more skilled, confident, and able to interrupt problematic practices in a wider set of circumstances.

4. Counter by bringing your knowledge of context to bear. For example, when you hear the term "IDU" applied to people, you might say, "I have been reading about the overwhelming number of people who use injection drugs who also have trauma histories."

Avoid Imposing Your Own Interpretations

As people are commodified and their health and illness experiences decontextualized into discrete problems to be solved, there is also the tendency to narrate and interpret people from our own vantage points—to impose our own understandings on them. Labeling plays an important role in this process. For example, the wife of the patient who has been in the hallway for 2 days who repeatedly asks when a bed will be found becomes "the nagging wife." The patient who is sullen, angry, does not do what he or she is asked to do, does not act as expected, requires more time to move than others, and requires more pain medication than the nurse thinks is needed becomes "the difficult patient."

These imposing practices have significant consequences for the well-being of patients and families. For example, Cleveland's review of the experience of parenting in the NICU identified a number of studies in which mothers expressed fear of being labeled by nurses as "difficult" with the consequence of decreasing their involvement in their infant's care. In particular, they worried about being perceived as "pushy." "They feared that voicing their opinions would increase their infant's vulnerability" (Cleveland, 2008, p. 680). Denison, Varcoe, and Browne (in press) found that women labeled as "native" were discouraged from seeking health care for themselves or being with their children when hospitalized because of experiences of being judged negatively and encountering racism by nurses.

Buber's (1958) distinction between I-It and I-Thou relationships is helpful in understanding the difference between imposing understandings where people are commodified and objectified by expert knowers and contextual, culturally safe understandings of people that are meaningful and respectful. An "I-It" relationship involves a relationship between a person and an object. Yalom (1980) describes that when relating to "It" people hold back a part of themselves. From this detached stance, they inspect, categorize, analyze, and make judgments about the "other." In this way, I-It relationships are instrumental relationships that lack mutual responsiveness. Within the scientific, biomedical world of health care, such instrumental relationships have tended to be the norm. As Parse (1998) describes, within the biomedical view, practice focuses on diagnosing, treating, and/or preventing disease. For this reason, nursing becomes instrumental; the nurse inspects, categorizes, makes judgments about and treats the "disease."

In contrast, the I-Thou relationship involves a mutual process where nurses orient to people and families as human beings in the midst of meaningful experiences (Buber, 1958; Yalom, 1980). That involves inquiring into those experiences to know what is significant to particular people and families and to determine how nursing care might be most effective and responsive. Privileging individuals' and families' narratives is a key strategy toward integrating understanding of context and culture.

Pay Attention to Practice Contexts

Nursing encounters with individuals and families occur in diverse contexts, and those contexts shape people's experiences of health and health care and enable and constrain nursing practice. Understanding the situations of particular people provides a basis for you to act to produce situations that will better enhance their health. Paying attention to patterns within practice contexts provides a basis for you to produce situations that affect multiple individuals and families. For example, if in caring for Mrs. Zhang you realize that many patients who do not speak English are not being offered interpreter services, then you can facilitate better use of such services. Or, if there are not adequate services available, you can participate in improving that situation.

Practice contexts also are important to nurse well-being. When nurses practice in contexts in which they feel unable to practice in accordance with nursing values, particularly values for fairness, they can experience high levels of distress (Epstein & Hamric, 2009; Hamric, 2010; Harrowing & Mill, 2010; Pauly, Varcoe, Storch, & Newton, 2009; Silen, Svantesson, Kjellstrom, Sidenvall, & Christensson, 2011; Varcoe, Pauly, Storch, Newton, & Makaroff, 2012; Varcoe, Pauly, Webster, & Storch, 2012). Such distress can lead to poor mental health for nurses and lead some nurses to leave their positions or to leave nursing altogether (Kulig et al., 2009; Taylor & Barling, 2004; Ulrich et al., 2007). Working to produce situations and practice contexts that are more conducive to health promotion therefore has beneficial effects for nurses.

THIS WEEK IN PRACTICE
Inquiring into
Context and Culture

This week when you are in practice, pick any individual, family, or family member with whom you can have a conversation. Be transparent with the person or people you choose, and tell them that you want to learn as much as possible about how people's circumstances affect their health.

Follow their lead as to what is important. If a question is needed beyond telling them about your interest, perhaps open with a question such as, "What circumstances led up to you being here?" Listen to what is of significance and importance to them. Listen to how history, sociopolitical influences, economics, and physical contexts have shaped and continue to shape their experiences. Listen to how they are using language and available discourses and how language and discourses have been used with them. General questions such as, "What led to that?" "What was your situation then?" "How were you living at that time?" and so on can direct attention to multiple contexts. Pay attention to what circumstances were within their control, what circumstances were potentially modifiable, and who could have modified them.

After your conversation, consider what you learned. What did you learn about this particular individual or family? What did you learn about the immediate health care context? What did you learn about yourself? Pay attention to how long your conversation was. How much did you learn in a few minutes? In 10 minutes?

YOUR RELATIONAL INQUIRY TOOLBOX

Add the following tools to your relational inquiry toolbox:
- Discern the relevance of context to health, health care, and nursing action in each situation.
- Look at culture contextually by looking beyond values and beliefs associated with particular groups.
- Look for the problematic effects when the idea of culture is used in a decontextualized way.
- Use the text box questions to analyze how social structures and inequities are shaping health and health care.
- Integrate your knowledge of historical contexts and economic dynamics to further your understanding of how health is being socially produced.
- Examine how social determinants are shaping health and creating health inequities.

continued on page 189

```
YOUR RELATIONAL INQUIRY TOOLBOX  continued
```

- Pay attention to the effects of labeling and constructively respond to labeling practices.
- Consciously integrate the ideas of cultural safety in practice.
- Pay attention to multiple differences and the connection between those differences.

REFERENCES

Allen, D. G. (1999). Knowledge, politics, culture, and gender: A discourse perspective. *Canadian Journal of Nursing Research, 30*(4), 227–234.

Anderson, J. M., Perry, J., Blue, C., Browne, A. J., Henderson, A., Khan, K. B., et al. (2003). "Rewriting" cultural safety within the postcolonial and postnational feminist project: Toward new epistemologies of healing. *Advances in Nursing Science, 26*(3), 196–214.

Arnaert, A., Seller, R., & Wainwright, M. (2009). Homecare nurses' attitudes toward palliative care in a rural community in Western Quebec. *Journal of Hospice & Palliative Nursing, 11*(4), 202–208.

Bales, K. (2012). *Disposable people: New slavery in the global economy* (2nd ed.). Berkeley, CA: University of California Press.

Beagan, B. L., Chapman, G. E., Johnston, J., McPhail, D., Power, E., & Vallianatos, H. (in press). *The family table: Intersections of class, place, gender and food practices*. Vancouver, British Columbia, Canada: UBC Press.

Beddoes, Z. M. (2012, October 13). Special report: The world economy. *The Economist*. Retrieved July 26, 2013, from http://econ.st/QNGakg

Bergum, V. (2013). Relational ethics for health care. In J. Storch, P. Rodney, & R. Starzomski (Eds.), *Toward a moral horizon: Nursing ethics for leadership and practice* (2nd ed., pp. 127–142). Toronto, Ontario, Canada: Pearson.

Brown, H. (2008). *The face to face is not so innocent: The relational construction of interpersonal spaces of maternal-infant care* (Doctoral dissertation). University of Victoria.

Browne, A. J., & Fiske, J. (2001). First Nations women's encounters with mainstream health care services. *Western Journal of Nursing Research, 23*(2), 126–147.

Browne, A. J., Varcoe, C., Smye, V., Reimer-Kirkham, S., Lynam, M. J., & Wong, S. (2009). Cultural safety and the challenges of translating critically oriented knowledge in practice. *Nursing Philosophy, 10*, 167–179.

Buber, M. (1958). *I and thou*. New York: Scribner.

Butler, J. (n.d.). *From and against precarity*. Retrieved July 26, 2013, from http://occupytheory.org/read/from-and-against-precarity.html

Carveth, J. A. (1995). Perceived patient deviance and avoidance by nurses. *Nursing Research, 44*(3), 173–178.

Chopoorian, T. L. (1986). Reconceptualizing the environment. In P. Moccia (Ed.), *New approaches to theory development* (pp. 39–54). New York: National League of Nursing.

Cleveland, L. M. (2008). Parenting in the neonatal intensive care unit. *Journal of Obstetric, Gynecologic, & Neonatal Nursing, 37*(6), 666–691.

Conference Board of Canada. (2009). *Child poverty*. Retrieved November 13, 2011, from http://www.conferenceboard.ca/hcp/details/society/child-poverty.aspx

Conroy, K., Sandel, M., & Zuckerman, B. (2010). Poverty grown up: How childhood socioeconomic status impacts adult health. *Journal of Developmental & Behavioral Pediatrics, 31*(2), 154–160.

Corak, M. (2006). Do poor children become poor adults? Lessons from a cross-country comparison of generational earnings mobility. In J.

Creedy & G. Kalb (Eds.) (Ed.), *Dynamics of inequality and poverty* (pp. 143). Oxford, United Kingdom: Elsevier.

Corley, M. C., & Goren, S. (1998). The dark side of nursing: Impact of stigmatizing responses on patients. *Scholarly Inquiry for Nursing Practice, 12*(2), 99–118.

Culley, L. (1996). A critique of multiculturalism in health care: The challenge for nurse education. *Journal of Advanced Nursing, 23*, 564–570.

Culley, L. (2006). Transcending transculturalism? Race, ethnicity and health-care. *Nursing Inquiry, 13*(2), 144–153.

Davis, D. L., & Walker, K. (2010). Rediscovering the material body in midwifery through an exploration of theories of embodiment. *Midwifery, 26*(4), 457–462.

Denison, J., Varcoe, C., & Browne, A. J. (in press). Aboriginal women's experiences of accessing health care when state apprehension of children is being threatened. *Journal of Advanced Nursing.*

Epstein, E. G., & Hamric, A. B. (2009). Moral distress, moral residue and the crescendo effect. *The Journal of Clinical Ethics, 20*(4), 330–342.

Evans, G. W., & Kim, P. (2007). Childhood poverty and health: Cumulative risk exposure and stress dysregulation. *Psychological Science, 18*(11), 953–957.

German, D., & Latkin, C. (2012). Boredom, depressive symptoms, and HIV risk behaviors among urban injection drug users. *AIDS and Behavior, 16*(8), 2244–2250.

Gray, P., & Thomas, D. (2002, November). *Whose cultures count when it comes to cultural competence?* Paper presented at the Critical and Feminist Perspectives in Nursing Conference, Portland, ME.

Grief, C. L., & Elliott, R. (1994). Emergency nurses' moral evaluation of patients. *Journal of Emergency Nursing, 20*, 275–279.

Hall, J. M. (1999). Marginalization revisited: Critical, postmodern, and liberation perspectives. *Advances in Nursing Science, 22*(2), 88–102.

Hall, J. M., Stevens, P. E., & Meleis, A. I. (1994). Marginalization: A guiding concept for valuing diversity in nursing knowledge development. *Advances in Nursing Science, 16*(4), 23–41.

Hamric, A. B. (2010). Moral distress and nurse-physician relationships. *American Medical Association Virtual Mentor, 12*(1), 6–11.

Hardin, P. K. (2001). Theory and language: Locating agency between free will and discursive marionettes. *Nursing Inquiry, 8*(1), 11–18.

Harrowing, J., & Mill, J. (2010). Moral distress among Ugandan nurses providing HIV care: A critical ethnography. *International Journal of Nursing Studies, 47*, 723–731.

Hedges, C. (2012). *Days of destruction, days of revolt.* New York: Nation Books.

Hodgson, G. (2011). *A big idea whose time has yet to arrive: A guaranteed annual income.* Ottawa, Ontario, Canada: Conference Board of Canada.

Johnson, M., & Webb, C. (1995a). The power of social judgement: Struggle and negotiation in the nursing process. *Nurse Education Today, 15*, 83–89.

Johnson, M., & Webb, C. (1995b). Rediscovering unpopular patients: The concept of social judgement. *Journal of Advanced Nursing, 21*, 466–475.

Kelly, M. P., & May, D. (1982). Good and bad patients: A review of the literature and a theoretical critique. *Journal of Advanced Nursing, 7*, 147–156.

Kemp, C. L., Ball, M. M., Perkins, M. M., Hollingsworth, C., & Lepore, M. J. (2009). "I get along with most of them": Direct care workers' relationships with residents' families in assisted living. *The Gerontologist, 49*(2), 224–235.

Khalil, D. D. (2009). Nurses' attitudes towards "difficult" and "good" patients in eight public hospitals. *International Journal of Nursing Practice, 15*, 437–443.

Kleffel, D. (1996). Environmental paradigms: Moving toward an ecocentric perspective. *Advances in Nursing Science, 18*(4), 1–10.

Kulig, J. C., Stewart, N., Penz, K., Forbes, D., Morgan, D., & Emerson, P. (2009). Work setting, community attachment, and satisfaction among rural and remote nurses. *Public Health Nursing, 26*(5), 430–439.

Lerner, S. (2010). *Sacrifice zones: The front lines of toxic chemical exposure in the United States.* Cambridge, MA: MIT Press.

Liaschenko, J. (1994). Making a bridge: The moral work with patients we do not like. *Journal of Palliative Care, 10*(3), 83–89.

Liaschenko, J. (1995). Ethics in the work of acting for patients. *Advances in Nursing Science, 18*(2), 1–12.

Lustig, N., Lopez-Calva, L. F., & Ortiz-Juarez, E. (2012). *Declining inequality in Latin America in the 2000s: The cases of Argentina, Brazil, and Mexico.* Washington, DC: Center for Global Development.

Lynam, M. J., & Cowley, S. (2007). Understanding marginalization as a social determinant of health. *Critical Public Health, 17*(2), 137–149.

Maas, B., Fairbairn, N., Kerr, T., Li, K., Montaner, J. S. G., & Wood, E. (2007). Neighborhood and HIV infection among IDU: Place of residence independently predicts HIV infection among a cohort of injection drug users. *Health & Place, 13*(2), 432–439.

Malone, R. E. (1996). Almost "like family": Emergency nurses and "frequent flyers." *Journal of Emergency Nursing, 22*(3), 176–183.

Maupin, C. R. (1995). The potential for noncaring when dealing with difficult patients: Strategies for moral decision making. *Journal of Cardiovascular Nursing, 9*(3), 11–22.

Milanovic, B. (2012). *Global income inequality by the numbers: In history and now.* Washington, DC: World Bank.

O'Connor, N. (1993). *Paterson and Zderad humanistic nursing theory. Notes on nursing theory.* Newbury Park, CA: Sage.

Papps, E., & Ramsden, I. (1996). Cultural safety in nursing: The New Zealand experience. *International Journal for Quality in Health Care, 8*(5), 491–497.

Parse, R. (1998). *The human becoming school of thought. A perspective for nurses and other health professionals.* Thousand Oaks, CA: Sage.

Pauly, B., Varcoe, C., Storch, J., & Newton, L. (2009). Registered nurses' perceptions of moral distress and ethical climate. *Nursing Ethics, 16*(5), 561–573.

Peternelj-Taylor, C. (2004). An exploration of othering in forensic psychiatric and correctional nursing. *Canadian Journal of Nursing Research, 36*(4), 130–146.

Podrasky, D., & Sexton, D. (1988). Nurses' reactions to difficult patients. *Image: Journal of Nursing Scholarship, 20*(1), 16–21.

Polashek, N. R. (1998). Cultural safety: A new concept in nursing people with different ethnicities. *Journal of Advanced Nursing, 27*, 452–457.

Ramsden, I., & Spoonley, P. (1994). The cultural safety debate in nursing education in Aotearoa. *New Zealand Annual Review of Education, 1993*, 161–174.

Razack, S. (1998). *Looking white people in the eye: Gender, race, and culture in courtrooms and classrooms.* Toronto, Ontario, Canada: University of Toronto Press.

Reimer-Kirkham, S., Smye, V., Tang, S., Anderson, J., Blue, C., Browne, A. J., et al. (2002). Rethinking cultural safety while waiting to do fieldwork: Methodological implications for nursing research. *Research in Nursing & Health, 25*(3), 222–232.

Reimer-Kirkham, S., Varcoe, C., Browne, A. J., Lynam, M. J., Khan, K. B., & McDonald, H. (2009). Critical inquiry and knowledge translation: Exploring compatibilities and tensions. *Nursing Philosophy, 10*, 152–166.

Rogers, C. (1961). *On becoming a person.* Boston: Houghton Mifflin.

Santiago, C. D., Wadsworth, M. E., & Stump, J. (2011). Socioeconomic status, neighborhood disadvantage, and poverty-related stress: Prospective effects on psychological syndromes among diverse low-income families. *Journal of Economic Psychology, 32*(2), 218–230.

Silen, M., Svantesson, M., Kjellstrom, S., Sidenvall, B., & Christensson, L. (2011). Moral distress and ethical climate in a Swedish nursing context: Perceptions and instrument usability. *Journal of Clinical Nursing, 20*(23–24), 3483–3493.

Smye, V. L., & Browne, A. J. (2002). "Cultural safety" and the analysis of health policy affecting Aboriginal people. *Nurse Researcher, 9*(3), 42–56.

Solar, O., & Irwin, A. (2010). *A conceptual framework for action on the social determinants of health: Social determinants of health discussion paper 2 (policy and practice).* Geneva, Switzerland: World Health Organization.

Stephen, M. (2013, January 10). Martin Stephen: I had a stroke of good luck with my stroke, *The Telegraph.* Retrieved from http://www.telegraph.co.uk /health/9793218/Martin-Stephen-I -had-a-stroke-of-good-luck-with-my -stroke.html

Stephenson, P. (1999). Expanding notions of culture for cross-cultural ethics in health and medicine. In H. Coward & P. Ratanakul (Eds.), *A cross-cultural dialogue on health care ethics* (pp. 68–91). Waterloo, Ontario, Canada: Wilfried Laurier University Press.

Stevens, P. E. (1989). A critical social reconceptualization of the environment in nursing: Implications for methodology. *Advances in Nursing Science, 11*(4), 56–68.

Stevens, P. E. (1992). Who gets care? Access to health care as an arena for nursing action. *Scholarly Inquiry for Nursing Practice, 6*(3), 185–200.

Stevens, P. E. (1994). Lesbians' health related experiences of care and noncare. *Western Journal of Nursing Research, 16,* 639–659.

Swendson, C., & Windsor, C. (1996). Rethinking cultural sensitivity. *Nursing Inquiry, 3,* 3–12.

Taylor, B., & Barling, J. (2004). Identifying sources and effects of carer fatigue and burnout for mental health nurses: A qualitative approach. *International Journal of Mental Health Nursing, 13*(2), 117–125.

Ulrich, C., O'Donnell, P., Taylor, C., Farrar, A., Danis, M., & Grady, C. (2007). Ethical climate, ethics stress, and the job satisfaction of nurses and social workers in the United States. *Social Science & Medicine, 65*(8), 1708–1719.

UNICEF Innocenti Research Centre. (2012). Measuring child poverty: New league tables of child poverty in the world's rich countries. Florence, Italy: Author.

UNICEF Office of Research. (2013). Child well-being in rich countries: A comparative overview. *Innocenti report card 11.* Florence, Italy: Author.

Varcoe, C., & Browne, A. J. (in press). Culture and cultural safety: Beyond cultural inventories. In C. D. Gregory, L. Raymond-Seniuk, & L. Patrick (Eds.), *Fundamentals: Perspectives on the art and science of Canadian nursing.* Philadelphia: Lippincott Williams & Wilkins.

Varcoe, C., Browne, A., & Anderson, J. (2010). Cultural considerations in health assessment. In T. Stephen, L. Skillen, R. Day, & L. Bickley (Eds.), *Canadian Bates' guide to physical examination and history taking for nurses* (pp. 27–50). Philadelphia: Lippincott Williams & Wilkins.

Varcoe, C., Pauly, B., Storch, J., Newton, L., & Makaroff, K. (2012). Nurses' perceptions of and responses to morally distressing situations. *Nursing Ethics, 19*(4), 488–500.

Varcoe, C., Pauly, B., Webster, G., & Storch, J. (2012). Moral distress: Tensions as springboards for action. *HEC Forum: An Interdisciplinary Journal on Hospitals' Ethical and Legal Issues, 24*(1), 51–62.

Whitehead, M., & Dahlgren, G. (2006). *A discussion paper on concepts and principles for tackling social inequities in health: Levelling up part 1.* Copenhagen, Denmark: World Health Organization (Europe).

Wood, P. J., & Schwass, M. (1993). Cultural safety: A framework for changing attitudes. *New Praxis in New Zealand, 8*(1), 4–15.

Yalom, I. D. (1980). *Existential philosophy.* New York: Basic Books.

Young, M., & Mulvale, J. P. (2009). *Possibilities and prospects: The debate over a guaranteed income.* Ottawa, Ontario, Canada: Canadian Center for Policy Alternatives.

5 All Nursing Is Family Nursing

LEARNING OBJECTIVES

By engaging with the material in this chapter, you will be able to:

1. Share your insights into the nature of your own current approach to family nursing practice.

2. Define and describe family from a relational perspective.

3. Discuss a range of perspectives on what constitutes family nursing.

4. Explain how relational inquiry can enhance your effectiveness as a nurse caring for diverse people and families in any health care context.

5. Compare and contrast three models of care that shape the contexts in which family nursing is practiced: family-centered care, patient-centered care, and person-focused care.

In this chapter, we focus specifically on family nursing. We explore a relational understanding of family and examine how "family nursing as relational inquiry" is integral to all nursing practice. As you'll discover, a relational inquiry approach expands your ability to work with diverse people and families across all clinical settings.

EXPANDING YOUR REFERENCE POINTS FOR NURSING

As we have described in the first few chapters, when you bring a relational inquiry approach to your practice, you extend your reference point for who constitutes your patient and what you consider when determining your nursing obligations. One way your view expands is to consider how family is influencing any health care situation regardless of clinical setting or who your particular patient population might be.

Carie Semeniuk, a nurse who works in an adult intensive care unit (ICU) setting, recently took a relational inquiry course that I (Gweneth) taught. In the first "To Illustrate" box, she describes how integrating relational inquiry into her practice shifted her reference point for action; in particular, she came to see how family was integral to her everyday work.

TO ILLUSTRATE
Rethinking Family Nursing
in the ICU

I am very much a "doer" of nursing. I am skill-driven and . . . I didn't think my practice in the ICU setting fit under the umbrella of family nursing. I realize (having now taken the relational inquiry course) that I was very naïve in my true understanding of the concepts surrounding family nursing.

When getting report on my critically ill patient while working at the bedside, I used to ask, "How is the family?" I would do this with a negative tone to my voice, because what I realized I was really wondering was if they would be hindering my nursing care, requiring too much of my attention. I was not really inquiring to see how they were coping or wanting to know anything about them. Undertaking a relational inquiry, I have had to start at the beginning and look at myself. What are my beliefs, my values, what is important to me in my career as a registered nurse? I realize I was protecting myself by putting on this persona of being too busy, not allowing relationships to take place.

Now I get report, and I ask about the family. I research the kardex, social work notes, nursing notes, and find out everything I can about the family. Then I introduce myself, and I take 5 minutes to listen to their story, their fears, their questions. Whatever it is they want to share. I listen and then engage in relational inquiry by asking questions like What has your experience been like here in the ICU? What resources are in place for you to help you through this time? Sometimes I feel myself pulling away, but I have promised myself to give those 5 minutes.

Last week, a young female patient I had cared for passed away. The husband saw me in the hallway and hugged me. Through his tears, he thanked me for sitting with them in the mornings before I started my tasks. He had felt that because his wife was so ill, very few nurses took the time to talk to him or listen; they were always so busy doing things.

Carie's story is an all too familiar one. Often, nursing care is directed toward individual patients and their immediate physical health statuses and needs. Although families may be present, they are often treated as a backdrop to the "actual" patient. Who the nurse views as the recipient of care determines how, when, and even if family members are considered relevant to the care process.

We emphasize the importance of family nursing as an essential reference point in relational inquiry practice because, as Duhamel (2010) observes, even though family nursing has been taught in most nursing curricula for over two decades, family nursing is still visibly absent in many clinical settings. Many nurses do not consider family relevant to their care. It is this absence of family nursing that we wish to address and challenge in this chapter and will continue to address throughout the book as we consider nursing in contemporary health care settings.

As part of this chapter's exploration into family nursing, we will be offering definitions, concepts, and theories to expand your understanding. However, our first goal is to bring your attention to your own practice, to help you explore the ways in which family and family nursing might be relevant and important to the care you provide in your day-to-day nursing work. Returning to the metaphor of a camera, we invite you to view your current practice from a number of different vantage points. Then, in line with our pragmatic approach, we'll provide an opportunity for you to consider the consequences of your current views of family and family nursing and the theories and knowledge that shape those views. Gaining this kind of clarity is vital to effective nursing practice.

As part of this self-assessment, we will introduce perspectives that we believe can help you expand your understanding of family and enhance your nursing capacity for respectful and responsive family nursing practice across all clinical sites of care.

What Is Family Nursing?

If you peruse the nursing literature, you will find a range of perspectives on what constitutes family nursing. Kaakinen, Harmon Hanson, and Denham (2010) describe family nursing as "a scientific discipline based in theory" with family health care nursing being "an art and a science that has evolved as a way of thinking about and working with families" (p. 3). These authors contend that there are four different approaches to care within family nursing. What distinguishes the four approaches and how family nursing is enacted varies according to *who the designated patient is*, or who the focus of care is deemed to be:

- *Family as context.* This first approach focuses on assessment and care of an individual within the context of family. Within this approach, the individual is the designated client/patient, and the family is considered "either as a resource or a stressor to their [the individual's] health and illness" (Kaakinen et al., 2010, p. 10).

- *Family as client.* In the second approach, each individual family member is considered to be a client; thus, each individual is assessed and health care is provided for all family members. Kaakinen and colleagues (2010) suggest that family physician practice exemplifies this family as client approach.

- *Family systems.* In the third approach to family nursing, both the individuals in the family and the family unit are the focus of care. The family unit is understood to be an interactional system. In this family systems approach, it is assumed that affecting one part of the system (one family member) will affect the whole family unit (Wright & Leahey, 2012).

- *Family as a component of society.* In the fourth approach to family nursing that these authors identify, family is a component of society. In this approach, family is viewed as one of the many institutions within society that as a unit interacts with other institutions to exchange or receive services.

These different approaches illustrate how the term "family nursing" can be used to refer to quite different forms of nursing practice. Considering the different approaches to family nursing outlined by Kaakinen and colleagues (2010), it becomes evident that (a) what constitutes "family nursing" varies at the point-of-care, and (b) the question of who is the designated recipient of care becomes crucial in terms of determining your nursing actions and obligations. On who and what do you focus your nursing practice? Do you see the individual in the bed with a specific disease condition as your patient? Is your patient a group of individual family members who present at the primary health care clinic with various health challenges? Or perhaps you see both the individual members and the family system as the focus of your care and you subsequently center attention on promoting the well-being of both individuals and the family unit. Might your focus of nursing care be the family as a societal institution? *This question of who constitutes your patient at the point-of-care is a vital one for you to consider as a nurse since who and what you consider your focus of care to be shapes how (and even whether) you view family nursing as relevant to your own everyday nursing work. Moreover, the answer to this question serves as your reference point for any nursing action, and it shapes your nursing assessment and how you determine your nursing obligations and actions.*

What Informs Your Everyday Practice?

Theorizing is a vital part of any nursing practice since it creates the opportunity for you to learn from your experiences and enhance your responsiveness. We will be exploring this process of conscious theorizing more fully in Chapter 7. At this point, we want to draw attention to the theories and other forms of knowledge that are informing your current understanding of family and family nursing.

Parker and Smith (2010) describe theories as "mental patterns or frameworks created to help understand and create meaning from our experience, organize and articulate our knowing, and ask questions leading to new insights. As such, theories are . . . human inventions" (p. 7). The theories we invent and work from profoundly shape what we see, how we interpret what we see, and how we act.

According to Segaric and Hall (2005), one major contributing factor in nurses not integrating family nursing into their practice is the persistent lack of conceptual clarity in family nursing theory and the confusion around family and family nursing concepts. Similarly, Bauman (2000) contends that what is missing in the field of family nursing is the development of family theories specific to nursing. For example, when one looks historically at the evolution of family nursing, one sees that the field was developed using theories borrowed from the social sciences, biology, and psychotherapy. Writers in the field of family nursing have borrowed structural functional theory, developmental and family life cycle theory, family systems theory, symbolic interaction theory, family stress theory, structural determinism, and so forth to outline approaches to family nursing practice. While these theories can be helpful in understanding the phenomenon of family, Bauman asserts that we need family theories specific to nursing.

We believe what is most important is that you consider and enlist theories and other forms of knowledge that are most useful to your nursing practice at the point-of-care. Thus, the question orienting our discussion of family nursing throughout this book is: What can help us provide high-quality nursing care to people and families? We invite you to bring this pragmatic question to the contemporary nursing realities within which you work. As Rolfe (1998) contends, any nursing theory might be "out of touch with the needs and realities of clinical practice. . .[academics might be] generating theories and models which either have no relevance to practicing nurses, or else which are impossible to translate to practice" (p. 1317). Thus, the theories and frameworks we use and/or "invent" to inform our family nursing work need careful scrutiny.

Identifying the Views, Knowledge, and Theories Informing Your Practice

In this chapter specifically, we are inviting you to explore different ways of knowing family and wider possibilities for theorizing and responding as a family nurse. We'll consider how a relational consciousness expands your view—how it might help you to see family and family nursing with fresh eyes. But before setting out, it's important to know where you're starting from. Some core questions we invite you to consider include:

- What reference points am I using for my nursing practice, and how do those reference points limit my view of family?
- Are my current views of family and family nursing adequate given the people I care for and the nature of nursing work?
- Is the knowledge and theory I am enlisting to inform my actions supporting high-quality nursing practice?

To begin your consideration of family nursing in everyday practice, I invite you into my (Gweneth) cousin Janet's experience as she describes living through the loss of one child and the illness of another. Janet tells her story in her own words.

TO ILLUSTRATE

Janet's Living Family Experience

My name is Janet, and I am the mom of four boys. In 2005, we lost our second son to a tragic accident in our small community. He was 15. Our other sons were 17, 13, and 9 at the time. In true mama bear fashion, I did my due diligence. I read all the literature pertaining to grief and loss of a sibling. We went to counselors and attended grief groups. My kids were fairly "classic" in their responses to their brother's death. My 17-year-old son suffered survivor guilt, undertook risky behaviors, and had a hard time talking about his brother. In spite of this, he was able to complete high school and leave home to attend university. In February 2007, he experienced his first psychotic episode—translate that to mean that our whole family experienced his first episode.

continued on page 198

Since then, he has had successful work experiences, gone to university, played hockey, snowboarded, wakeboarded, and run a triathlon and a half marathon. He has attended weddings and funerals and family holidays. And he has had seven more admissions and three diagnoses (which frankly have not significantly altered the treatment plan).

He has had some amazing experiences with the health care system. Some amazingly wonderful—some amazingly horrible!

My son is a bright, athletic, musical, funny young man with family and friends who love him and want to support him. He has goals, aspirations, and dreams similar to any young man's. Again, when my son became ill, I did my due diligence and researched everything I could. Most everything I read suggested that people with strong family and friend support were the most likely to recover. Imagine my surprise then when during his hospital admission, I was told that I couldn't possibly be informed of how my son had slept because of the privacy act that governed the information the hospital was allowed to release. Imagine my surprise when the unit manager lectured me on the merits of the policy and why they could be sued if it was not strictly adhered to. Imagine my outrage when a nurse said, "Ma'am, you have no idea how many times I have 'wrestled' with your son to keep him from eloping from the hospital." No, I don't, because you won't even tell me how he slept.

To put this in perspective, at no time has my son ever asked for information to be withheld. In fact, at one point, his outpatient program had a signed consent to share information with us. When he relapsed and was admitted as an inpatient, we were told that the consent did not apply. This was within the same health district. And he was mute at the time, so he could neither give nor rescind consent.

My son is nothing if not clever. As a certified patient, he has eloped from an unlocked unit several times (left without permission). On each occasion, the onus was pretty much put on us to find him and return him. Imagine his 78-year-old granny finding him on her doorstep in hospital PJs miles from the hospital and having to walk him back into the unit with the police, and then to have no staff member even look up as they walked past the desk.

Imagine the bleakness of being told that our beautiful boy, the apple of our eye, was basically a "salvage operation."

These are true stories, and if they happened to my family, they have happened to others. I could go on, but now I would like to paint you some different pictures. Some of these things may seem small or even trivial but really, they are not; it takes very little to instill hope.

There was the time when a nurse stayed after her shift encouraging my son to take his injection. One time when I was concerned because I couldn't find my son, his social worker told me that he often stopped by

continued on page 199

TO ILLUSTRATE *continued*

Janet's Living Family Experience

the outpatient waiting room to read the newspaper and have a coffee. The social worker told me he would call me if he saw him, and he did. Being told that I can call anytime to see how he's doing is huge and actually makes [the staff's] job easier because it reduces the number of times I feel desperate to call.

One of my favorite stories is when a support staffer told me that my son has my smile. Firstly, it made me feel welcome. Secondly, it let me know that someone had made him smile!

Frankly guys, he was mine before he became yours, and he will be mine again. Please give us some tools in our toolbox to help him manage his goals so that he can have a meaningful role in life, no matter what that looks like. Help me (and all families) hold his hope for him until he can hold it for himself. If I could send one message with you, it would be this. Remember to treat each person as if he or she were your son, your daughter, your mother, or your dad.

My son is currently an inpatient in another health district. A few nights ago when I phoned to check on him, the nurse said, "Hi, Janet, I'm glad you called. Let me tell you about his day." Imagine how well I slept after that.

Janet's story highlights the multiple dimensions of any illness experience. Her story illustrates the way in which one person's illness is not just experienced by that individual. While Janet's son was the one with the diagnosed medical condition, the illness was a family experience. It also speaks to how, as nurses, we may see only one small snapshot of a much larger moving picture; whether a person or family is living with a chronic health challenge or experiencing an episodic illness, the diagnosis and treatment is only one small aspect of their living experiences, of their lives. Janet's examples of how seemingly minor things ("He has your smile," or "Good to hear from you") can make a profound difference to the well-being of a mother who lives in fear of losing another child and how other seemingly minor things (watching others see only "the mental patient" or "a salvage operation") can have an incredibly detrimental impact. While Janet's story speaks to many things, perhaps more than anything it speaks to the importance of stepping out of individualist ideology to see people and families in the midst of their experiences, to see beyond the label and beyond the designated "patient" to look at the living experience of family. As Bauman (2000) states, we need to move beyond thinking of nursing as a one-on-one service and the skin as the boundary of the client. People are relational beings whose experiences of health and healing are complex and multifaceted and intricately connected to others in their lifeworlds. Seeing people as distinct entities separate from one another does not allow us to see the intricate, living, relational whole of people and their illness situations.

As you consider Janet's story in light of the theories and models that inform your own nursing practice, ask yourself how adequate your knowledge and approach is. Bauman (2000) describes that ideally, family nursing theory needs to guide nurses "to consider families' quality of life as complex, changing and interwoven" (p. 289). Whether the health concern is some form of illness, an eating concern, exposure to health hazards, violence, addictions, or end-of-life issues, a family focus is essential (Bauman, 2000). Thus, within nursing, family "needs to be understood as a locus of meaning, purpose, and life-affirming rituals" (Bauman, 2000, p. 289). Yet often when I (Gweneth) ask nurses I teach to undertake an examination of their family nursing practice and the theories and reference points that inform that practice, they find themselves a bit disconcerted—both in terms of how they have and/or have not considered "family" in their practice and also in terms of what they have done or not done as a nurse given their limited understandings. In contrast to Bauman's description, many have not understood family as a locus of meaning (an important site where life meanings are lived and created) or considered family focus as essential to their nursing work. I (Colleen) have noticed that nurses are particularly challenged to see family as central to those in their care and to nursing practice when they work in settings where literal families often are not in the foreground or have limited direct effect on nursing work.

Within Janet's story, it is possible to see the importance of meaning and living experience and its impact on well-being. While Janet's son is the one with the illness, the entire family is living that illness experience. Yet how did the various nurses caring for Janet's family "see" that? Enlisting the hermeneutic phenomenologic (HP) and critical lenses from Chapter 2 and the relational understandings of context and culture, can you identify any filters that were narrowing their views?

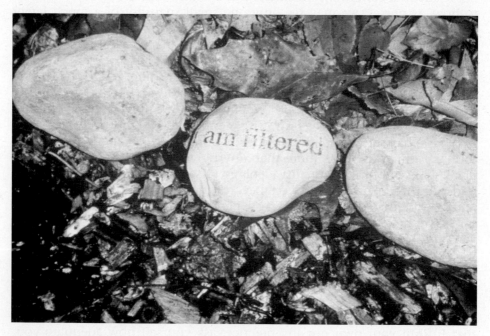

"I am filtered." (Leaves, rocks, and photo transfer by Connie Sabo.)

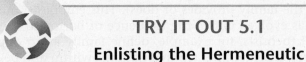

TRY IT OUT 5.1
Enlisting the Hermeneutic Phenomenologic and Critical Lenses

Reread Janet's story to enlist the HP and critical lenses you read about in Chapter 2. Can you see how Janet and the nurses were interpreting her son differently? How might Janet's background of losing a child shape her experience of being barred access? How might the meaning of her son leaving the unit in the middle of the night in a psychotic state be different to her than to the nurses?

How might the HP lens help us make sense of the differences among the nurses—that one saw Janet's son as a "salvage operation" while another noticed his smile; that one refused to give information while another offered it?

How might the critical lens help us to consider how the normative practices in health care and the larger society are shaping the care and treatment? For example, how might the stigma of mental illness be shaping how Janet's son is treated? If he suffered from asthma, do you believe that the privacy policy might be interpreted differently? How might a critical lens lead you to examine how nurses are enacting their power and operating within power relations that influence health care settings? Finally, what discourses of family (e.g., supportive families, difficult families) may be operating?

As you consider Janet's story, we invite you to think about your own nursing practice. How is your current nursing approach family oriented? Within Janet's words, you can hear quite clearly the difference among the various nurses and how their approaches resulted in different health experiences for Janet, her husband, children, 78-year-old parents, and for myself (Gweneth), since even the tone of my cousin's voice on the phone from 1,500 miles away conveys how the current health care reality is affecting her and her family's well-being.

As Janet identifies, research has shown that social support is one of the primary factors affecting the well-being of people living with mental health challenges. This is also the case for health in general (Thoits, 2011; Uchino, 2009; Umberson & Montez, 2010). With that in mind, how do you take family into consideration when caring for people? If your designated patient has no family involved, visible or known, do you ignore family, or do you extend your view to consider what other kinds of support might be important and available? If the person does have a literal family in view, do you extend yourself and include them in your "care" picture? How might you extend your view beyond existing conceptualizations of family to enable more responsive nursing practice? One way to start is to consider your definition of family.

WHAT IS FAMILY?

As we detailed in Chapter 1, traditionally, family nursing theorists have defined family in a literal sense—as a configuration of people who are connected in some way (e.g., legally, socially, biologically). The majority of definitions describe "family" according to structure (who is in the family) and function (what the family provides or does). This emphasis on structure and function has evolved out of the influence of borrowed theories. Structural-functional theorists, for example, define family as an open sociocultural system and focus on interactional patterns within and between families and other social systems (Friedman, Bowden, & Jones, 2003; Kaakinen et al., 2010). Systems theorists theorize family as a system of interacting parts (Wright & Leahey, 2012). How do *you* define family?

TRY IT OUT 5.2

The Meaning of Family

Try to find someone whose experience of family is different from your own and someone whose experience is similar to your own.

In preparation, spend a few minutes thinking about how you might go about this. What comes to mind with regard to how you might choose someone? For example, how would you identify someone who would potentially have had a different family experience than your own? What criteria of difference would you use? It may occur to you to choose someone from a different ethnic or racial background. However, are you sure that those characteristics would mean they had a different family experience? Is it possible that someone who looks different from you physically may have experienced family in ways closer to your own than someone who appears similar to you?

After you have decided how you will choose the two people, consider how you might approach them. How would you talk to them to come to know what family means for them and how they experience family? For example, looking through an HP lens, how would you engage in order to move the conversation beyond the factual description of the literal family to the experience of family? What questions might you ask? What questions would you ask if you were to enlist the critical lens to assist you? What questions might you pose, for example, to understand the economic and political circumstances of the person's family? How would you learn about how power played out within the family and between the family and wider circumstances?

After your conversation, discuss your findings with your classmates or colleagues. For example, it might be interesting to discuss how many people you each had to go through to find someone "similar" or "different." What were the differences? What were the similarities? How did the experience of talking with the person inform your understanding of family? What questions were raised for you? What were the surprises?

Family in Its Scripted Form Shapes Nursing Practice

When thinking about family in the context of nursing, it is important to consider how we script families—that is, how we think about and describe them to others. Often, normative ideologies about what constitutes a "good" family and an "unfortunate" or "not so good" family impact how we narrate and script people and families, the assumptions we make about their family experiences, and how we interpersonally relate to them. In Chapter 1, we described how media representations of family offer particular Eurocentric "truths" of family. For example, marketing people depict family (usually mom, dad, and the two children) as a warm, nurturing, safe haven, and they speak of "getting back to family values" as though all families share the same values (Doane, 2003).

When you've been bombarded by such images and value messages, how have they affected you? Have you begun to assume that these values and images are true? Do you expect families to function according to them? Do you view families who reflect these values and images as healthy, normal, and well-functioning? Do you view families who do not reflect them more negatively? If you were to listen to your language, would you find yourself using labels such as broken family, single-parent family, extended family, gay/lesbian family, and so forth?

It would be surprising if you haven't found yourself using these kinds of labels at some point, because many were coined by academic "experts" and are widely used among human service professionals. For example, recently I (Colleen) was working with nurses from the Nuu-Chah-Nulth Tribal Council (an indigenous government). One of the nurses said, "Extended family is *not* our word. All our nation is family. All are related— hishuckishtsawalk [everything is one]." This brought me up short. I realized that I use the term *extended family* in a way that is intended to distinguish it from nuclear family but ends up implying that the nuclear family is the norm. The nurse's challenge to this limiting practice drew my attention to the fact that having been taught the terms in nursing school, I had taken them up without question, assuming they were relevant to all people and families. Realizing the limitations of that distinction, I was inspired to inquire further into what I took for granted—what I thought I "knew"— and examine what I did *not know* about family for Nuu-Chah-Nulth people. In doing so, I could see how Nuu-Chah-Nulth people enacted family differently from my experience and that I have a limited understanding of the depth of those differences.

Given the multicultural, global community in which we live and the differing values, customs, and the variety of life experiences people have, what constitutes "family" and how it is experienced is diverse. A relational inquiry approach guides you to look beyond the labels, the dominant ideologies, the "normal" surface indicators, and "either/or" thinking of good/not good, privileged/disadvantaged, etc., so that your understandings of people and families may be broadened. For example, consider my (Gweneth) family of origin. My parents divorced when I was 6 years old, and my mother, with an eighth-grade education, raised me and my three siblings without my father. A nurse doing a risk assessment using surface indicators such as economics, social status, education, parent involvement, etc., could have described my family as broken, disadvantaged, single-parent, low-income, and/or high-risk. However, to really understand my family experience, a nurse would have had to look beyond these surface indicators. Because my mother had a very small income, we grew up in a very small house in a low-income neighborhood mostly populated by immigrant families. Family closeness was a given as was an intimate family relational experience that went beyond our nuclear family. The boundaries between our nuclear family and our extended family were permeable. My grandparents, aunts, uncles, and cousins were central people in my daily life. Similarly, while we did not have money for music lessons or any other activities, I just had to walk into any of my friends' homes to experience international cuisine and a rich array of different languages, traditions, and ways of being. Thus, living in a diverse community, my understanding of family was a constantly changing experience of different combinations of people and relations. To me, difference was normal. Thus, I found it intriguing to learn years later when I was in graduate school to become a psychologist that I had come from a "high-risk family" and had been a "disadvantaged child." What was even more interesting, however, was that as I practiced as a psychologist and worked with many people who had come from "good" families (according to dominant ways of thinking), I could see the ways in which some of their privileges had contributed to their current psychological challenges.

While there is no question that we live in an inequitable world and many people are profoundly disadvantaged compared to others, relational inquiry directs us to carefully consider the distinctions and judgments we are making about people and families. For example, when I (Gweneth) was raising my own three children in a two-parent family with many of the economic, social, and educational privileges that I never even knew existed when I was a child, I realized that, paradoxically, in some ways I had had a more privileged family and childhood experience than my three children were having. They did not have an extended family around that was rooted in a larger, multicultural community. We lived in a rather monochrome neighborhood compared to the textured neighborhood of my childhood. As such, they did not get to experience the rich diversity of people I had known as a child. Given these complexities, how do we determine what constitutes a disadvantage or a privilege? And what criteria are we using to distinguish between a healthy, "functional" family and an unhealthy, "dysfunctional" family? Moreover, what leads us to believe we have the right to use such disrespectful and judgmental labels as "dysfunctional" with any person or family?

TRY IT OUT 5.3

How Do You Script Family?

Take a few minutes and write a response to the following:
1. List four words that come to your mind when you think of the word "family" and three defining features of your "family."
2. Based on this reflection, what are two things you learned in your own family of origin that shape how you think of families? Can you think of other things that have influenced how you think of family (images in advertisements, the geographic areas in which you have lived, experiences with friends, etc.)?

continued on page 205

TRY IT OUT 5.3 *continued*
How Do You Script Family?

3.   Look at what you have written, and ask yourself, "What movie would I make about family?" Who would be the central characters? Who would be the star? What would the storyline be? Would there be heroes and heroines? Compare your movie with the movie you think someone else in your family would make.

4.   As you look over your responses to the above questions, consider how your personal view of family might be shaping your nursing practice. For example, what have you *not* been considering about people and families as you go about your nursing work? What questions have you *not* been asking or inviting? To what might you now pay more attention in order to enhance your ability to care for people and families?

Family as a Relational Living Experience

A number of years ago, I (Gweneth) was inspired to take a deeper look at how I was scripting family when I attended a conference where one of the keynote speakers was Ryan, a young man who was about 19 years old.

TO ILLUSTRATE
Five Minutes of Family

At the time of this presentation, Ryan was working with a grassroots initiative helping children who were currently living on the street to reconnect with mainstream society. At the beginning of his talk, Ryan discussed growing up in foster care, of eventually living on the street, and of what "made the difference" and helped him "get on with his life." While Ryan had many important insights to offer the professionals sitting in the audience, he particularly emphasized how vital each moment of connection was to a child who had never known deep connection. I was so struck by his words that I actually wrote them down:

> *"What do I know of love? I only know of unlove, being bought on a street corner, being given a cigarette by a guard to beat up another kid . . . Remember that connection with you might be the only experience of love that kid has ever had. Although a five-minute connection may not seem important to you, it has a different meaning to a kid who has never had anyone care. It can make a big difference."*[1]

---

[1] This story which has previously been published in *Nursing Philosophy* has been reprinted with permission from Blackwell Publishing.

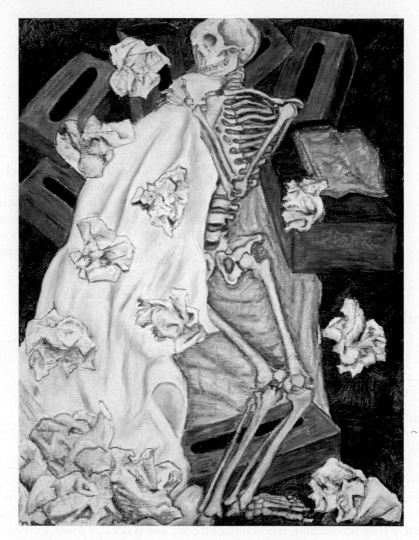

"Unlove." (Oil Bar on Rag Paper by Danaca Ackerson.)

As I listened to Ryan's words, I knew that the reason they were having such an impact on me was because they were echoing the deeper stirrings I had experienced about family and why I had actually oriented my nursing work toward family health promotion. Although Ryan had never had or known family in the literal sense, he was speaking of what I had come to know about family both as a person and in my work as a nurse. Ryan was speaking about what it is that makes actual families so vital.

Family is supposedly the societal medium through which people

- Are seen as individuals
- Experience that they matter and that other people matter
- Experience being loved and loving others
- Experience being valued and how to value others

- Experience a sense of belonging and connection to something more than themselves
- Are cared for and supported when they go through life-threatening or life-altering situations

However, Ryan was highlighting something deeper: the power of a loving connection, no matter how brief or who was involved. In essence, Ryan's story drew my attention to the fact that many people live in this world without a family and/or without a family's care. The awareness of these harsh realities moved me to think beyond family in its literal sense. Ryan said that although he had never lived or experienced an actual family, he still needed to experience deep, loving connection with others. He still required relational experiences where he had the opportunity to come to know that feeling of being seen and cared about, to learn how to care about and for others, to experience being part of the human family—to belong and be a part of something bigger. It was this *relational experience of connectedness and support* that was significant to his health and healing—not necessarily a literal family.

Certainly, what Ryan had to say was not new. It has been well documented through research that relational/social support promotes health (Thoits, 2011; Uchino, 2009; Umberson & Montez, 2010). However, as I listened carefully to Ryan's story and to my own resonance with what he was saying, I was able to more fully articulate my unease at the limitations of my own practice and the limitations of existing conceptual understandings of "family" in nursing. For example, I could see how thinking of family as a configuration of people was limiting my view. If my goal was to promote relational experiences of care and well-being for all of my patients, regardless of whether they had a literal family involved, I needed to change my reference point for my nursing practice.

Through the above experience, I revised the "theory" of family that was guiding my practice and the way I was scripting family. Theorizing "family as a relational, living experience" (Hartrick, 2002), I began to scrutinize my practice and ask myself how I might *support the opportunity for people to have that relational experience—to feel and have the experience of being cared for and about*. In doing so, I began paying more attention to each moment of nursing action as a potential relational, health-promoting experience. Looking beyond the individual in the bed or the family unit, my focus of attention became more consciously and intentionally relating to who was and was not in the room. For example, for individuals who did not have family involved in their lives, I became much more intentional in considering ways to respond to that "family situation." That entailed simple things like paying closer attention to how I interacted with the patients so they had relational experiences of feeling cared for and about as they laid in their hospital beds alone. I also extended my view to relate more consciously to present families and to consider the well-being of both individual family members and the family as a whole.

The field of family nursing has actually been developed based on the understanding that (a) families exert real effects on people, and those effects can be positive and/or negative; and (b) families are changeable, and so nurses should intervene to ensure families are as "healthy" as possible. However, Ryan's story draws attention to something beyond that understanding and approach—namely, the embodied, relational experience of family. Given that family is a central organizing structure for society, we are highly influenced by "family" regardless of the extent to which we are involved with a literal family; family is an experiential social reality. This means that by virtue of living in the world, we and our health experiences are highly influenced by our family experiences. Even when the experience of family is marked by absence, as it is with Ryan, the ideas and importance of family are always influential. Ryan's story draws attention to the importance of family in his life. He didn't have one. Given the responsibilities we bequeath to families, this absence had major implications for Ryan's health and well-being.

With what is happening in contemporary health care contexts, extending our definition of "family" in this relational way is becoming increasingly important. One simple example is how health care cutbacks have translated into strategies for early discharge. These strategies rest on the assumption that people have families to look after them while still in acute healing stages. They also assume that families are able, willing, and have the resources to do so. Regardless of who is in the room, my relational inquiry approach (and the HP and critical lenses I enlist as part of that approach) enables me to extend my proximal view to consider the contextual aspects and what other possibilities might be enlisted to provide support and care as people live through their illness situations. Intentionally practicing in this relational-inquiry way, one becomes more effective in meeting the nursing goal of promoting health and well-being for all.

Ryan's story challenges us to see the absence of family as integral to our nursing care. At the same time, we need to consider how literal families are integral to our nursing care. We invite you to pay close attention to how you are (and are not) fostering the experiences we hope people can have in actual families including

- The experience of being seen, being valued, and feeling of value
- The experience of learning about themselves in all of their complexity
- The experience of belonging and being cared about
- The experience of having the capacity and strength to cope with vulnerability and adversity
- The opportunity to develop their own relational capacities to nurture growth and wellness in themselves and in others

We also invite you to draw on discussions in Chapters 2 and 4 to help you consider and pay closer attention to the societal and health care norms and structures that are shaping your understandings of family and family nursing practice.

Regardless of who the designated patient is, a relational orientation enables us to extend our view and scrutinize how existing conceptualizations of family might be constraining us (Hartrick Doane & Varcoe, 2005b). This scrutiny is supported through intrapersonal, interpersonal, and contextual inquiry. Intrapersonally, what understandings of family are shaping you? What understandings of family can you see playing out and being promoted interpersonally? How does the context in which you live and work shape understandings of family?

Family is an integral experience to us all because it is a central structure within society. Yet, it can be quite an interesting experience to actually think about family and open up the space to see it with fresh eyes. For example, when talking with other people, it is possible to see just how much our own background shapes our understandings and views in addition to our interpretations of family. Yet, even if two people come from similar backgrounds, their experiences might not be the same. For example, two people may grow up in the same family, but differing circumstances that occur may result in one sibling having one family experience and another quite a different one. Or, as we explained in Chapter 4, people may be from the same ethnic/cultural group, yet differences of economics, education, language, and so forth can profoundly shape family experiences quite differently for any two people.

In this chapter, we are inviting you to try out this relational inquiry approach to family and family nursing—to "see" family nursing as relevant to all people (e.g., to see the absence of family as integral to your nursing care) and to also extend your view to actual families and family members to consider how they might be integral to your nursing care. We invite you to pay close attention to how you are (and are not) fostering the experiences we hope people can have in actual families. Questions for you to consider include: How might you foster people's and families' experiences of being seen, being valued, and feeling of value? How might you act to promote a sense of belonging and being cared about? How might you support people's and families' capacities and strengths to cope with vulnerability and adversity? How are the societal and health care norms and structures that are shaping understandings of family and family nursing practice constraining possibilities?

FAMILY NURSING AS A PRACTICE OF RELATIONAL INQUIRY

You now recognize that to promote well-being in any nursing situation, you need to consciously attune and respond to how family is being experienced and how it is affecting that particular nursing situation, including the health and well-being of those involved. Relational inquiry as an approach to nursing practice offers a way of doing that—a way of knowing, choosing, and enacting responsive, effective family nursing practice.

Simply put, *family nursing as relational inquiry supports you to consider the adequacy of your nursing approach in light of the purpose and commitments of everyday nursing at point-of-care.* Using a relational inquiry approach, you become conscious of the values, assumptions, theories, and other forms of knowledge that are informing your work as a nurse, and you check to ensure they are adequately aligned to the imperatives of nursing situations and the values and obligations toward which you are working (such as the well-being of people and families).

Looking with Fresh Eyes as You Practice

Taking a relational inquiry approach and theorizing family nursing in everyday practice through a relational orientation enables us to look with fresh eyes as we go about our everyday nursing work. Specifically, it extends the reference points for family nursing as well as the types of knowledge and the theories we enlist to inform our work. While many of the family nursing approaches that have been developed have much to offer, we believe that theorizing family and family nursing through a relational lens can further enrich family nursing practice. For example, existing models of family nursing tend to emphasize and provide direction for assessing *actual* families around numerous domains. Yet, that form of practice is not necessarily central to many nurses' work. In most health care settings, the designated patient is usually an individual as opposed to the family unit. Thus, those models are not necessarily aligned with the way practice is organized and enacted within many contemporary health care settings. Even in sites where "family-centered care" is espoused (e.g., in pediatric, maternal/child, community health, neonatal ICU), focused in-depth assessment of families is often not central to most nurses' work. Moreover, later in the chapter, we will be exploring how even in settings that espouse a "family-centered approach," the way family nursing is enacted may not be relationally responsive.

Given this contextual reality, rather than outlining available family nursing knowledge that you "should" know and use, we are focusing our attention on helping you consider point-of-care family nursing practice and how to enlist available knowledge to work effectively. What are the contexts in which you practice? Who are the people/families you care for in your practice setting? Inspired by pragmatism, we invite you to take a concerted look at the contemporary health care settings in which you work and to consider the varied forms your nursing care might need to take to respond to the needs and realities *of people and families* at point-of-care (Hartrick Doane & Varcoe, 2005a, 2005b). As we described in Chapter 1, relational inquiry is focused on both responding to the needs and realities of particular situations and acting to affect those situations—to produce situations of a desired kind. Further exploration into your own reference points for family nursing can support you to move beyond limited understandings of family and family nursing and more consciously choose theories and approaches that can support your family nursing action.

TRY IT OUT 5.4

Models of Family Nursing

A range of family nursing models is available to inform your practice. Here, we invite you to explore some of these considering their relevance to your own family nursing practice. As you look at the different models, ask yourself what *you* think of the different ways family nursing is understood and approached. How would the way family is conceptualized and understood in a particular model inform your own nursing action?

Go to the International Family Nursing Association website (http://nternationalfamilynursing.org/resources-for-family-nursing/practice/

continued on page 211

TRY IT OUT 5.4 *continued*

Models of Family Nursing

practice-models) and choose one specific model to explore. As you read about the model, consider the following questions:

- How is family defined?
- How does the model orient you as a nurse?
- Who is the designated client/patient?
- What does the model direct your attention toward?
- What does it take for granted or assume about family, health, and/or nursing?
- What does it lead you to question?
- What does it lead you to take for granted?
- What questions does it *not* lead you to ask?

Enlist the HP and critical lenses from Chapter 2 to help you expand your view and consider what else might need to be brought into the picture for you to be a responsive nurse. Next, think about your current or most recent practice context. Consider these questions:

- How does the model you chose align with the realities of that health care setting?
- How might the model expand your own practice within that setting?
- What would the model lead you to do differently?
- Are those actions responsive and the "best," given the nature and particularities of the patients in that setting? Are the actions the model outlines "adequate?"
- Are there aspects that would not be addressed?
- How does the model theoretically and/or practically align with the realities at point-of-care?
- Is there a fit between point-of-care imperatives and the model?
- What are the implications of that alignment/misalignment for your own understanding and practice of family nursing?

Bringing a Pragmatic Attitude to Family Nursing

Family nursing as relational inquiry differs somewhat from the majority of other family nursing approaches. As a form of practice, it is not grounded in a prescribed framework. Rather, it is grounded in an attitude and a way of relating, being, and proceeding. That is, it is grounded in a *way* of nursing. This way of nursing involves looking beyond categorical ways of thinking and prescribed indicators to attune to people and situations. It also involves enlisting *multiple* modes of inquiry, forms of knowledge, and relational strategies to look with fresh eyes at each situation. Deeply rooted in a pragmatic approach to theory and knowledge development, relational inquiry is an approach that seeks to not limit or confine our understanding of people/families and define some situations as family nursing situations and others as not, but to expand possibilities for understanding and action. With a relational inquiry approach, rather than practicing from one fixed model of family nursing, you engage in a pragmatic inquiry into people, situations, knowledge, and action. You continually ask yourself:

- Who is this person or family?
- What is informing and shaping my understanding intrapersonally, interpersonally, and contextually?
- Are our ways of describing families and family health/illness adequate to the situation and supporting us to be as responsive as possible?
- What understandings of family am I privileging?
- How adequate is my knowledge and practice for the situation at hand?
- Do available theories and the knowledge in use in this situation address and inform the situational concerns and challenges?
- What other knowledge might be helpful?

As such, relational inquiry enables you to open up to new theoretical possibilities rather than narrowing down or selecting one explanation or direction. Family nursing practice becomes a process of inquiry and choice as we purposefully question the adequacy of our knowledge and the action we and others are taking. In this way, family nursing becomes an embodied, reflexive process of responsive action. Below, Carie Semeniuk offers another story from her ICU experience, describing the impact of relational inquiry on her family nursing practice.

TO ILLUSTRATE

Black Socks and a Mother's Love

Last month, a young boy was admitted to ICU with an ecstasy overdose. His family showed up a day later and didn't seem very engaged in his care. I was frustrated with them and didn't understand how a mother could not be sitting crying at her son's bedside in this situation. Nurses were commenting about the lack of family support on shift handover and in rounds. I remember telling myself to take a step back and look at the situation without any preconceived ideas or feelings.

Later that day, I brought the mom in a cup of tea when she arrived at the bedside. I asked her how she was doing. She got up and left the room, leaving a black pair of socks on the bed. A few hours later, she came back into the room and asked me where the socks were. I explained I had put them on her son's feet as they felt cold. She noticed that and she grabbed my arm. She asked me if I had children and I said yes, I have two sons. She began telling me about her journey as a mother. Her son had been an addict since age 12 and had suffered from mental illness since age 6. He had stolen from them and abused her and his sister physically. Her marriage to her husband had ended as a result of the stress. Since age 6,

continued on page 213

TO ILLUSTRATE *continued*

Black Socks and a Mother's Love

---

he never allowed her to hug him or have any emotional connection; her only physical connection with him had been to put socks on his feet because they were always cold.

She cried and cried, and I sat there and listened. She was hurting, and I felt awful that I had judged her. I didn't know how her reaction in this situation was driven by the context of her life experiences with her son. I couldn't relate to her experience, or understand her ideas of family because of my own experience and beliefs. Her actions were "normal" to her, and her choices were constrained by her life circumstances.

Practicing under a relational inquiry approach enables me to accept differences and understand they are not always choices, just products of the context of people's lives. Not judging people because they are different from me and letting go of my own bias and preconceived ideas of normal has significantly improved my nursing practice. Connecting with patients and families across these differences has opened my eyes up to a whole new world. It has made me a better listener, has allowed me to be open to relationships that I would have never been open to before.

Carie's story illustrates how relational inquiry provided a grounding for her practice by ironically enabling her to step out of her "knowing" of family. As she looked beyond her own idea of what constituted a healthy family or a good mother, her eyes were opened "to a whole new world." Not only did her knowledge base expand (she gained knowledge and understanding that could inform her care of the family), but she was able to extend her own ability to respond and care for patients and families. Carie's story also points to the importance of viewing families' experiences as far more complex than the simple dichotomies of good/bad or nurturing/dysfunctional.

As Carie describes in her story, our theories and frameworks can at times actually limit our responsiveness as nurses. Relational inquiry offers a way of enabling us to theorize our practice in the midst of practice situations. It enables us to conceptualize family relationally and (a) focus on the consequences of ideas and theories, (b) draw upon multiple theories and knowledge perspectives examining their contradictions and complementary contributions in light of diverse people and families, and (c) remake our theory/practice in sync with the point-of-care nursing situations within which we find ourselves.

FAMILY NURSING PRACTICE IN CONTEXT

In Chapter 4, we emphasized the importance of understanding how context is relevant to your nursing actions. As part of that discussion, we examined how context is embedded and embodied in people, language, and actions and how context shapes the kind of nurse you strive to be, what you view as important, and the actions you take to meet your nursing obligations.

We have just explored how the societal context and your own particular sociohistorical background shape how you experience and relate interpersonally to family. At this point, we turn our attention to how the health care context shapes family nursing. Of particular importance is who is deemed to be the designated patient or client in your particular health care context. Given that nurses work across a variety of settings, the designated client varies. However, within the health care world, there are three particular discourses and models of care we feel it is important to examine when considering family nursing practice. These are family-centered care (FCC), patient-centered care (PCC), and person-focused care (PFC). We consider each in light of a relational inquiry family nursing approach.

Family-Centered Care

The FCC movement has its roots in pediatrics. It appears to date back to the 1950s and 1960s when researchers and clinicians started to look at the emotional and psychological impacts of separating children and infants from their mothers (Harrison, 2010). Shields (2010) explains that until the 1950s, parents were actually seen negatively when it came to care of hospitalized children, and there was routine exclusion of parents. (Does this resonate when you think about how you have seen family members treated in other health care settings?) It was not until researchers started to notice significant differences between infants and children separated from their mothers and those whose mothers were involved in their care that the relationship between children, parents, and health care professionals was reconsidered (Shields, 2010). This led to the introduction of FCC, which was broadly defined by the tenet that family is a constant in a child's life, whereas health care providers and systems fluctuate and are temporary.

Over time, FCC models have been refined and now include several elements such as that used by the American Academy of Pediatrics (AAP) (Committee on Hospital Care and Institute for Patient- and Family-Centered Care, 2012). These models include such things as the importance of respecting and honoring differences in families, collaborating in care, sharing information, providing support, and ensuring flexibility in access to services (Committee on Hospital Care & Institute for Patient- and Family-Centered Care, 2012; Gooding et al., 2011; Harrison, 2010). FCC is increasingly being taken up in maternity care, long-term care (Boise & White, 2004), and critical care settings (Davidson, 2009). Overall, FCC seems to be focused in clinical areas where designated patients are viewed as unable to advocate for themselves.

Franck and Callery (2004) suggest that "the major constructs of FCC common to all theoretical models are: Respect for the child and family; recognition of the importance of the family to the child's well-being; and partnership between the health care team and the child/family" (p. 270). However, at point-of-care, there is great variation in how these abstract constructs are interpreted and operationalized (Franck & Callery, 2004; Shields, 2010). For example, although there is apparent consensus about the value of FCC in pediatric care, it is implemented in different ways across different settings. Franck and Callery (2004) offer the example of parental involvement; in some hospitals, parental involvement means merely allowing parents to be present, whereas in other settings, it means expecting parents to perform nearly all of the child's routine care. The care of the parent and family also varies in practice and in the conceptual literature. Despite FCC principles being encouraged since the 1950s, unclear conceptual definitions and inconsistent implementation of FCC remains (Franck & Callery, 2004, p. 265). Moreover, Shields (2010) observes that "while FCC seems ideal and is found in a plethora of policies and documents . . . no rigorous evidence exists about its benefits (or otherwise)" (p. 2630). Given the lack of theoretical clarity and the lack of empirical evidence that FCC is feasible and/or even ethical, Shields (2010) raises the following questions: (1) Is FCC relevant now? (2) Is it relevant only in Western countries? (3) What does it mean to implement FCC? (4) Is FCC implemented effectively? (5) Does it make a difference? (p. 2632).

Our own experience as nurses has also led us to question whether FCC is always relationally responsive and positive for families. For example, Shields (2010) cites research in which parents felt pressure from health care providers to provide care for their children in the hospital but were not able to do so because of work or other commitments. Some parents did not feel comfortable interacting with the health care staff. In short, a rigid implementation of the FCC approach in some settings may actually serve to reduce responsive care since generalized policies that set parameters on how families "should" be involved may not be equitable and/or responsive to a particular family's situation.

To actually be family-centered, this can often be challenging given the competing interests that may be at play. For example, while ensuring families who want to provide care to their loved one is responsive and health-promoting, expecting all families to do so and/or downloading care to family members under the appearance of being "family-centered" is an area of growing concern. For example, Shields (2010) refers to research done in countries where parents participated in care, not by choice, but because of insufficient staffing. While parental involvement in decision making and care planning is important, socioeconomic factors such as class, employment realities, and so forth shape how parents are included—with health care providers at times assuming that less educated parents may not have sufficient understanding to participate in the decision-making process (Shields, 2010). Even in Nordic countries where FCC is considered to be well implemented, parents still found it challenging to negotiate care with health care staff (Shields, 2001). Similarly, in a multicountry study (Shields, Hallstrom, & O'Callaghan, 2003), major differences occurred between parents and health care providers in terms of what parents needed. Shields (2010) highlights the disconnect between what clinicians feel is FCC and what parents actually experience.

FCC within the context of maternity settings in a Canadian setting has also been questioned. For example, researchers interviewed women and compared their experiences to the philosophy of FCC that maternity care systems supposedly practiced (Jimenez, Klein, Hivon, & Mason, 2010). Titling their findings "The mirage of change," the researchers describe the disjuncture between women's experiences and the FCC model. In particular, the researchers concluded that women's birth experience "continues to be undermined by a system of care that does not prioritize women's informed choice" (p. 166). While the FCC approach has tended, in theory, to emphasize the welcoming of family into the experience and mitigate the medicalization of birth in the institutional setting (and some maternity units have labor rooms that look more like hotel rooms complete with double beds to create a "home-like" environment), less attention is paid to what this means beyond the elimination of visiting hours and nice wallpaper. As Jimenez and colleagues describe, the most important factor in true FCC is the relational process between women/families and caregivers and how that relational process supports shared, informed decision making, knowledge, and choices.

Kelly Gray, a nurse who has worked in a range of settings that espouse FCC models of care, describes her experience in the next "To Illustrate" box.

TO ILLUSTRATE
Kelly's Experience of Family-Centered Care

Having been a nurse in women's and infant health for just over 15 years, I have seen the FCC model become the standard in the field. While the FCC model is widely accepted, the challenge lies in the interpretation of the model and in implementation. Working in different regions and settings across the United States and Canada has given me a snapshot of various ways this model is taken up. For some, FCC meant newly renovated "home-like" rooms to minimize the medicalized feeling of birthing in a hospital. Thus, rooms were created complete with beds for partners or support people so that the family could remain together, visiting hours were eliminated, and increased support was provided for "alternative" birth plans (e.g., water birth). For others, the FCC model began and ended at the décor, and still for others, despite challenges of physical layout and resource restraints, the FCC philosophy was fully embraced by a change in how nurses oriented their practice and related to women and families.

Perhaps one of the biggest questions in implementation of FCC (at least in my clinical area of obstetrics/maternity) is that of what constitutes shared decision-making. While shared decision-making is an espoused tenet of FCC, I have found that women are often given "choices" within a very small range of options—options that are acceptable to the care providers. For example, since "risk" is something that obstetric care providers (nurses and physicians alike) define according to their own values and norms, the choices women are presented with most often fall within the acceptable range of risk that the care provider is willing to take on. So if a particular family's values are different from those of the health care provider, their preferences may be excluded from the decision-making options.

While questions about the FCC model had arisen in my nursing practice, my personal experience has also led me to really think hard about FCC. It was during my first pregnancy that the stark difference between the standard obstetrical care that I'd worked within and what I was experiencing as a patient in a midwifery practice showed me the limitations

continued on page 217

TO ILLUSTRATE *continued*

Kelly's Experience of Family-Centered Care

of FCC as it is currently enacted. Being cared for by a midwife, "routine" tests and exams were all discussed prior to being ordered. They were presented to my partner and I as recommendations but by no means were they presented as required or mandatory. We were given time to talk, ask questions, and discuss the impact of results—what we would learn from this routine exam, what were the benefits, what were the challenges. No longer were my opinions "nice to haves;" they were seen as integral to my care. I was given choice and control over my care.

The differences I noted three years ago with my first baby are now heightened all the more as I have been receiving "shared care"—care by both a midwife and an obstetrician—as I'm expecting twins. I now have a unique vantage point of watching and experiencing two systems, both of which would, I am sure, pronounce themselves FCC advocates. Outside of the differences that come from a system that views birth as a normal physiologic process and one that is trained to respond to abnormal processes, there are often subtle ways in which I have noted differences when it comes to FCC or women-centered care. For example, each prenatal visit requires that a woman's weight and presence or absence of protein and glucose in the urine be assessed. In the midwife's office, I do this myself; I am seen as capable and competent to weigh myself and dip my own urine in the privacy of the bathroom. At the obstetrician's office, I am handed a little paper cup and asked to go to the washroom out the door, around the corner, and down a corridor and then carry my little paper cup all the way back and through the waiting room to the office assistant who will then dip my urine before taking me into the exam room where she will weigh me on a scale that says, "Do not touch scale, ask for assistance"—very small acts but significant in meaning.

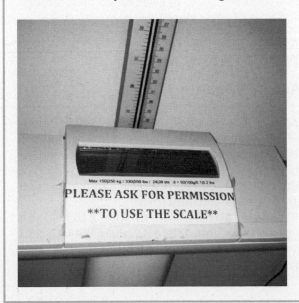

Do not touch.

continued on page 218

TO ILLUSTRATE *continued*

Kelly's Experience of Family-Centered Care

My personal experiences of FCC have led me to consider the implications for my current practice in the area of infertility. Granted, the field is very unique. First, many of the decisions that women and couples undertake are what are known as patient preference-sensitive decisions. In other words, there is not a medical imperative to choose treatment; a woman or couple can choose to forgo treatment or to opt for less or more aggressive treatments. Second, infertility treatment is not usually covered by health insurance, creating a for-profit business model which in most regions is quite competitive. This, in many ways I think, has influenced the evolution of the way we deliver care. Though the FCC tagline is not used, clinics had to become more responsive to patients' requests and wishes to include their partners in treatments. Recently, the literature in the field has started to adopt the PCC language with studies coming out of Europe, outlining ways for clinics to be more patient-centered including the very business-motivating finding that the number one reason women switched clinics was a lack of PCC—and that women would even be willing to sacrifice pregnancy rates for improved PCC. These studies have only come out in the past year but it will be interesting to see how this will impact care delivery in the field. One of the most frequent concerns I hear from patients is the way the fertility treatment "takes over your life" and the ways it becomes "regulated" and "scheduled to the nth degree." Perhaps a more PCC approach could work to individualize the treatment process more—daily blood tests at 0600 or 0900 instead of the very strict 0730 and personal health records so women could access their treatment information when they wanted. I wonder if in 15 years' time, I'll be having the same reflections.

TRY IT OUT 5.5

Acts of Meaning

In her description, Kelly describes how "small acts" conveyed a fundamental difference in how FCC was implemented between her midwife and obstetrician. Reread Kelly's description of urine testing and how it was handled differently in the different settings. Also reread her description of how profit-oriented infertility clinics have been responsive to families and compare that to the obstetrical settings she describes.

As you read, enlist the HP and critical lenses from Chapter 2 to help you look beneath the surface to consider the different values, beliefs, and assumptions that underpin the different forms of practice. How has practice been shaped by the fact that only those families with considerable

continued on page 219

> ### TRY IT OUT 5.5 *continued*
>
> ### Acts of Meaning
>
> economic resources (which intersect with social resources) can access fertility technologies? How might the two forms of obstetrical practice be experienced differently by different people?
>
> For example, looking through an HP lens you might notice how Kelly's description of what the two different approaches were like for *her* stands out. "*In the midwife's office, I do this myself; I am seen as capable and competent to weigh myself and dip my own urine in the privacy of the bathroom.*" Kelly's words reveal the *meaning* she made of the midwife's approach; it helped her feel capable and competent. Yet, might that same approach be experienced differently or have different meaning for someone else who is not a nurse and/or is not familiar with handling urine or wanting the responsibility to test the urine for protein? Similarly, how might the approach at the obstetrician's office where people are "*handed a little paper cup and asked to go to the washroom out the door, around the corner, and down a corridor, and then [asked to carry the] little paper cup all the way back and through the waiting room to the office assistant*" be experienced differently depending on people's sociocultural backgrounds?
>
> Consider how the HP and critical lenses might assist you in each of these settings to provide responsive FCC. For example, what would you need to consider, and what questions would you want to ask patients who came to the midwife's office to ensure FCC? Similarly, how might you make the approach at the obstetrician's office more family-centered? How would you analyze the influence of the population served by the different practices—for example, in Kelly's context, primarily highly educated urban women access midwifery. How might the lenses help you modify your own approach to be as responsive as possible in FCC situations?

Patient-Centered Care

A second discourse and model of care that is contextually relevant to how patient/family nursing is delivered (or not) is PCC. The patient-centered discourse spans a range of contexts and is touted as the goal in a number of differing initiatives in health care. Kitson, Marshall, Bassett, and Zeitz (2013) describe how national and international health organizations and lobby groups are all emphasizing the philosophy and practice of PCC "as being the core of new and effective models of care delivery" (p. 5). For example, in primary care, there is an emerging concept in the United States and Canada called the "primary care medical home," which refers to a patient-centered primary care model (Rittenhouse, 2009). A PCC orientation has been used to design a more patient-focused transfer process in emergency settings (Cronin-Waelde & Sbardella, 2013). Similarly, there are organizational/administrative strategies aimed toward improving PCC (Abdelhadi & Drach-Zahavy, 2012) and informatics strategies such as designing electronic medical records to reflect PCC (Krist Ah, 2011; Reti, Feldman, Ross, & Safran, 2010).

However, as with FCC, although there is an implicit assumption that everyone agrees on the core elements of PCC, there is actually wide variance in how PCC is understood and implemented (Kitson et al., 2013). From a review of the literature, Kitson and colleagues (2013) found three main elements underlying a PCC approach to care: (a) patient participation and involvement, (b) a collaborative relationship between the patient and health care provider, and (c) the context in which care is delivered. This research also revealed that as with the FCC approach, making PCC a reality at point-of-care is a challenge.

Considering PCC in light of family nursing, what is significant is how PCC discussions are often quite distinct from discussions of FCC. Although some of the pediatric literature on PCC incorporates the family in order to put the child more in the center of the care process (Rosen, 2012), "the family" is noticeably absent from PCC discussions. Often, PCC simply means personalized medicine and, as such, focuses attention on moving from generalized care to personalized care of an individual with a disease condition. The PCC discourse also emphasizes a consumer approach to health care aimed at improving patient satisfaction. Thus, in reading the PCC literature, it is possible to see the underpinnings of individualist ideology. Since you may work in a context where PCC is the organizing and espoused model of care, it is important to consider how this ideology is shaping your practice. Moreover, how might taking a relational inquiry approach enable you to modify your own actions to attend to family when practicing within a PCC context?

Person-Focused Care

Within the discussions of PCC, there is another term, person-focused care (PFC), that at times is used in tandem with PCC and at other times used very distinctly (Starfield, 2011). Providing an overview of the differences in these two terms, Starfield contends that PCC most often centers on the management of diseases whereas PFC considers disease and illness as part of the life-course experience with health. Starfield states that (a) whereas PCC privileges professionally defined conditions, PFC allows for specification of health concerns by the people living with those concerns, and (b) whereas PCC is concerned with the evolution of the disease, PFC is concerned with people's illness experience and the disease process. In a similar vein, Slater (2006) asserts that the key difference between PCC and PFC is in the implication of patient or client. This author argues that "patient" is a reductionist view through which a person is reduced to his or her illness or disease, while PFC allows for a broader view of the whole person.

Implications for Point-of-Care Family Nursing

While the discussions in the literature and the distinctions that are being drawn between FCC, PCC, and PFC are interesting, what is far more important is the implications of these discourses for point-of-care nursing practice. Specifically, what stands out from the research related to all of these discourses and the models of care they give rise to is the awareness that what clinicians view as family-centered or patient-centered may not be what patients and families experience, want, or need (MacKean, Thurston, & Scott, 2005). Also, when these models are implemented, there is often no explicit look at relationships of power and the power inherent in any prescribed model of care. For example, if you consider Kelly's description of the way urine testing is done in the midwife's office and how it is done in the obstetrician's office, power is a central consideration. On the surface, it would seem that the midwife is equalizing the power relation and supporting women to be more in charge by testing their own urine. Yet, that well-intentioned approach may not be *experienced* as power-generating for a woman who may not want to participate in that way. This leads to a central working principle underlying relational inquiry practice—namely, "it all depends." For example, while any approach may have the intention of interrupting the traditional power hierarchy and support more shared decision making and so forth, given the diversity of people and families, one cannot assume that simply adopting a model and changing policies will accomplish that. To be truly FCC requires that the particularities of people and families be considered. This is where relational inquiry comes in. Given that you work in health care contexts where practice is organized in differing ways—ways that are variously responsive to the needs of particular people and families—relational inquiry supports you to critically consider how the goals and values of responsive, health-promoting care are being supported and to make ongoing adjustments to your approach in order to support effective, high-quality care.

Working *with* People and Families

So how does one best care for people and families when illness has disrupted their everyday life? Within contemporary health care settings, a large amount of our nursing work with people and families occurs when they are experiencing extenuating circumstances that have challenged their everyday lives. Given that reality, there are four particular imperatives: (a) joining people and families on the "roller coaster," (b) including family in the care picture, (c) recognizing and acknowledging the caregiving work families are doing, and (d) asking what support a particular person or family might need.

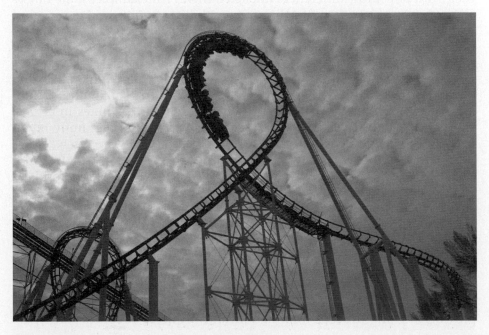

Roller coaster.

Nelms and Eggenberger (2010) describe how many families use the roller coaster metaphor when describing their experience of illness. In acute care, people and families may be in the midst of an acute illness situation. One family member may be requiring some form of medical intervention, and you may interact with other family members as part of that care process. Similarly, in residential settings, the nature of your interactions will vary depending on whether family members live in the same city, how often they visit, and so forth. The amount of time you spend with people and families may be brief or lengthy. So how will you know how best to care for them? As they live in the midst of uncertainty, confusion, and vulnerability, as they grapple with how to cope with the unknown outcomes of treatments, vacillating symptoms, doubts about treatment decisions, unexpected events, and so forth (Nelms & Eggenberger, 2010), one important question to ask yourself is: How might I be with them on the roller coaster in ways that are as responsive and health-promoting as possible? (The five Cs we described in Chapter 3 can be helpful here.)

Another central imperative is to see family as part of the care picture; whether there is a present family or not, family needs to be considered. For example, earlier in the chapter, you read Janet's story of living with a chronic mental health challenge and how the nurses' responses to her made such a difference. Similar to Janet's description, in their research into families' experience of having a loved one in the ICU, Nelms and Eggenberger (2010) describe how important the nurse's response was to family members during a critical illness. "As one family said, 'We've had kind of bad experience with a nurse, and after we talked about it, we realized that she was there for John [the patient], but we didn't feel she was there for us. I guess that is part of her job to be there for him and take care of him, but what about remembering that we are there too!'" (p. 472). Within this research, the families described significant differences between how nurses treated them and how those differences impacted them. For example, some nurses allowed open access, were "forthcoming with information, and never asked family members to leave no matter what the official visiting policy stated; others kept the family members waiting for long periods of time and were reticent to share information" (p. 162).

As you include family in the care picture, it is also imperative that you recognize and acknowledge the caregiving work actual families are doing within the illness situation. In their research with families in critical care areas, Vandall-Walker & Clark (2011) found that while family members tend to be scripted as bystanders at the bedside, they are often "working" hard. Family members work as monitors, decision-makers, advocates, and providers of direct care, and they work to provide numerous forms of support (emotional, economic, legal, etc.) (Vandall-Walker & Clark, 2011). Nelms and Eggenberger (2010) describe that on top of all of this caregiving work, families also felt they had to work hard to make connections with nurses. That is, family members intentionally worked hard to be seen in a good light by nurses by being courteous, accommodating, and diplomatic in order to ensure good care for their loved ones.

Along the same vein, Vandall-Walker and Clark's (2011) research found that families have to "work" to break down barriers put up by health care providers, "work" to access information, and "work" to be able to participate in the care process. How do you collaborate with families in the caregiving work? Do you consider yourself to be the primary caregiver or the only person providing care? Do you look to see what kind of care the "patient" and/or the family members are providing and/or are wanting? Vandall-Walker and Clark (2011) describe that often the most compelling need for many family members is to be able to be there for and with their ill relative. They also described the tension between the need to be there for the ill person and simultaneously look after themselves. While being with the ill person over long periods of time was costly to their own health, their willingness to leave and care for their own health was dependent on their feeling confident in the care being provided to the ill person (Vandall-Walker & Clark, 2011).

Similarly, ensuring that family is considered in the care picture also needs to happen when there is no literal family. How often are people discharged home with no support (instrumental or otherwise)? Considering resources that a person without family might need and exploring options with that person given the health/illness situation is an important aspect of "family nursing" care.

Overall, it is imperative that as a nurse you consider the well-being of all people involved in any nursing situation. For example, is the person alone and without family? Do family members want to be involved in the care of their ill loved one but are not sure how? Are family members struggling with the unknown and in need of information? Do they need their own suffering and vulnerability acknowledged? Do they need to inform you to ensure you are knowledgeable enough to offer good care? Some family members may have been caring for their relative with a chronic illness condition for several years and need to ensure you are aware of that person's specific routines and preferences. Similarly, some families may have specific practices that are important to them. For example, in their research into public health nursing, Falk-Raphael and Betker (2012) describe how a nurse on a new baby visit was concerned about care because the baby's head had not been washed. It was only on further inquiry that the nurse learned that not washing the head for a period of time after birth was an important cultural practice for the family.

A relational inquiry approach to family nursing helps you see people and families in their contexts, avoid simplistic assumptions, and take multiple and diverse influences into account as you provide care. Earlier in the chapter, you read Carie Semeniuk's stories of working in the ICU and how taking a relational inquiry approach in her practice changed the way she worked as a nurse. Reflecting on that change, Carie writes:

> I always knew my values and beliefs were my own and a reflection of my life and experiences. I never realized the impact that had on my nursing career. When examining my practice, I realized I assume what I deem as normal is just that—"normal." I assume families should behave in a certain way when losing a loved one; this belief stems from my values and how I would behave. Learning about relational inquiry, I understand now that it is OK to have differences. It is connecting across these differences that matters.

Taking a relational inquiry approach moves us beyond thinking we know or have to know. It helps us extend our knowledge and action by specifically turning family nursing and action into a question. How is family relevant in this particular situation? Who do I need to include in my care? How might I need to extend my view? What would be the most responsive and effective action? We will continue to explore these questions throughout the coming chapters.

THIS WEEK IN PRACTICE
Who Is the Designated Patient?

This week, undertake an inquiry in your clinical setting. If you are not currently working in a clinical setting, think back to the most recent setting in which you worked as a nurse. The focus of your inquiry is to observe who the "unit of care" is and how you work in concert with that contextual reference point. Is the unit of care the individual with a specific medical diagnosis (e.g., is the appendectomy the unit of care)? How is "family" worked with or not? How does the specific setting within which you are working shape who *you* deem the client to be and how *you* understand and approach "family?" How is the "family nursing" handled or not? Does the usual degree of presence or absence of literal family make a difference? Represent the "unit of care" and its relation to "family" visually, if you can. Share your observations with another nurse.

YOUR RELATIONAL INQUIRY TOOLBOX

Add the following tools to your relational inquiry toolbox.
- Look to see how family is being scripted (by you, by social norms, by the particular health care context).
- Check how aligned your family nursing actions are to the specific needs of patients and families at point-of-care.
- Scrutinize the adequacy of your family nursing theories and models in light of your point-of-care practice.
- See family in every nursing care picture.
- Scrutinize how your particular health care setting is limiting or supporting responsive family nursing practice.

REFERENCES

Abdelhadi, N., & Drach-Zahavy, A. (2012). Promoting patient care: Work engagement as a mediator between ward service climate and patient-centred care. *Journal of Advanced Nursing, 68*(6), 1276–1287.

Bauman, S. (2000). Family nursing: Theory-anemic, nursing theory-deprived. *Nursing Science Quarterly, 13*(4), 285–290.

Boise, L., & White, D. (2004). The family's role in person-centered care: Practice considerations. *Journal of Psychosocial Nursing and Mental Health Services, 42*(5), 12–20.

Committee on Hospital Care & Institute for Patient- and Family-Centered Care. (2012). Patient- and family-centered care and the pediatrician's role. *Pediatrics, 129*(2), 394–404.

Cronin-Waelde, D., & Sbardella, S. (2013). Patient-centered transfer process for patients admitted through the ED boosts satisfaction, improves safety. *ED Management, 25*(2), 17–20.

Davidson, J. E. (2009). Family-centered care: Meeting the needs of patients' families and helping families adapt to critical illness. *Critical Care Nurse, 29*(3), 28–34.

Doane, G. A. (2003). Through pragmatic eyes: Philosophy and the resourcing of family nursing. *Nursing Philosophy, 4*(1), 25–32.

Duhamel, F. (2010). Implementing family nursing: How do we translate knowledge into clinical practice? Part II: The evolution of 20 years of teaching, research, and practice to a Center of Excellence in Family Nursing. *Journal of Family Nursing, 16*(8), 8–25.

Falk-Rafael, A., & Betker, C. (2012). The primacy of relationships: A study of public health nursing practice from a critical caring perspective. *Advances in Nursing Science, 35*(4), 315–332.

Franck, L. S., & Callery, P. (2004). Re-thinking family care across the continuum of children's health care. *Child: Care, Health and Development, 30*(3), 265–277.

Friedman, M. M., Bowden, V. R., & Jones, E. G. (2003). *Family nursing: Research, theory and practice* (5th ed.). Upper Saddle River, NJ: Prentice Hall.

Gooding, J. S., Cooper, L. G., Blaine, A. I., Franck, L. S., Howse, J. L., & Berns, S. D. (2011). Family support and family-centered care in the neonatal intensive care unit: Origins, advances, impact. *Seminars in Perinatology, 35*(1), 20–28.

Harrison, T. M. (2010). Family-centered pediatric nursing care: State of the science. *Journal of Pediatric Nursing, 25*(5), 335–343.

Hartrick, G. A. (2002). Beyond polarities of knowledge: The pragmatics of faith. *Nursing Philosophy, 3*(1), 27–34.

Hartrick Doane, G. A., & Varcoe, C. (2005a). *Family nursing as relational inquiry: Developing health-promoting practice.* Philadelphia: Lippincott Williams & Wilkins.

Hartrick Doane, G. A., & Varcoe, C. (2005b). Toward compassionate action: Pragmatism and the inseparability of theory/practice. *Advances in Nursing Science, 28*(1), 81–90.

Jimenez, V., Klein, M. C., Hivon, M., & Mason, C. (2010). A mirage of change: Family-centered maternity care in practice. *Birth, 37*(2), 160–167.

Kaakinen, J. R., Harmon Hanson, S., & Denham, S. (2010). Family health care nursing: An introduction. In J. R. Kaakinen, V. Gedaly-Duff, D. Padgett Coehlo, & S. Harmon Hanson (Eds.), *Family health care nursing.* Philadelphia: F. A. Davis.

Kitson, A., Marshall, A., Bassett, K., & Zeitz, K. (2013). What are the core elements of patient-centered care? A narrative review and synthesis of the literature from health policy, medicine and nursing. *Journal of Advanced Nursing, 69*(1), 4–15.

Krist Ah, W. S. H. (2011). A vision for patient-centered health information systems. *Journal of the American Medical Association, 305*(3), 300–301.

MacKean, G. L., Thurston, W. E., & Scott, C. M. (2005). Bridging the divide between families and health professionals' perspectives on family-centered care. *Health Expectations, 8*(1), 74–85.

Nelms, T. P., & Eggenberger, S. K. (2010). The essense of family critical illness experience and nurse-family meetings. *Journal of Family Nursing, 16*(4), 462–486.

Parker, M. E., & Smith, M. C. (2010). *Nursing theories and nursing practice* (3rd ed.). Philadelphia: Davis Plus.

Reti, S. R., Feldman, H. J., Ross, S. E., & Safran, C. (2010). Improving personal health records for patient-centered care. *Journal of the American Medical Informatics Association, 17*(2), 192–195.

Rittenhouse, S. S. M. (2009). The patient-centered medical home: Will it stand the test of health reform? *Journal of the American Medical Association, 301*(19), 2038–2040.

Rolfe, G. (1998). The theory-practice gap in nursing: From research-based practice to practitioner-based research. *Journal of Advanced Nursing, 28*, 672–679.

Rosen, P. (2012). A paradigm in pediatrics to deliver family and child-centered care. *International Journal of Person Centered Medicine, 2*(4), 878–882.

Segaric, C. A., & Hall, W. A. (2005). The family nursing theory-practice gap: A matter of clarity? *Nursing Inquiry, 12*(3), 210–218.

Shields, L. (2001). *The delivery of family-centred care in hospitals in Iceland, Sweden and England: A report for The Winston Churchill Memorial Trust*. Retrieved from http://www.churchilltrust.com.au/res/File/Fellow_Reports/Shields%20Linda%202000.pdf

Shields, L. (2010). Questioning family-centered care. *Journal of Clinical Nursing, 19*(17–18), 2629–2638.

Shields, L., Hallstrom, I., & O'Callaghan, M. (2003). An examination of the needs of parents of hospitalized children: Comparing parents' and staff's perceptions. *Scandinavian Journal of Caring Sciences, 17*, 176–184.

Slater, L. (2006). Person-centredness: A concept analysis. *Contemporary Nurse: A Journal for the Australian Nursing Profession, 23*(1), 135–144.

Starfield, B. (2011). Is patient-centered the same as person-focused care? *The Permanente Journal, 15*(2), 63–69.

Thoits, P. A. (2011). Mechanisms linking social ties and support to physical and mental health. *Journal of Health and Social Behavior, 52*(2), 145–161.

Uchino, B. N. (2009). Understanding the links between social support and physical health: A life-span perspective with emphasis on the separability of perceived and received support. *Perspectives on Psychological Science, 4*(3), 236–255.

Umberson, D., & Montez, J. K. (2010). Social relationships and health: A flashpoint for health policy. *Journal of Health and Social Behavior, 51*(1S), S54–S66.

Vandall-Walker, V., & Clark, A. M. (2011). It starts with access! A grounded theory of family members working to get through critical illness. *Journal of Family Nursing, 17*(2), 148–181.

Wright, L. M., & Leahey, M. (2012). *Nurses and families: A guide to family assessment and intervention* (6th ed.). Philadelphia: F. A. Davis.

6 Ways of Knowing to Support Relational Inquiry

LEARNING OBJECTIVES

By engaging with the material in this chapter, you will be able to:

1. Explain relational inquiry as a process that both supports and requires different ways of knowing and different forms of knowledge.

2. Compare an objective Cartesian view of knowledge with a relational view.

3. Explain why both knowing and not knowing are integral to safe, competent nursing practice.

4. Explain how the HP and critical lenses can enhance knowing and not knowing within relational inquiry.

5. Explain how knowing and not knowing can be practiced at intrapersonal, interpersonal, and contextual levels.

6. Articulate key questions to be used with four interrelated modes of inquiry and forms of knowledge: empirical, ethical, aesthetic, and sociopolitical.

7. Explain how to integrate multiple modes of inquiry and forms of knowledge into nursing practice.

In this chapter, we explore how relational inquiry is a process that both supports and requires different ways of knowing and different forms of knowledge. Contrasting the Cartesian and relational views of knowledge, we briefly explore how knowing and not knowing can work together to broaden our knowledge base. We explore the specific ways of knowing that have been discussed in the nursing literature, illustrating how these differing ways of knowing produce different kinds of knowledge—all of which are required for nursing practice. As we examine the practice of knowing, we ask you to think about the nature of knowledge and how you relate to knowledge so that you might more effectively choose and respond in practice. Assuming a relational orientation and enlisting the hermeneutic phenomenologic (HP) and critical lenses, we consider the continuous ongoing process of knowing/ not knowing at the intrapersonal, interpersonal, and contextual levels.

APPROACHES TO KNOWLEDGE AND KNOWING

In Chapter 4, we contrasted a relational understanding that considers the body and mind to be inseparable, with the "Cartesian" view that considers the body and mind to be separate entities (the mind is the distinct knowing aspect of people). In this chapter, we build on that discussion to consider the differences between an objective Cartesian view and a relational view of knowledge more generally, showing how nursing requires approaches to knowledge beyond the Cartesian view.

A Cartesian View of Knowledge

A Cartesian epistemology (theory of knowledge) has underpinned much of Western science and thus has had a strong influence on how we think about knowledge and knowing within the health care world. Cartesian epistemology emphasizes empirical study (research that relies on observation) and has served to generate a wealth of knowledge used in treating illness and disease. A Cartesian approach favors "objective" knowledge and assumes that we can separate rational, logical thought from emotional knowing and "objective" knowledge from "subjective" knowledge. Given the assumption that truth and knowledge are detached and separate from human beings and contexts, from a Cartesian view, objective truth is not only considered possible but desirable. Within a Cartesian view, "objective truth" is assumed to be universal (there is one truth/reality) and generalizable (between people and contexts). That is, it is assumed that people can determine "the truth" by looking at the "facts"— what can be seen, heard, smelled, tasted, or verified in some concrete way. It assumes those facts are the same regardless of who is doing the knowing. For example, from this perspective, it is assumed that it doesn't matter which nurse assesses an individual or family because that assessment is objective; therefore, any two nurses would come to the same "truth" and conclusions about that individual or family. Similarly, from a Cartesian perspective, it is presumed that the facts are unchangeable from context to context, so what is known about a particular phenomenon is transferable to all situations. For example, if a nurse is determining how to prevent the negative consequences of incontinence through a Cartesian lens of objectivity, the nurse would be attempting to come to the one "right" or "true" approach that would likely transfer from one situation to the other and from one patient to another.

In thinking critically about this Cartesian view of knowledge as objective and universal, it is likely that you can identify times when this assumption does not hold up, times when there has seemed to be more than one "truth." For example, if you have ever asked people to tell you about a movie they have seen, you will have likely heard different things from different people about the same movie—different versions regarding what the movie was about, whether it was good or not good, and so forth. Even movie critics who bring their expert, objective view will come to different conclusions. They each offer a different "truth" about the movie, and you are left with multiple truths to sort through when deciding whether you will see the movie or not.

We have found nursing work to be similar. That is, rather than being able to determine one clear truth, we most often find ourselves in complex situations where there are multiple truths (interpretations, experiences, perspectives). Even how and what clinical evidence is gathered, recorded, and interpreted varies between clinicians. For example, when I (Gweneth) was in private practice as a psychologist and received referral letters from physicians or other health practitioners, I found that their descriptions and interpretations of particular clients often differed from my own. Yet, because the Cartesian view of knowledge has dominated the scientific world, including the world of nursing, knowledge and practice are often accepted as though there is one objective truth or certainty to find and follow. If you observe how many nurses and other health care professionals go about their work, it becomes apparent that health care knowledge and practice is often grounded in the notion of a Cartesian objective truth. For example, people are assessed by expert (objective) professionals whose job it is to come up with an accurate problem, definition, or diagnosis (objective truth).

The Limitations of Objective Knowledge

While there is no doubt that objective knowledge (such as biomedical knowledge) is vital for competent nursing action, from a nursing practice perspective, "objective" knowledge alone is insufficient.

TO ILLUSTRATE
Just Tell Her to Let It Go

My (Colleen's) mother died of leukemia. Or rather, she died of a catastrophic bowel infection in the presence of severely compromised immunity secondary to leukemia. Or perhaps she died of shame. My mother received a diagnosis of leukemia about 6 months before she died. Like so many families, we struggled with how to live well in the face of a terminal diagnosis, and I clung tightly to the promise of "about a year" that we received from the hematologist. Thus, when she was suddenly hospitalized with a severe bowel infection, my family and I were not as well prepared as you might imagine. What was particularly difficult for me as a nurse was the quality of my mother's nursing care. One particular incident stood out for me.

Despite the fact that my mother was a nurse herself, she was quite modest in terms of her own physical privacy. In her last few days, she was horrified at the idea of losing control of her bowels. The nurses on her unit did not seem to comprehend that my mother was dying. They saw her diagnosis of bowel infection and treated her as someone who would shortly be discharged. Worse, they were often impatient and abrupt. For example, my mother had severe chills and rigor and asked for yet another warm blanket as she shivered uncontrollably. "You've got enough blankets," was one nurse's impatient reply. On the day before she died, despite her weakened state, my mother asked me to help her to the toilet, humiliated at having been diapered. Knowing I could easily assist her and desperately wanting to help my mother have a little bit of control in her situation. I stopped a "busy nurse" to ask where I could get a portable toilet. "Oh, she's got a diaper. Just tell her to let it go."

This story of a moment in my mother's health care experience at the end of her life highlights how important the smallest of nursing acts can be, how important the knowledge that informs each moment is, and how each moment should be informed by multiple forms of knowledge. What knowledge did the nurses draw upon? What knowledge was missing? What ways of knowing predominated? What knowledge and whose knowledge predominated? Incontinence is an everyday occurrence that nurses deal with, and some knowledge informing nursing practice (e.g., the importance of preventing excoriation and breakdown by keeping skin clean and dry) seems routine. At first glance, the knowledge base informing nursing practice related to incontinence does not seem complex. However, if you look a little deeper, you can see that empirical knowledge (such as evidence about the physiologic effects of incontinence and about the fluid dynamics and physics of absorbent materials) is not adequate to responsive nursing care in particular situations.

In the example of my mother's impending incontinence, the objective truth was that diapering would absorb urine and feces in a way that minimized effort. Yet, as Thayer-Bacon (2003) contends, this kind of objective knowledge is surface knowledge and, as such, most often reveals only what can be externally accessed. For example, the nurse did not inquire as to what meaning diapering might have to my mother and how it might symbolize her ultimate loss of control with her impending death. Objective knowledge is knowledge "about" things (Thayer-Bacon, 2003) and thus does not penetrate into inner depths and/or ever-changing aspects of health and healing. In addition, because objective knowledge arises from a detached observer (the objective nurse), it is often decontextualized and depersonalized knowledge. As James (1907) contended, the detached "objective" way of approaching knowing and knowledge may result in the ability to name objects, but it does not allow us to come to know human experience in any depth. Although five different people on your unit may be incontinent, their experiences will vary according to their particular situations. Thus, given our commitment as nurses to provide responsive, "good" care, we must move beyond objective knowledge.

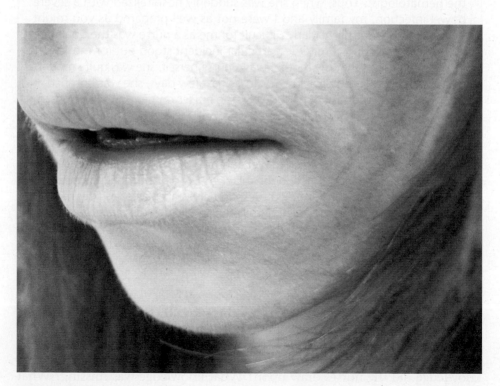

Knowledge about things. (Photograph by Gweneth Doane.)

Often, an objective approach to knowledge severely constrains our ability to know and respond to people's unique health and healing processes. Therefore, in this book we have intentionally and explicitly moved beyond a Cartesian view of knowledge and in particular beyond the notion of objective truth. Specifically, the relational inquiry approach to nursing that we present challenges many of the assumptions of Cartesian thought. A relational consciousness implies understanding health and healing as simultaneously physical, mental, emotional, social, and spiritual—as an interwoven "whole" experience. Therefore, nursing practice that is relational and responsive to the uniqueness of people and families must be informed by multiple forms of knowledge including empirical, ethical, aesthetic, and sociopolitical knowledge. To that end, in this chapter, we introduce these as both ways of knowing and forms of knowledge.

A Relational View of Knowledge

In a relational view, knowledge is understood to be "socially constructed by embedded, embodied people who are in relation with each other" (Thayer-Bacon, 2003, p. 10) and the world. A relational epistemology highlights the inseparability of mind and body and thus of people and their worlds. We emphasize this relational understanding of knowledge because it stands in contrast to the Cartesian epistemology that underpins most of the health care world.

A Relational View Is Grounded in Pragmatism

As we described in Chapter 1, pragmatism provides the grounding for relational inquiry practice. In Chapter 1, we identified three key features of a pragmatic view of knowledge: Knowledge is limited, active, and useful. From a pragmatic perspective, because knowledge is understood to be limited, fallible, and incomplete, any theory or expert truth is considered to be in need of continual scrutiny. That is, regardless of *what* is known about a particular patient, disease, or situation, knowledge (and what we think we know) is always up for question and in the process of revision. In other words, knowledge is active. Because knowledge is evaluated by the extent to which it is useful, we are compelled to ask: How *adequate* is our knowledge? What *don't* we know? What *other* knowledge might be drawn upon to extend our understanding and action? Moreover, we're compelled to recognize the fundamental assumptions that shape our knowledge as we engage in various forms of inquiry and draw on multiple forms of knowledge (see Box 6.1).

With this pragmatic grounding, you can see that to be competent and effective as a nurse, you must consciously assume a stance of inquiry while working between knowing and not knowing, which are of equal importance. Moreover, as we said in earlier chapters, you must develop the capacity of curiosity and intentionally inquire into the knowledge you are enlisting at any particular moment. You must consider at what levels you are enlisting knowledge (intrapersonal, interpersonal, and contextual) to determine the best action. In short, a pragmatic grounding assumes the need for multiple ways of knowing and forms of knowledge. Relational inquiry offers a way for that knowledge to be accessed.

BOX 6.1
Pragmatic Assumptions about Knowledge in Nursing

- Knowledge is never certain, universal, or complete; however, there are more adequate understandings.
- Knowing cannot be separated from the knower because even "facts" are created and interpreted by people.
- Because knowledge is always shaped by the people using it and those people are situated in and constituted by particular situations, all knowledge is socially and relationally mediated and constructed.
- Knowledge (e.g., nursing theory, biomedical research, etc.) is of value to the extent that it enables our actions to be as responsive and effective as possible.
- Knowing is about action—about being informed enough to choose the best action.
- To ensure good action, all knowledge needs to be scrutinized within the realities of nursing situations to determine if the existing knowledge is adequate or if other knowledge is required.
- Multiple forms of knowledge are needed to know and practice competently and responsively.
- Depending upon the particular situation, some knowledge may be more helpful and adequate than other knowledge.
- Knowledge is not static; rather, being knowledgeable requires an ongoing process of inquiry.
- Relational inquiry supports consideration of the *adequacy* of our knowing in terms of our overall nursing purpose and commitments.
- Central to this pragmatic approach to knowledge is a relational epistemology.

Because the knower is always central to the knowing process, it is essential that as nurses, we continually inquire into the knowledge we and others bring to any situation, as well as the values underlying that knowledge. Whose values dominate? What knowledge is valued by different knowers? Similarly, our inquiry encompasses the power dynamics operating in any situation. Who is wielding more power in the situation, and how are those power dynamics shaping the knowledge being deployed? Finally, our inquiry requires that we ask about the limitations of our knowledge and what more we might need to learn in order to be as responsive as possible to patients, families, communities, and their respective particular circumstances to thereby promote their well-being.

A Relational View Is Enhanced by Using the Hermeneutic Phenomenologic and Critical Lenses

The lenses we introduced in Chapter 2 serve as pragmatic tools to expand relational consciousness and guide the inquiry process to enlist multiple ways of knowing and forms of knowledge. The HP lens continuously draws your attention to people's living experiences and how they interpret and live in those experiences as well as how people are situated and constituted within particular social conditions. For example, by enlisting the HP lens, you not only are able to identify the physical symptoms of an illness but also how those symptoms are affecting a person's day-to-day functioning. You can develop an insider view of the illness—gain knowledge of what is particularly meaningful, what matters most to the person and/or family, look for connections between symptoms, or discern significant patterns in symptoms (e.g., how and when a person with asthma uses an inhaler, what shapes those decisions and how all of that is affecting the efficacy of the prescribed treatment and the person's health and well-being). The critical lens draws your attention to the sociopolitical, economic, physical, and language contexts within which people are situated and constituted and how structures and power continuously shape their experiences. For example, what is shaping people's decisions about how they participate in any health care that is offered? Do they have the money to fill expensive prescriptions or the resources to create a dust-free environment for their child?

Relating as a Knower

The process of knowing (a patient, an illness situation, the best clinical action to take, etc.) that we outline in this book rests upon and is supported by a practice of relating and inquiring. To start our explorations into *knowing as a practice of relational inquiry*, we begin by turning your attention to the intrapersonal level—to yourself as a knower.

As we have described, from a pragmatic perspective, we are limited as knowers by the *selective interests* that we bring to any experience or situation. Thayer-Bacon (2003) describes selective interest as the bias or attitude that exists in each thought we have. Our selective interest determines the questions we ask and even the way we go about answering our questions. Selective interest causes us to notice certain things and not others as well as to attend to certain experiences and not others.

Thaler and Sunstein (2009) describe how people develop particular reference points based on their own social locations and backgrounds that shape their interpretations of the value or meaning of something. The authors offer the example of envisioning the size of a city you have never been to. If you are from a small town (say 10,000 people), and that is the reference point that serves as your anchor, you might consider a city of 200,000 people big. However, if you are from New York City, you might consider that same city of 200,000 people small. How you interpret and "know" a city all depends on the reference point from which you start.

Importantly, people make adjustments to their perspectives in relation to the particular reference point from which they start. So, if nurses are anchored in the biomedical milieu of disease treatment, and if that serves as their reference point for knowledge, their choices and adjustments are made from there. For example, if we are steeped mostly in valuing empirical and biomedical knowledge which continue to be dominant in nursing (Chinn & Kramer, 2011), we relate "knowing" and "knowledge" to that reference point. So if that is the case on a given medical unit, nurses there will view one another as knowledgeable based on the extent to which they have knowledge of pathophysiology, pharmacology, and other biomedical treatments. More importantly, in terms of our nursing assessment/inquiry, that reference point guides us to ask only certain questions and frame those questions according to empirical knowledge and/or biomedical conditions despite the presence of other potentially important factors.

Since knowing begins from particular reference points, in relational inquiry, we explicitly want to help you to (a) become consciously aware of the reference points that are shaping your "knowing practice" and (b) structure and revise your reference points and your "choice architecture" (Thaler & Sunstein, 2009) so that you can move beyond your habitual reference points and limited selective interests. For example, consider the World Health Organization's (1986, p. 1) socioenvironmental definition of health—"a resource for living . . . the extent to which an individual or group is able to realize aspirations, to satisfy needs, and to change or cope with the environment." Next, consider the traditional medical definition of health as "the absence of disease or infirmity." Your reference point for knowing a patient would differ tremendously according to which definition you anchor your nursing practice in. Anchoring in a socioenvironmental perspective of health would extend your reference point for knowing (and the knowledge you would enlist as a nurse) far beyond empirical knowledge of disease. Thinking about this process highlights the importance of consciously considering the reference points you are using as a knower and how they shape how you interpret, "know," and choose to provide care.

TO ILLUSTRATE
I'll Be Tying Him up Soon!

The following story was told to us by a student who participated in an ethics research study (Storch, Hartrick Doane, Rodney, Varcoe, & Starzomski, 1999–2001; Varcoe et al., 2004):

"[When I was in my first year] there was an old fellow that was restrained. And he so badly did not want to be restrained. His wrists were tied to his chair; his hips were tied to the chair. And if he wasn't, he would slide out of his chair. So to everyone it seemed that was a worthwhile reason for going against his wishes. As a student—and I was pretty fresh as a student then—it really bothered me. . . . Because I just didn't think that was a good enough reason to go against his wishes. I felt like, 'Isn't there something else we can do so we're—so both sides see, you know, compromise?'. . . I thought it was just me . . . you know, fresh mind, oh, I'll get used to it, I'll be tying him up soon. I'll see why it's good. You know. But now I think, 'Well, wait a minute here, what I was thinking was important.' And now I would say something. And I would have rationale from the ethical point of view. And I would be able to lay it out so people could really see the dilemma."

This story highlights both the power of reference points and how inquiry is needed at all levels to enlist multiple forms of knowing for safe, competent nursing practice. For example, as a result of the patient safety mandate, the practice of "tying patients up for their own well-being" was the normative reference point from which the nurses on the unit worked. However, the student who was new to the unit and to the profession did not have that same reference point. She did not *relate* tying someone up to patient well-being. Thus, she questioned the decision and wondered about the possibility of other choices. She shared the patient safety concern, yet seeing the man in such distress led her to question the nursing action. She later describes that in her third year, when she learned about ethical theory, she realized that her own intrapersonal response offered important knowledge. That is, she realized that her own response wasn't because she was "fresh-minded." Her intrapersonal response and her question of what was right was an ethical question—a question of the best nursing choice and action. Apparently, no one except the student saw restraining the man against his wishes as an ethical problem. Yet when one stops to critically consider that norm (as the student did), the potential harm of such action becomes evident. For example, even though as a first-year student, the nurse in the story may not have been familiar with the literature that outlines the harmful effects (including interrelated physiologic, psychological, and ethical effects) of restraints (Goethals, Dierckx de Casterlé, & Gastmans, 2012; Shorr et al., 2002), or have knowledge of ethical theory, her own personal response to the situation offered a form of knowledge and a site for inquiry. Her response served as a site for questioning and extending the knowledge being used to promote patient safety.

Seeing the Reference Points that Shape Your Choices

By inviting you to more consciously question and choose how you relate in situations, we are attempting to nudge you toward more effective choice and knowledge making (Thaler & Sunstein, 2009). Yet we also are aware that to change the reference points and the choice architecture from which people operate is not a simple process because they are often taken for granted and unquestioned. However, thinking about this anchoring process in terms of your work as a nurse highlights the importance of consciously considering the reference points you are using as you make choices. In what are you anchoring your knowledge choices, and how does that shape the knowledge you enlist as a nurse and how you subsequently act?

Each of you will vary in what you bring to nursing. For example, I (Colleen) teach in a nursing program in which students already have degrees in a range of areas: arts, psychology, science, and so on; each brings different starting points, but all need to develop their knowledge in relation to the dominance of the Cartesian way of seeing the mind and body separate, the emphasis on biomedicine and physiology, and the pervasive concern with corporate efficiency.

When we teach practicing nurses and ask them to examine their nursing actions to see what is informing their practice as a nurse, the most common thing we hear after they have done so are exclamations of surprise and shock. As we assign the nurses various observation and inquiry exercises and ask them to look beyond the surface of their behaviors and critically consider what is leading to specific actions (what reference points are underneath the behavioral tip of the iceberg), they begin to see how they are being informed by values, normative practices, and organizational imperatives that often are inconsistent with their own nursing commitments and purpose. As one nurse recently put it to me (Gweneth) in a conversation, "My allegiance as a nurse did not align with my own values or what I wanted to provide for my patients." At the same time, they begin to see how they are privileging certain forms of knowledge while ignoring others.

TRY IT OUT 6.1

Identify Your Allegiances and Reference Points

Pick some common concern in nursing: incontinence, pain management, unconsciousness, child abuse, infection control, medication administration, bathing, or suctioning. Pick something to which you have been introduced in your education to date or with which you have some experience. If possible, pair up with someone with a similar concern of interest. In point form, write *for 1 minute*, everything you know about it.

So, for example, if we had done this about incontinence when we were in nursing school, we might have included points such as:

- Early, regular toileting
- Maintain skin integrity
- Prevent excoriation
- Bladder training, if possible

Then, see if you can discern any pattern. What is your reference point for entering into knowing in relation to this phenomenon? What are your allegiances? Do you have a similar pattern to what can be seen in the points we have identified? Which focus on physiologic concerns and empirical evidence? Or do you have a wider view already?

If we were to do this activity today, we'd include many other points that would attend to knowledge beyond pathophysiology and ways of knowing beyond empirical inquiry. For example, we'd include functioning in day-to-day life, wondering what it is like to live with incontinence, to be sexually active, and so forth.

If you have a partner with whom you can compare notes, see how your patterns, allegiances, and reference points are similar or different, and see if you can explain those similarities and differences. Undoubtedly, your reference points and allegiances with respect to any given phenomenon will arise from your personal experiences, your educations, and the ways in which you have thought about the issue.

TO ILLUSTRATE

Orienting to Fetal Alcohol Syndrome

A few years ago when I (Colleen) was teaching first-year nursing, I asked students to do an activity similar to Try It Out 6.1. I had asked the class to analyze a phenomenon of their choice to examine what historical, economic, political, social, and cultural influences shaped people's experiences of that phenomenon. One student (I will call her Lana) picked fetal alcohol syndrome. I have a strong sociopolitical understanding of fetal alcohol syndrome (FAS). I am aware from my research that FAS is overdiagnosed in Aboriginal children and that, in Canada, most social support goes to infants and young children diagnosed with FAS, whereas when those children reach adulthood, they receive little support.

Lana, however, had a different set of allegiances and reference points. She had selected FAS because she had an adopted younger brother (I will call him Dean) with FAS. Although her family was otherwise Caucasian, her little brother (who was about 7 years old at the time) was Aboriginal.

Lana had a difficult time doing the assignment. Upon its completion, she told me that it had prompted her to realize how angry her mother (and to some extent her entire family) was at Dean's birth mother. The family tried to limit any contact between Dean and his birth mother, and Lana came to see that they were (perhaps unwittingly) turning Dean against her. Through her inquiry, Lana began to question what circumstances might have led Dean's birth mother to excessive drinking and how this might be linked to race-based policies and policy-enforced poverty (the consequences of colonization for many indigenous people). She also began to question what might be best for Dean. Lana's inquiry led her to raise such questions with her mother and indeed caused significant conflict between her and her mother. However, despite this, Lana told me that it was one of the most profound learning experiences she had ever had; she dramatically shifted her own allegiances and reference points in relation to FAS and indeed to many other phenomena as well.

Examining your own reference points and allegiances is an important starting point for inquiry. As we have suggested, all knowing is personal, so knowing and not knowing begins with yourself. To continue our discussion of knowing as a practice of relational inquiry, we now consider how our own ways of knowing shape how we relate interpersonally as knowers and how our intrapersonal and interpersonal practices as knowers are shaped contextually.

Knowing and Not Knowing as Ways of Relating

Knowing is a very important part of high-quality, competent nursing practice. Repeatedly, research has shown that people want nurses to be knowledgeable about their health and illness conditions (Kvåle &

Bondevik, 2010; Van der Elst, Dierckx de Casterlé, & Gastmans, 2012). However, as we have shown, taking an expert stance and privileging knowing can actually limit our nursing knowledge and action because it closes down inquiry and obscures knowledge that may be important to being effective. Returning to the example of my mother's impending incontinence, the nurse who told her to "just let it go" took the stance of expert, telling us in one short sentence what "should" happen. Yet, on what was she basing that choice and action? When I (Gweneth) heard this story, I found myself asking some targeted knowledge questions. For example, even if one were to argue that patients need to be diapered because of limited health care resources (as some nurses and administrators would), if one considers the decision objectively, the question of knowledge competence comes into view. Empirically, I wonder about the iatrogenic effects of leaving urine and feces on the skin given Mrs. Varcoe's weakened state. Thus, I find myself wanting to gather more empirical knowledge to find out if any studies have been done about the effects of diapering in already immune-compromised elderly patients. Similarly, the story draws my attention to *how important it is to relate one form of knowledge to another.* For example, to make a competent, evidence-based clinical decision, I would need to relate the latest empirical knowledge about the potential iatrogenic consequences of diapering elderly patients with bowel disease with particular patient knowledge (e.g., Colleen's mother's past history of urinary tract infections that might indicate an increased susceptibility to future infections or, in this situation, knowledge that she is expected to die within days, making further infection less of a concern).

As nurses, we are encouraged to primarily relate as expert knowers. Indeed, often an expert stance of knower is required. In relational inquiry, it is not a question of whether we enlist our expert knowledge but why, how, and when we do. Most importantly, relational inquiry directs us to (a) purposefully examine the knowledge we are enlisting and the knowledge we may not be enlisting and (b) consider how to most effectively relate different forms of knowledge to gain the fullest knowledge possible. For example, recently while living in Mexico, my (Colleen's) partner asked me to look at a man who had been stung by a scorpion. His arm was reddened and swollen around the sting to about twice the circumference of this other arm. More concerning was that he seemed vague and distracted and his speech seemed a bit slurred. He was clearly in pain but was refusing to be taken to medical care. He had taken an antihistamine, but I was concerned about the severity of his reaction. Knowing that over 1,000 people die of scorpion stings per year in Mexico, and not knowing how his reaction compared, how to ascertain the virulence of a specific scorpion, or what he was like prior to the sting, I assumed an "expert" stance, telling him what I knew of the risks and "ordering" him to go to a clinic. Subsequently, however, I learned more—what shape and color the most toxic scorpions are, how to administer more specific first aid for scorpion stings, and so on.

As this story suggests, relating as an expert knower has its place and is useful, but it is always limited. The pragmatic view that considers all knowledge as incomplete, fallible, and subjective means that you need to relate simultaneously through both knowing and not knowing. *It is not feasible to bring all possible knowledge to bear on any given situation; however, it is possible to enlist multiple forms of knowing simultaneously to ensure your knowledge is as adequate as possible.* And how you *do* that, how you know or don't know, is by engaging in multiple modes of inquiry and simultaneously and intentionally linking different domains of knowledge. In the situation above, I (Colleen) recognized the limits of my empirical knowledge. At the same time, although it was not a prominent feature in the story as I told it, I was thinking using other modes of inquiry. For example, based on sociopolitical knowledge, I observed that the man appeared to have adequate means to afford medical attention. He was from the United States on vacation and had expensive sports equipment and a fairly new truck. Had it been the Mexican gardener (who was also present and earned a subsistence-level wage without medical coverage) who was stung, I would have needed to consider a more adequate response—one that did not immediately send him off to a clinic for expensive medical attention that he might not be able to afford. In particular, I would have been less willing to err on the side of caution recommending medical attention based on my incomplete empirical knowledge.

Relating through knowing and not knowing simultaneously in all instances assists you to continually question the limits of your knowledge and continuously inquire to expand that knowledge. Doing so at all levels can be aided by explicitly seeking to integrate multiple forms of knowledge and by using multiple ways of knowing and modes of inquiry.

Forms of Knowledge and Ways of Knowing that Inform Nursing Practice

Throughout the past three decades, there has been an intense interest in the question of "knowing" in nursing (how we know and what we know). One important catalyst for this interest was in 1978 when Carper proposed that there are at least four "ways of knowing" in nursing: empirical, aesthetic, ethical, and personal knowing. She described the empirical pattern of knowing as the dominant form and as involving factual and descriptive knowing aimed at the development of abstract and theoretical explanations. Carper saw the aesthetic pattern of knowing as related to understanding what is of significance to particular patients (and we would say, particular families, communities, and situations) and identified empathy—"the capacity for participating in or vicariously experiencing another's feelings" (p. 15)— as a central mode of aesthetic knowing. She described the ethical pattern of knowing as requiring knowledge of different philosophical positions regarding what is good and right, and as involving the making of moral choices and actions. Finally, Carper drew on Buber to describe personal knowing as encompassing knowledge of the self in relation to others and in relation to one's own self.

Carper's (1978) typology challenged empirical knowledge as *the* knowledge base for nursing and widened understanding of knowledge and knowing in nursing. Carper's work stimulated lively investigation and debate about knowing in nursing (e.g., Benner, Tanner, & Chesla, 1996; Chinn & Jacobs-Kramer, 1988; Chinn & Kramer, 2011; Wainwright, 2000; White, 1995) and inspired nurses to consider ideas about knowing that authors in other disciplines had generated. Chinn and Jacobs-Kramer (1988) offered a detailed critical analysis of Carper's work to facilitate integration of these patterns of knowing into clinical nursing practice (White, 1995). Nurses have continued to modify and develop understandings of "knowing" in nursing through both theoretical and research-based investigations (Archibald, 2012; Banks-Wallace, 2000; Grant, 2001; Liaschenko, 1997; Liaschenko & Fisher, 1999; Schaefer, 2002; Wainwright, 2000). Most recently, Chinn and Kramer (2011) articulated a typology of empirical, ethical, personal, and aesthetic knowing with emancipatory knowing integrating all forms of knowing. They write that "emancipatory knowing is the human capacity to be aware of and to critically reflect upon the social, cultural, and political status quo and to figure out how and why it came to be that way." Fully discussing this rich literature is beyond the scope of this book, but there are two developments that are of key importance to relational inquiry practice: (a) the position of personal knowledge and (b) the importance of sociopolitical knowing. Notice as you read further how these developments are compatible with a pragmatic grounding and complement the HP and critical lenses.

The Position of Personal Knowledge

There is controversy in how to think about personal knowing. Although some see it as a distinct way of knowing, we agree with those who see personal knowing as underlying all ways of knowing. Thus, we do not consider personal knowledge as a mode of inquiry but as a broad reference to the fact that all knowing rests in individual people.

Personal knowledge has only recently come to be valued in nursing. Since Carper's (1978) description of patterns of knowing in nursing, increased attention has been focused on personal knowing. Nursing scholars have divided into at least two camps regarding what they think about personal knowledge in nursing. In one camp are the followers of Carper, who have accepted her notion that personal knowing is a separate category and one of at least four fundamental patterns of knowing in nursing. In another camp are those such as Benner (1984), Smith (1992), and Sweeney (1994), who build from Polanyi's work (1962) on personal knowledge to argue that personal knowing is not a separate category but penetrates all forms of knowing. For example, Smith asserts that knowing is the weaving of threads that may originate from sources such as science, the arts, life experiences, and encounters. She says that while the sources of knowledge may be similar or different, the threads we select from those sources are personal choices. Consequently, all "knowing" is personally shaped. We agree with Smith that "in this way, all 'knowing' is fundamentally and primarily personal knowing" (p. 2). As we described in previous chapters, as a person you bring different forms of knowledge together in your own unique way—filtering them through your own personal framework of understanding, past experiences, values, beliefs, and so forth. Thus, all knowing is personal because it arises from your own particular perspective.

In concluding that all knowing is "personal knowing," Smith (1992) and Sweeney (1994) both argued that the category of knowledge that Carper called personal knowledge is actually self-knowledge (what we would call intrapersonal knowing). Chinn and Kramer (2011) take a similar stance, saying that while "in a sense all knowing is personal knowing," they treat personal knowing as "a process of self-knowing that is shaped by . . . relationships with others and that also shapes . . . relationships when caring for others" (p. 109). Self-knowledge involves knowledge of oneself including awareness of one's values, beliefs, socio-environmental location, and so forth. Self-knowledge allows us a clearer view into how we are making our personal choices of knowing. Cultivating self-knowledge is part of the process of "reflexivity," which we described in Chapter 2 as the active, purposeful reflection on one's beliefs, values, thoughts, and actions, and thoughtful action as a consequence of that reflection.

As we have outlined earlier, when we develop and pay attention to self-knowledge, we have the opportunity to see how we personally shape all our knowledge, to question reflexively and perhaps move beyond the habits of mind (habits of knowing) that constrain our understandings. That is, by developing and paying attention to self-knowledge, we can begin to see and more purposefully decide how we are personally shaping knowledge. At the same time, as we open up to knowing ourselves more fully, we simultaneously expand our knowing of others. We are able to expand and move beyond our own selective interests and to better see the taken-for-granted assumptions and contextual elements that may limit our view of individuals, families, and the world.

In line with a pragmatist view, understanding that all knowledge is personal suggests that our knowledge cannot be seen as incontestable knowledge or "truth." For example, just because we experience particular patients as "challenging" does not mean they *are* challenging. As hermeneutic phenomenology informs us, our lived experience is interpreted within and through our own reference points, selective interests, ideologies, values, taken-for-granted rights and wrongs, and so forth. For this reason, it is important to critically examine what we think we "know" as well as what is shaping our knowledge. This inquiry process of reflexively scrutinizing our knowledge and how we are "knowing" promotes our ability to expand our interpretations and "know" in new ways.

The Importance of Sociopolitical Knowing

While reflexive consideration of personal knowing is vital to nursing practice, reframing one's own knowing may be insufficient for transforming larger practice patterns that are shaped by the dominant societal interests and ideologies. For example, one nurse alone cannot change policies and ways of thinking that lead to a patient being transferred from emergency to die on a different unit within an hour of transfer as in the story told in Chapter 1. Personal interests can lead to individual resistance to practices and policies that constrain socio-environmental health promotion, but collective changes are required to transform the structures that dominate practice. It was this understanding that led White (1995) to argue for adding sociopolitical knowing to Carper's original typology.

White (1995) noted that the context appeared to be missing from both Carper's (1978) analysis and Chinn and Jacobs-Kramer's (1988) analysis and extension of Carper's work. White remarked that Chinn and Jacobs-Kramer's reconceptualization was an adequate description of the nurse–patient relationship and the persons of nurse and patients but that the sociopolitical context of people and their interactions was missing. Thus, White advocated adding sociopolitical knowing to the typology of ways of knowing in nursing. She argued that the other patterns address the "who," "how," and "what" of nursing practice, but sociopolitical knowing addresses the "wherein," drawing attention to the broader context of practice and causing "the nurse to question the taken-for-granted assumptions about practice, the profession, and health policies" (White, 1995, pp. 83–84).

Importantly, White (1995) pointed out that the sociopolitical context of relations fundamentally concerns cultural identity. She noted that one's cultural location influences one's "understanding of health, disease, language, identity, and connection to the land" and that such knowing is related to "deeply embedded historical connections to and dislocation from land and heritage" (White, 1995, p. 84).

Similarly, Banks-Wallace (2000) argues that racial/ethnic identity and class are significantly influential on women's ways of knowing. Banks-Wallace draws upon a "womanist" understanding of ways of knowing to suggest how health interventions can be made far more effective in assisting African-American women to incorporate health-promoting behaviors. By "womanist" she means understanding based on women's experiences of the combined effects of being both an African American and a woman. This is a specific example illustrating the importance of understanding the intersectionality of oppressions as discussed in Chapter 4. Banks-Wallace points out that most "cultural-based" interventions in health care focus attention upon appropriate language rather than considering whether the knowledge being offered is relevant and valid for the group being targeted. She uses the example of health promotion interventions to address issues such as cardiovascular disease, obesity, and hypertension (e.g., weight loss, diet, blood pressure monitoring) for African-American women that do not take into account the experience of living under the chronic stress of "feeling like they are nothing" in American society. To us, this highlights the importance of informing our practice through sociopolitical knowing—of intentionally inquiring into and taking the context of individuals, families, communities, nurses, and health care into account. Therefore, relational inquiry always includes the contextual level.

Throughout this book, we continually draw your attention to the contexts and to the importance of personal and social locations to both individuals', families', and your own understanding of health and health care. We agree with White (1995) that a sociopolitical understanding can be a frame within which to understand other patterns of knowing and that this frame is essential to the future of nursing in the increasingly economically driven world. Indeed, in 2008, Chinn and Kramer (2008) introduced "emancipatory knowing" as a fifth pattern that connects and surrounds with the four patterns initially described by Carper.

Overall, this means that we approach practice with the understanding that all knowledge is dynamic and contestable and that to practice in an informed and "knowledgeable" manner requires paying attention and inquiring into self, other, and context "all at once." From a relational inquiry perspective, it is not simply a matter of being intentional toward people and families. You are not just trying to understand people; you are trying to "know" them in context, yourself in context, and yourself as you relate to individuals and families in context. Thus, a relational inquiry approach to knowing means intentionally inquiring into the self, other, and context all at once and bringing multiple ways of knowing and the forms of knowledge they produce together to determine best action.

USING MULTIPLE MODES OF INQUIRY TO SUPPORT RELATIONAL INQUIRY

As the literature in nursing illustrates, there are many different ways of conceptualizing forms of knowledge and ways of knowing. Building on previous descriptions in the nursing literature, we have chosen a typology of four modes of inquiry:

- **Empirical Inquiry**: Focuses on developing empirical knowledge through observation and experiment, including research, and is aimed at developing theoretical and conceptual understandings. Empirical inquiry is critical to nursing practice and continues to prevail as the underpinnings of nursing knowledge (Chinn & Kramer, 2011). Empirical knowledge provides objective evidence, facts, and understandings to nursing decisions.
- **Ethical Inquiry**: Focuses on clarifying values, commitments, and obligations. Ethical knowledge provides direction to nursing decisions to uphold values and obligations to which nurses are committed.
- **Aesthetic Inquiry**: Focuses on engaging the "art" of human existence including attending to deeper meanings, beauty, and creative resources. Chinn and Kramer (2011) define aesthetic knowing as "that aspect of knowing that requires an understanding of deeper meanings in a situation and on the basis of those meanings calls forth the creative resources of the nurse that transforms experience into what is not yet real but is envisioned as possible" (p. 127). Aesthetic knowledge provides direction to nursing in supporting attention to meaning in health and illness experiences.
- **Sociopolitical Inquiry**: Focuses on developing analyses of power relations. Sociopolitical knowledge provides contextual and political knowledge to nursing decisions.

We have chosen these modes of inquiry because we think they support nursing practice particularly well. Although for the purposes of description we discuss each separately, we want to emphasize their "relational whole." That is, they are not separate domains but are intricately related and form an inherent whole. For example, the questions we ask as part of an empirical inquiry are shaped by sociopolitical knowledge and the questions that arise from that knowledge. While the movement in health care toward evidence-based practice has tended to privilege empirical knowledge and evidence, all forms of knowledge and ways of knowing are required for optimizing the effectiveness of nursing practice. Moreover, because people "know" from their own reference points and can get habituated into using certain modes of inquiry, by consciously enlisting the four modes and using them to inform each other, you can develop a much more in-depth knowledge base to inform your nursing action.

TO ILLUSTRATE

Congestive Heart Failure on the Psychiatric Unit

At one point in my (Gweneth's) career, I transitioned from working in an adult intensive care unit (ICU) to an inpatient psychiatric unit. About a month after I started working on the psychiatric unit, I came on afternoon shift and was told that one of my patients who had been diagnosed with bipolar illness was "becoming increasingly manic." Mrs. Smith (a pseudonym) had been going around the unit in an agitated state, grabbing onto any nurse who passed by exclaiming, "My legs are burning up, my legs are burning up, someone has to do something or they're going to explode!" During report, I was told that the day staff had obtained an order for extra sedation since she was "obviously going to be a handful." Being new to psychiatry and feeling very much out of my element, I went in to greet Mrs. Smith. Not quite knowing what to do from a psychiatric perspective and having come from ICU where at the beginning of each shift, standard practice was to do a head-to-toe assessment of my patients, that physical once-over was still my comfortable "reference point" for action. Thus, when Mrs. Smith started complaining of her legs, without even really thinking about it, I launched into a physical assessment. I had noticed when I walked in the room that she looked flushed and her breathing seemed labored, but of course that could have just been from her agitation. However, given her distress and her insistence that I look at her legs, I asked her to lie down on the bed so I could check her over. Removing her slippers and lifting her robe, I was shocked at what I found. Her legs were probably about twice their normal size with pitting edema. On checking her vital signs, I found her blood pressure to be at a dangerously high level, her chest sounds to be of concern, and her heart rate racing and irregular. To make a long story short, within an hour, Mrs. Smith had been admitted to the cardiac unit with a diagnosis of congestive heart failure.

We tell this story to illustrate

- The integral connection between personal/contextual reference points
- The importance of knowing and not knowing
- How the HP and critical lenses, inquiry at all levels, and purposefully relating different forms of knowledge to one another work together to support responsive, competent nursing practice

Since Mrs. Smith was a patient in a psychiatric context and had a diagnostic label of "bipolar illness," those were the *reference points* through which she was viewed and "known." Although she had spent the day complaining about her legs, her calls for attention were interpreted through those reference points as merely symptoms of an escalating manic phase of her illness. My (Gweneth's) own response also illustrates how reference points shape knowledge and action. For example, still feeling out of my element as a psychiatric nurse, I turned my attention to something that I did know. I knew how to do a physical assessment, so that was my first relational mode of intervention. To be honest, while (intrapersonally) I certainly wanted to care for Mrs. Smith and respond to her concerns, my assessment (interpersonal) was mostly inspired by my desire to lessen her agitation and be able to demonstrate my confidence that her legs were fine. Contextually, as the newbie nurse, I was working from the assumption that the more experienced nurses knew more and that their assessment was right. Thus, it wasn't until I saw Mrs. Smith's legs that I realized that she knew more than we did and that our arrogance as knowers had resulted in harm.

What also becomes apparent in considering this situation is how the different ways of knowing shape each other. For example, the kind of empirical knowledge that was enlisted was shaped by the sociopolitical context of the psychiatric unit and what was considered "good" nursing (ethical knowing) and meaningful attention (aesthetic knowing) within that context. Similarly, in looking through the HP and critical lenses, it is possible to see how the ideology that separates physical illness from mental illness and expert knowledge over living experience led us to privilege our own knowledge and not respond to Mrs. Smith's living experience. In doing so, we completely misdiagnosed her condition and failed to meet our nursing obligations. In telling this story, I am aware that if I had been working in psychiatry longer and my reference point had shifted, I may not have approached the situation in the same way. For example, I might have no longer been in the habit of physical assessment. Similarly, I might not have been as aware of my lack of knowledge and so may not have looked at Mrs. Smith's legs. My knowing arrogance might have resulted in much further harm to Mrs. Smith. At the time, the experience left me questioning what I had missed "knowing" when I worked in the ICU and had practiced chiefly from that reference point.

Because not knowing is seen as a vital part of being a competent nurse, relational inquiry as a practice of knowing supports you to both be humble in what you think you know and confident in what you do not know. By working between knowing and not knowing and enlisting and relating multiple forms of knowledge to one another,

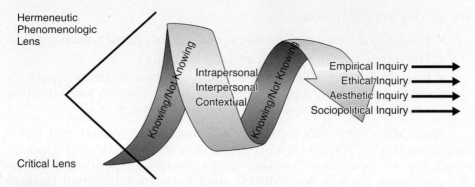

Fig. 6.1 A relational inquiry process.

you are able to extend both your knowledge and your competence as a nurse. This enlisting and relating "knowing" process is supported through four specific modes of inquiry—empirical, ethical, aesthetic, and sociopolitical.

In the case of Mrs. Smith, the empirical questions we as nurses asked were limited to the psychiatric knowledge domain because we assumed ourselves to "know better" than she did, and we also held the power. If we had inquired sociopolitically about how power was shaping the empirical knowledge we were and were not enlisting, our power-over-knowledge choices and the limited empirical knowledge we were enlisting would have been brought to our attention. Similarly, this sociopolitical inquiry would have raised questions about our ethical comportment and how we were responding aesthetically to Mrs. Smith's living experience (to the deeper meanings of her experience and her own knowledge resources).

For the purposes of examining each mode of inquiry, in what follows, we have treated each separately (keeping in mind their interrelatedness) before bringing them all together. Figure 6.1 shows how the HP and critical lenses work in concert with the pragmatic process of knowing/not knowing at all levels (intrapersonal, interpersonal, and contextual) and how the four modes of inquiry focus and guide the relational inquiry process. For example, although ethical inquiry focuses explicitly on values, commitments, and obligations, looking through a critical lens will invite you to think about which values are informing the empirical evidence that is developed, what empirical evidence is being drawn upon in particular situations, which forms of empirical evidence are valued over others, and so on (see Figure 6.2).

As Figure 6.1 suggests, each of these modes of inquiry are conducted at all levels simultaneously. In contrast to Carper (1978), we are not claiming that these are mutually exclusive nor are we claiming that they are complete. Rather, as Figure 6.2 and Table 6.1 suggest, these forms of inquiry overlap with each other and also with other ways of thinking about types of knowledge and ways of knowing. So, for example, White's (1995) idea of sociopolitical knowing provides a frame not only for generating sociopolitical knowledge but also for understanding how power dynamics influence empirical, ethical, and aesthetic knowledge and knowing. We also are not

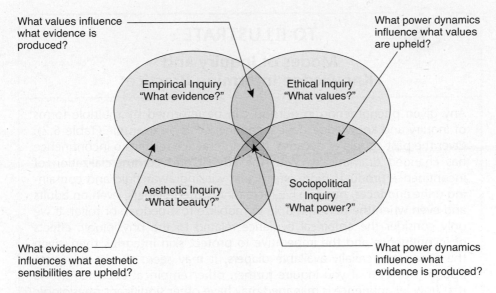

Fig. 6.2 Examples of interrelatedness among modes of inquiry.

claiming that the questions we pose are comprehensive and complete. Questions have been posed throughout this book, and undoubtedly, you have posed your own questions as you read earlier chapters. Rather, the questions we pose are used to illustrate *some* of the ways that relational inquiry practice informs and is informed by various modes of inquiry.

Table 6.1: Questions at Each Level within Different Modes of Inquiry

Mode of Inquiry	Empirical Inquiry	Ethical Inquiry	Aesthetic Inquiry	Sociopolitical Inquiry
Emphasis	What evidence?	What values?	What beauty in human existence?	What power dynamics?
Intrapersonal	What evidence do I have? What evidence do I need?	What values do I hold?	What aesthetic do I hold?	What orientation to power do I hold?
Interpersonal	What evidence informs my actions?	How do I enact my values with others?	How do I promote that aesthetic with others?	How am I enacting my power with others?
Contextual	What evidence dominates or is missing in this context (situation, health care organization, society)?	What values are promoted or discouraged in this context?	What aesthetic is encouraged or discouraged in this context?	What power dynamics support or constrain my practice in this context?

TO ILLUSTRATE

Modes of Inquiry and Knowledge Informing Practice

Any given phenomenon in nursing can be informed by multiple forms of inquiry and knowledge. Take incontinence as an example (Table 6.2). Over the past couple of decades, nursing practice related to incontinence has changed dramatically. With the advent and commercialization of incontinence products more effective at wicking away fluid and containing urine and feces, nurses have increasingly used diapers, even on adults and even when the person is able to mobilize to a bedpan or toilet. If we only consider the empirical evidence related to the physiologic effects of incontinence and the imperative to protect skin integrity, then given the new commercially available diapers, it may seem like an adequate option. However, if you inquire further, other empirical evidence shows that how incontinence is managed may have other significant physiologic effects. For example, when nurses use diapers instead of mobilizing a person to the toilet, they may lose the only opportunity they have to mobilize that person and hence lose the extensive physiologic benefits of mobilization. Further, for example, the use of a catheter or a diaper may affect the person's comfort in socializing. Simply leaving a person alone in bed rather than mobilizing that person misses an opportunity for the nurse to engage the person socially. Beginning with the intrapersonal, what reference points do you bring to your inquiry of incontinence? What experience do you have? What do you "know," and what is the source of that knowledge? How is your empirical knowledge also influenced by, for example, advertising media that might draw on empirical knowledge? What forms of knowledge dominate your current understanding, and where might you expand your knowledge?

Moving beyond empirical inquiry, asking questions about values and obligations (remember our discussion in Chapter 3 about relational obligations) related to incontinence draws attention to a range of values that are staples of nursing codes of ethics. On an intrapersonal level, what values do you hold that are relevant to the issue of incontinence (e.g., privacy, autonomy, respect)? On an interpersonal level, how do different practices affect different patients? How, for example, is a particular person's autonomy affected by diapering? Contextually, what values are upheld, and which values might collide or conflict? For example, you will notice that from unit to unit, different unit cultures arise so that different practices are considered acceptable whereas others are not. In our study of ethical practice in nursing (Doane, Storch, & Pauly, 2009) on one unit, nurses actively resisted the organizational imperative to introduce having men and women in the same rooms, whereas in other units they did not.

What nursing implications can be identified through inquiry regarding the aesthetics of practice? Again, at the intrapersonal level, to what aesthetic

Table 6.2: Multiple Modes of Inquiry and Knowledge Inform One Occurrence

Type of Inquiry	Empirical Inquiry	Ethical Inquiry	Aesthetic Inquiry	Sociopolitical Inquiry
Focus	What evidence?	What values?	What beauty in human existence?	What power dynamics?
Incontinence	• Physiology (e.g., muscle control) • Physiologic effects (e.g., impaired skin integrity) • Social effects (e.g., decreased socialization) • Effects of treatment (e.g., decreased mobility)	• Respect • Beneficence • Autonomy • Justice	• Embarrassment • Shame • Humiliation • Odors • Infantilizing • Appearance	• Nursing time • Diaper company interests • Trivializing nursing as "bedpan jockeys" • Elderly people have relatively less power
Nursing Implications	Optimize mobility Optimize social connections	Optimize autonomy, etc.	Minimize shame, etc.	Comprehensively optimize time use; influence policy

of human experience do you subscribe? Do you ever inquire into what is of deep meaning to your patients or how you might uphold their aesthetics? For example, in her study of nursing practice in relation to the body, Lawler (1991) described how nurses took action through "minifisms" ("Let's get this wee bit of blood cleaned up," "Oh, you've had a little accident") to minimize embarrassment, shame, shock, and so forth for patients. On a contextual level, what aesthetic is facilitated? For example, the nurse in Chapter 1 was providing care to a dying man within certain institutional conditions; while she might at some other time work to shift those conditions, in the immediate situation, the possibilities for facilitating a good death were constrained.

Finally, by asking questions about power, nurses can more comprehensively decide how to use their time and other health care resources. First, at the intrapersonal level, what orientation to power do you hold? To what extent do you see yourself and nursing as practicing primarily at the direction of the organizations within which you work? At the direction of physicians? Managers? Where do you see the limits of your professional autonomy, and what sets those limits? How do power dynamics shape how you evaluate empirical knowledge in action? For example, although many health care products are marketed as "time-saving," and health care organizations are oriented to short-term savings, the cost of incontinence pads and diapers plus the cost of the harms associated with their use may be greater than the cost of more nursing staff to mobilize patients or provide bedpans. Contextually, how do power dynamics shape your decision making? For example, in the immediate situation, with the pressure of several ill patients, a nurse might make an informed decision to diaper a patient who on another day would be mobilized. However, that decision would be a specific time-based one and one that was determined by the specific circumstances, rather than on an unquestioned normative practice.

TRY IT OUT 6.2

Map the Phenomenon of Your Choice

Return to the common phenomenon you selected in Try It Out 6.1. Using a blank version of Table 6.2, try mapping the knowledge that might come into play if you used each of the four modes of inquiry and looked at all three domains (intrapersonal, interpersonal, and contextual). Think as broadly as you can. For example, when I (Gweneth) think back to my own experience as a student in medication administration and how nervous I was having an instructor watch me, knowledge about how to center myself in stressful situations would have been helpful (intrapersonal domain). Interpersonally, I needed knowledge about how to respond when someone doesn't want to take their medication. For example, when a person is being given a psychotropic medication they don't want, how do you balance the person's autonomy with the issues that give rise to the need for the medication? At the same time, I needed contextual knowledge of how medication administration was organized in different settings with different safety or efficiency concerns. As you continue through this chapter and encounter the more detailed descriptions of each form of inquiry and the questions we pose, add them to your "map."

ENGAGING IN A RELATIONAL INQUIRY: MEET HELENE AND DANA

Here, we discuss in more detail the modes of inquiry from a relational perspective. As we do so, we draw on the experience of Helene and her partner Dana. Helene and I (Colleen) began our friendship about 20 years ago when together we developed a course entitled "Patient Education." At that time, Helene drew on her extensive expertise as a "patient" (as you will see), and her two master's degrees: one in medical social work and the other in teaching blind people (a degree she took in anticipation that she might herself become blind one day). Helene's partner, Dana, was with her throughout the events we describe below. In Figure 6.3, they are pictured together on their wedding day.

Helene, a 40-year-old woman, is admitted through emergency to a medical unit of a hospital with serious dehydration secondary to severe

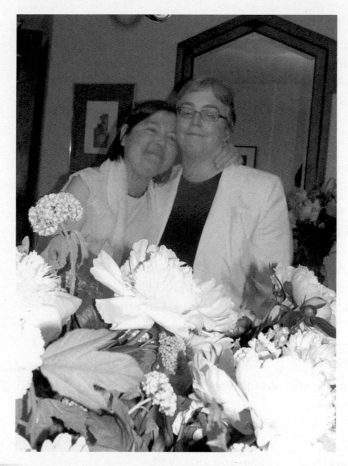

Fig. 6.3 Helene and Dana. (Photograph by Colleen Varcoe.)

diarrhea which has persisted over a period of several months. She is accompanied by her partner, Dana. Helene has diabetes, which was diagnosed at the age of 11. She has had chronic kidney disease for a number of years, but at present has a fully functioning transplanted kidney. After being on hemodialysis for several years, she had her first kidney transplant. This first transplant failed quite quickly. However, 3 years ago, Helene received a second renal transplant that continues to work effectively. At present, Helene is being admitted with the diagnosis of diarrhea and dehydration, NYD (not yet diagnosed). In addition to the above problems, Helene has had significant coronary artery disease, for which she had six bypass grafts in coronary artery bypass graft surgery about 6 years ago.

On admission to the medical unit, Helene is pale, thin, and tired-looking. In fact, she looks exhausted and distressed. She is quite weak and struggles to get on a bedpan which she requests as she is moved from the emergency stretcher to her bed on the unit.

On admission to the unit, Helene's vital signs are as follows:

Temperature: 37.7°C
Heart rate: 128 beats per minute
BP: 95/40

Helene's blood work is as follows:

FK506	13.3	[normal]
Sodium	148	[135–148 mmol/L]
Potassium	3.7	[3.6–5.0 mmol/L]
Chloride	129	[100–112 mmol/L]
Bicarb	7	[22–31 mmol/L]
WBC	9.5	[4.0–11.0 G/L]
HGB	160	[120–155 G/L]
MCV	93	[82–100 Fl]
RBC	5.2	[3.9–5.3 T/L]
HCT	0.48	[0.37–0.47]
Platelets	191	[125–400 G/L]
Neutrophils	6.9	[2.3–7.7 G/L]
Lymphocytes	1.5	[0.8–3.1 G/L]
Monocytes	1.1	[0.2–0.8 G/L]
Creatinine	183	[40–120 umol/L]
Urea	4.4	[2.5–8.0 mmol/l]
Magnesium	0.18	[0.70–1.05 mmol/L]
Glucose	3.6	[3.5–6.0 mmol/L]

Helene's monthly blood work for the 4 months prior to admission showed:

HGB	155, 163, 167, 165
WBC	6.0, 7.2, 6.1, 6.1
Platelets	179, 199, 204, 213
Creatinine	86, 79, 75, 76
Potassium	4.7, 4.4, 4.7, 4.4

On admission, Helene was on the following medications:

Mycophenolate 1 g BID
FK 506 (Tacrolimus) 3 mg BID
Prednisone 5 mg OD
Zocor 40 mg OD
Aspirin 325 mg OD
Insulin 23 units (N); R 2–5 units; and regular prn through the day

The above scenario is typical of admission information. Indeed, reading this, you know more of Helene's social history than you typically might for a newly admitted patient on a medical unit. One of the reasons we have chosen this particular clinical situation is because it is complex in terms of both Helene's biomedical conditions and her living experience. We wish to illustrate how even in such complex situations, relational inquiry can provide grounding for your nursing assessment and intervention and help you target your nursing action effectively. By enlisting the four modes of inquiry, you can determine the knowledge you have, the knowledge you need, and possibilities for action.

So where would *you* start? What strikes you about the history as presented above? Clearly, empirical data dominates, but what else do you notice? If you were to orient your nursing action in a socio-environmental definition of health, what would your first step be? For example, seeing Helene and having read her history and blood work, my (Gweneth's) attention is on her current physical state. If she can barely get on a bedpan, her choice and well-being are seriously compromised. Thus, my most immediate concern is to understand what is happening physically. I want to be clear about what is known and what empirical data might be missing—most specifically what might be contributing to her weakness. Thus, I would start with an empirical inquiry.

Empirical Inquiry

A relational perspective guides empirical inquiry in at least four important ways:

1. Through a relational approach, empirical inquiry must be conducted at the intrapersonal, interpersonal, and contextual levels.
2. A relational approach guides empirical inquiry to be more than application of evidence in a decontextualized manner; relational inquiry requires skillful use of generalizable data within a particular context.
3. A relational approach guides nurses to draw on a wide range of evidence beyond a focus on disease, illness, and treatment of physiologic problems; relational inquiry requires complex integration of multiple sources and forms of evidence.
4. Relational inquiry guides nurses to interpret empirical evidence and extend empirical inquiry in light of other forms of knowledge.

Empirical Inquiry at All Levels

Typically, empirical evidence is thought of as factual, undisputed, and objective. In that view, you as a knower are separate from the facts. However, as we have been discussing, from a relational inquiry perspective, you are integral to your own knowing. Starting at the intrapersonal level, what is your reference point in relation to Helene's situation? For example, what do you know about chronic kidney disease, and what do you know about kidney transplants? Do you know enough to skillfully interpret her blood work? Identifying the limits of your knowledge and inquiring further is fundamental to good practice, and it would be another crucial step in your care of Helene and Dana. So, if you did not have that knowledge, how might you get it? Who might you ask, "Is there anything I should know about a person with a renal transplant that would change how I interpret her blood work?" If you asked a physician such a question, what effect do you think doing so would have on your outlook?

Typically, empirical data is not seen as an interpersonal phenomenon. However, all evidence you gather shapes your interpersonal relationships. That is, while "standard" empirical data are often offered or collected, relational inquiry directs your attention to more *particular* features of a situation. So, for example, in thinking of next steps, what observations do you need to make about Helene to complement the vital signs and lab data above? Two people can have exactly the same hemoglobin for example, and one will look clinically different from the other. Further, how might this data play out in your care of Helene? For example, Dana is likely to question you about Helene's lab work results and medications (she always wants to know, and after all these years probably knows more than you do about lab values and how to interpret them in Helene's case). How would you interpret such questions? (As a challenge to your expertise? As overstepping Helene's autonomy? As an opportunity for collaboration and learning on your part?) What does your reaction tell you about your reference point in relation to "ownership" of empirical data? Who do you think owns and gets to use empirical knowledge? What will be important about your response? In turn, what does the empirical data suggest about what might be important to Helene and Dana? For example, you might think that Dana's insistence on knowing Helene's kidney function tests suggests that she is worrying that Helene's transplant is failing. Your knowledge that although being dehydrated is not good for kidney function, it will not necessarily provoke transplant failure, will allow you to respond to the concerns in a knowledgeable and meaningful way. Or do you interpret her questions as an indication of her lack of faith in your knowledge? How could you ascertain what is behind her question?

As you undertake your empirical inquiry, you are aware that empirical evidence is always contextual. The type of evidence that is generated is often a matter of routine. Gweneth's story about Mrs. Smith (whose legs were "burning") illustrates how the generation of certain evidence becomes routine in certain contexts. Knowing how the context shapes what evidence is produced and what evidence is valued and taken into account allows you to inquire as to what might be missing and what other empirical and other forms of evidence should be taken into account. For example, it may not be routine to generate certain kinds of empirical knowledge that Helene and Dana are asking for or with which you yourself are familiar. What would this mean for you as a competent nurse who is caring for Helene and Dana?

Relating Generalizable Data within a Particular Context

One of the crucial elements as you undertake your empirical inquiry will be that of translating what you know empirically into a useable form in particular situations. Using empirical data always involves moving from generalizable norms to specific situations. A relational inquiry approach helps you to do so more skillfully by avoiding the most common pitfall of assuming that population-based data can be applied directly to particular individuals. So, for example, I (Colleen) frequently encounter questions about whether "poor" people or "people living common-law" are more likely to experience intimate partner violence. This can be a dangerous assumption if applied to individuals. While it is true that there is a slightly higher incidence of violence at a population level in lower income levels or in common-law relationships, that does not mean that a *particular* woman with a low income or in a common-law relationship is likely to be experiencing violence; nor does it mean that a *particular* higher income, married woman is unlikely to be experiencing violence. Interpreting population data such as this requires constant inquiry. Rather than a simplistic idea that, for example, people who are married are less likely to be violent, you might entertain other explanations; perhaps women who experience violence in their relationships are less likely to commit to marriage.

To pick up on an example from Helene's situation, how do you interpret her blood pressure? You likely know that her BP is on the low end of normal, but inquiring further allows you to interpret this empirical data not just against population norms, but against the particular situation. For example, if you asked, Helene would tell you that her blood pressure tends to be in the range of 130/85, so you know that this current BP is exceptionally low for her.

Complex Integration of Multiple Sources and Forms of Empirical Evidence

As you proceed through your empirical inquiry, you will most likely find yourself presented with empirical evidence that draws your attention to certain features of any given situation. So, for example, because Helene's primary health problems at the moment appear to be dehydration, diarrhea, and significant acidosis, the data collected to date focuses on these issues and draws your attention to them. However, at the same time, you might find that attention to other evidence is being obscured. Thus, following a relational inquiry approach, you will need to ask what other data might be missing or what other interpretations should be considered. For example, a cursory inspection of her lab work tells you that her low blood pressure is at least in part due to dehydration. In particular, her elevated sodium, chloride, and hemoglobin suggest significant dehydration. Do you think that her hypotension is being masked to some extent by her concern and level of stress? Such analysis would leave you even more alert to the consequences of hypotension and provoke further inquiry. For example, does she become dizzy and faint when getting up?

When in a complex situation like this, the data and making sense of it can feel overwhelming, but focusing on the immediate "presenting experience" and what you know and don't know is a good place to start. By doing this, you will likely find that to provide good care to Helene, you can begin with her immediate experience and symptoms and work from there. For example, her dehydration and diarrhea must be understood in the context of diabetes and immunosuppression. Indeed, in addition to investigating various infections as causative, her physicians immediately began to investigate the possibility that diabetic neuropathy was the explanation for her diarrhea.

Because it is not your job as a nurse to determine "what is going on" to produce a medical diagnosis, as you look beyond the immediate symptoms, you can focus your attention on considering other questions that need to be asked to support the *nursing* aspect. For example, what other empirical information related to living with a chronic health condition might enhance your care for Helene and Dana? Study of the experience of living with chronic conditions such as diabetes or chronic kidney disease might be helpful in sensitizing you to the potential challenges they face and the capacities that might be supported. Researchers (e.g., Checton, Greene, Magsamen-Conrad, & Venetis, 2012; Jowett & Peel, 2009; Kneck, Klang, & Fagerberg, 2012; Yen et al., 2011) have extensively studied the experiences of diverse people living with chronic conditions, illustrating both the complexities of chronic illness and the ways in which health care providers are often disempowering despite good intentions. Similarly, research regarding the processes of renal transplantation decision making, particularly the challenging dynamics of families' experiences of being asked to consider organ donation (Gill, 2012; Gill & Lowes, 2008; McGrath, Pun, & Holewa, 2012) might provide some basis for "pattern recognition" in understanding Helene's experience. Empirical evidence about how nurses tend to relate to patients with chronic kidney disease might be helpful. For example, Aasen, Kvangarsnes, and Heggen (2012) recently described a study of nursing practice in dialysis units, showing how although they tended to exert power and control over patients, to a lesser extent, they also shared power with patients and transferred power to the patient's family members.

Relating to Empirical Evidence in Light of Other Forms of Knowledge

Another concrete step to take as part of your relational inquiry is to evaluate the empirical knowledge you have in light of other forms of knowledge. In relational inquiry, empirical knowledge needs to be purposefully "related" to other forms of knowledge and evaluated in light of that other knowledge. For example, Helene's current physiologic data and treatment must be evaluated in light of her values. At that point in time, Helene was weary of living and in fact was somewhat reluctant to come to the hospital, particularly because she knew that she would not be admitted to the renal floor where she was "known." She was continually balancing her value for her quality of life against her value for going on living, and in the back of her mind, always had the question of what if her transplanted kidney failed. So you need to consider the value and aesthetic questions you could ask to enhance your ability to care for Helene.

If you had some knowledge about families' experiences of transplantation and quality of life, you could use such knowledge to inquire further with Helene and her family. How did the decisions about transplantation get made in their family? Is there any relationship between this experience and their current level of social support? Such knowledge might also suggest sociopolitical inquiry. For example, how does a successful transplantation affect economic status through policies such as disability pension eligibility or health insurance eligibility? It is important to emphasize, however, that in relational inquiry practice, you do not merely ask any questions that might come to mind as a result of *your* knowledge and/or concerns. Rather, the *particular* questions that are asked are determined by listening to the meaningful experience of the patient or family and inquiring into each specific situation. So the questions you ask would be ones relevant to Helene and Dana and their immediate situation.

BOX 6.2

Questions for Empirical Inquiry

- What knowledge/evidence explicitly and implicitly is informing this situation/phenomenon?
- Whose knowledge/evidence is informing this situation/phenomenon?
- What knowledge/evidence is missing?
- Intrapersonal: What empirical evidence do you know and understand? What are the limits of your own knowledge? How are you relating empirical knowledge to other forms of knowledge?
- Interpersonal: How are you using your knowledge? What effect does your knowing/not knowing stance have on your patients, families, and colleagues? How might your interpersonal use of knowledge be enhanced by intentionally engaging other forms of knowledge and/or relating to other knowers (patients/families, colleagues, etc.)?
- Contextual: What knowledge dominates in this context? How does the context affect what evidence is gathered and used?
- HP lens: How is knowledge being interpreted? What knowledge or evidence is seen as significant? And how is the context of the knowers (including yourself) shaping what and how empirical evidence is known, valued, and deployed? What other forms of knowledge are drawn upon?
- Critical lens: How are power dynamics shaping what empirical evidence is produced, valued, understood, and employed? What and whose knowledge is valued and used?

Ethical Inquiry

As you care for Helene and Dana and undertake your relational inquiry, it is important to simultaneously bring ethical questions to bear. But how does a nurse "know" that his or her actions are ethical? A number of years ago, we were part of a team of researchers that undertook research into nursing ethics (Storch, Hartrick Doane, Rodney, Varcoe, & Starzomski, 2000-2007). Having found existing ethical theory and ethics education in nursing inadequate to offer nurses the knowledge and skills they require to navigate their way through the complex, ambiguous, and shifting terrain of everyday nursing practice, we undertook projects with the potential to inform ethical nursing theory, assist us in reconceptualizing nursing ethics, and inform our rethinking of ethics education in nursing. Through our work as a team, we came to believe that at the center of ethical practice is a particular way of relating in the world grounded in an ethic of social justice (as in Chapter 1) and the understanding that people, knowledge, decisions, and actions are relationally and contextually derived. This means, for example, that what constitutes ethical practice in one context or with one person or family may not be ethical in another. It also became evident that inquiry was integral to ethical practice in nursing (Hartrick Doane et al., 2009).

Ethical Inquiry in Everyday Nursing Practice

A relational inquiry approach offers inquiry processes to assist in deciding how to "do good." As we discussed in Chapter 3, principle-based biomedical ethics—meaning principles such as autonomy, beneficence, maleficence, and so on—have been widely used to understand ethics in medicine (Andorno, 2012; Evans, 2000; Wolf, 1994) and also have dominated nursing ethics (Rodney, Burgess, Phillips, McPherson, & Brown, 2013). However, nurses and others are progressively developing ethical theory particular to nurses and nursing issues. For example, Snellman and Gedda (2012) recently argued that nursing's "value ground" is anchored in two ethical principles that differ dramatically from biomedical principles. They see the principle of human value and the right to experience a meaningful life as the two grounding principles for nursing. They argue that the principle of human value asserts that every human being is of equal value and thus has the same human rights and the right to have them respected with no one person being superior to the other. Considering these two principles in light of Helene and Dana, attention would turn to how they are being valued as people and how the care you and others on the health care team are offering is in sync with their wishes.

There are several important interrelated trends in ethical theory that are particularly helpful to ethical inquiry in nursing. First, "relational" ethics highlights how all nursing work is carried out in what Rodney, Brown, and Liaschenko (2004) have called a relational matrix. That is, various authors have challenged the idea that moral agents are independent decision-makers and have shown how nurses make ethical decisions *in relation* to others (Austin, Goble, & Kelecevic, 2009; Bergum, 2013; Bourque Bearskin, 2011; Falk-Rafael & Betker, 2012; Hartrick Doane & Varcoe, 2007; Pergert & Lützén, 2012; Rodney et al., 2013; Woods, 2012). Thus, this relational theorizing of ethics directs us to ask questions about that relational matrix. For example, what are the reference points that are being used to determine "good" nursing? And how are reference points constructed through the relational matrix? For example, how does the convergence of intrapersonal, interpersonal, and contextual elements shape the reference points used for deciding what constitutes "good" nursing action for Helene and Dana? Thinking back to the example of the first-year student who walked into a relational matrix in which restraining a patient was considered to be "good" care, how might an ethical inquiry have enabled her to voice her concerns in a way that corresponded (remember the five Cs in Chapter 3) with the situation?

A second trend in ethical theory that is helpful to ethical inquiry is the development of contextual ethics (which is related to relational ethics). Contextual ethics has supported understanding that moral choices are shaped by context (Abma, Baur, Molewijk, & Widdershoven, 2010; Allmark, 2013; Ells, Hunt, & Chambers-Evans, 2011; Fox & Swazey, 2010; Hoffmaster, 2001; Sherwin, 2011; Varcoe, Pauly, Storch, Newton, & Makaroff, 2012; Varcoe, Pauly, Webster, & Storch, 2012; Widdershoven, Molewijk, & Abma, 2009; Winkler, 1993). That is, just as an individual or family can only be understood in context, contextual ethics emphasizes that the ethical issues that arise and the decisions that are made can only be understood within context. Considering the incontinence example and the practice of diapering patients, the ethics of that action and what constitutes "good" action is context-dependent. For example, on one day, given the contextual realities (several acutely ill patients and minimum staffing), it might be the best decision. However, on other days on the same unit, it might not. Ethical inquiry through a contextual/relational perspective highlights the temporal aspect of ethics and how what constitutes "good" nursing can only be determined in a particular situation. For example, at this point in time, Helene is weary of living, whereas on another admission, she may be in a different contextual life space.

Third, contextual ethics informed by feminist and postcolonial ideas has emphasized that race, sex, gender, class, history, colonialism, and other features of the sociopolitical context must be taken into account in understanding and making moral choices in nursing and health care (Brown, Rodney, Pauly, Varcoe, & Smye, 2004; Shaha, 1998; Sherwin, 1998). For example, in my research in emergency, I (Colleen) saw nurses deciding what care patients deserved in concert with their colleagues as well as in relation to unit norms (Varcoe, Rodney, & McCormick, 2003). In concert with emergency unit culture, nurses labeled patients who repeatedly returned to emergency as "frequent flyers" (see Malone, 1996) and judged those patients to some extent according to the opinions of their colleagues and in accordance with organizational pressure to get patients out of the unit quickly. Further, class and race-based assumptions were evident in those judgments, for example, when nurses racialized violence. In more recent research in emergency contexts, we saw how patients anticipated and attempted to counter racialized judgements by nurses and other care providers (Varcoe, Browne, Wong, & Smye, 2009). By understanding that such practices are not merely a consequence of either interpersonal relationships or the context acting upon individuals (Allen & Hardin, 2001), nurses can make choices that contribute to shaping health care culture differently.

A fourth trend in ethical theory has been the linking of ethics and spirituality. As Niebuhr (1972) and Hague (1995) have described, morality is a spiritual endeavour and spirituality is a moral endeavour. Simmington (2004) contends that an ethical environment is one in which "the total well-being of our patients, including their spiritual well-being, is honoured and advocated" (p. 466). Simmington asserts that healing and wholeness are spiritual concepts and that movement in the direction of healing and wholeness is movement in the direction of evolving spirituality. Subsequently, to practice ethically, nurses must question whether the social, cultural, and religious trends that inform ethical decision making are supporting people's spiritual life and/or if they are interfering with spiritual expression. "To act ethically . . . is to do all we can to remove barriers that interfere with the ability of individuals, groups, and the collective to live their lives fully . . . while our own spiritual journey, and those of the people we walk beside, may not be without pain, it is up to us to ensure that it is also not without joy" (Simmington, 2004, p. 480). This illustrates the integral connection between ethical and aesthetic inquiry and also sociopolitical inquiry. Another example would be the decision to tie up the elderly man. Might the decision have been shaped by bias related to age? From a critical relational view, we might ask: If it had been a young person, would the normative practice of tying patients up have been enacted? Or how is it that the nurses saw restraints as their only option? Had economic and/or policy decisions been made based on the valuing of certain types of care over others (e.g., valuing pharmacologic or high-tech interventions over care for the elderly—both of which are promoted by profit motives) or based on the geographical location of this particular health care agency? Is the nurse–patient ratio here a reflection of larger political and economic decisions shaped by such values? Given the multitude of factors that affect and shape nursing actions, relational inquiry as a practice of knowing supports the questioning of knowledge, values, and norms that dominate particular situations.

As nurses, we enlist knowledge to ensure that our nursing actions promote health and healing. Thus, a question you need to bring to your practice is: How do I determine what actually constitutes "healing/health-promoting" practice in Helene and Dana's situation? Ethical inquiry is ultimately an inquiry that is oriented toward that question. Ethical inquiry involves questions about "what is good" and "how shall I do good?" In nursing, this translates into "What is good care?" and "How shall I do good in my nursing practice?" An ethical inquiry is oriented to the question *What would be the most responsive, respectful, and effective way to ensure good and safe nursing care?*

Relating Ethical Knowledge to Other Forms of Knowledge

Interestingly, through our research into nursing ethics, we found one of the most significant aspects limiting nurses in their ethical practice was the way they separated ethical knowledge from other forms of knowledge (Hartrick Doane et al., 2009). In particular, they did not realize the significance of their nursing knowledge to ethical knowledge and/or relate one form of knowledge to another to inform their nursing practice. For example, many nurses assumed that to make an ethical decision, they required philosophical knowledge of formal ethical theory. While this formal knowledge of ethical theory is certainly helpful, the nurses did not see how their nursing knowledge enhanced their capacity to make "good" (ethical) decisions. Yet their *nursing* knowledge and knowledge of the health care setting offered a strong foundation for their ethical practice. It was this larger knowledge of *nursing* and the health care context that enabled them to think their way through situations and toward more ethical ways of responding. At the same time, there were other forms of knowledge that supported the nurses to determine "good" practice. So although you might not have studied formal theory to help you know what is ethical, within a relational inquiry approach, you can enlist empirical, aesthetic, and sociopolitical knowledge to inform ethical practice.

A pragmatist orientation and both the HP and critical lenses are based on the assumption that *knowledge can never be separated from values or ideology*; scientific research and theories (and the practices to which those give rise) are embedded in societal norms, values, and expectations. Knowledge is value-laden because those who have developed theories and knowledge have lived and participated in society and thus have been influenced and shaped by taken-for-granted societal truths and expectations. The form of knowledge that is drawn upon and also how knowledge is used is also shaped by values and ideology. Therefore, research evidence, theories, and models need to be considered and questioned through an ethical inquiry so that we do not (in the name of scientific, evidence-based practice) inadvertently see only the meanings and truths relevant to our normative reference points, existing theories, models, and values. Ethical inquiry directs our attention to the question of which values and normative reference points are being privileged. So as you care for Helene and Dana and undertake an ethical inquiry, you would be considering the values that are at play and shaping how knowledge is being used and enlisted. This inquiry enables knowledge that may be of great importance and relevance to providing effective nursing care not to be overlooked. Further, inquiry into what values are operating also helps us attend to how our own values are shaping us in any given situation and how we may be limiting our responsiveness to people who may not fit our values. Ethical inquiry also helps us attend to how we may be imposing oppressive societal values and expectations on people who may not fit dominant social values and norms.

By inquiring into what is of meaning (aesthetic) and value (ethical) to Helene and Dana, you are able to work contextually to ensure that knowledge informs the care they receive. This illustrates how the relevance of other forms of knowledge comes to the forefront by centering ethical inquiry on the question: *What would be the most responsive, respectful, and effective way to ensure good and safe nursing care?* For example, by asking this question in the situation with the elderly man who was restrained, it becomes apparent that if restraints are deemed as one potential nursing option, it would be important to ask, "What positive and negative effects might the restraints have?" For example, Shorr and colleagues (2002) cite literature that shows that in addition to the loss of autonomy and dignity, choking, agitation, confusion, decubitus ulcers, and even death may be caused by restraints. Thus, to proceed ethically, it is important to ask if there are other possibilities for care.

Goethals and colleagues (2012) show how nurses' decision making related to restraints are primarily motivated by safety, but context- and nurse-related factors hindered nurses from making ethical decisions on the appropriate use of physical restraints. They argued that nurses needed to carefully balance different options and associated ethical values. For example, are there calming strategies that could be used? Are there reasons for the man's behavior that could be addressed? For example, the evidence suggests an important relationship between urinary tract infections and delirium (Boockvar & Lachs, 2003; Eriksson, Gustafson, Fagerström, & Olofsson, 2011; Hufschmidt, Shabarin, Rauer, & Zimmer, 2010), particularly in older people. Have such possibilities been considered? Is there someone (a family member, a staff member, volunteer) who has a calming effect on the patient and who could sit with him? If not, do resources need to be sought to make different treatment possible? This example calls attention to the minute-to-minute decisions and actions in which nurses engage as they go about their everyday work and illustrates the importance of understanding these decisions *in relation to* all other aspects of nursing—and in particular, to the values and normative practices that give rise to those actions. Ethical inquiry involves looking beyond normative nursing practices to consider how we *should* practice, what values deserve our allegiance, to who and what we are obligated and responsible, how we should enact those obligations, and the principles and guidelines with which to ground our judgments and actions. Ethical inquiry brings attention to the way in which every minute of nursing practice involves ethics and an understanding of ethics as a deeply personal process that is lived in the complexity and ambiguity of everyday nursing work.

We believe that the relational inquiry process of nursing that we have described throughout this book provides a theoretical and practical foundation for ethical practice in nursing—for "doing good" in practice. As with all forms of inquiry, ethical inquiry requires attention at the intrapersonal, interpersonal, and contextual levels (Box 6.3). Ethical inquiry requires paying attention to your own values and how they are living in your practice. For example, how do your own age, social location, and experiences shape how you see the elderly man in restraints? Similarly, if you are heterosexual, how do your own normative assumptions and values shape how you relate with Helene and Dana? For some heterosexual nurses, providing care to same-sex couples requires careful examination of personal values. How does your particular racial identity and experience shape your relationship to racializing discourses? If you agree with Snellman and Gedda (2012) that the value ground of nursing includes the idea that all humans are of equal value, then how do you align all your values with that premise? At the interpersonal level, ethical inquiry leads you to ask about how values are being played out in relation to others. What constitutes a good relationship? Is it a matter of taking control and acting as expert, or are their other options? Directing the question "What is a good relationship" toward the "other" suggests the importance and possibility of understanding what people and families want from a health care relationship. Directing the question toward the context means analyzing both what would be a good relationship in that particular context and what would be a good context for high-quality nursing care. For example, what is considered a good relationship with a dying person within the culture of a palliative care unit might be quite different than within the culture of a prison. Quite different practices may be "normalized" and taken for granted within each of these contexts. Such questions surface the ways in which individuals, families, and contexts influence "good relationships" so that rather than operating in an unconscious way, nurses can more deliberately and intentionally make choices about how they take up ideas and practices. That is, it extends your choice architecture and the reference points from which you work.

Given that autonomy and self-determination are fundamental to any code of ethical practice, the question "How are autonomy and self-determination to be fostered?" is routine. However, a relational understanding of autonomy means that any person's or family's autonomy and choice can only be understood in context. This means, for example, that understanding a person's wish to die requires understanding that wish in context and in relation to what it is that ultimately concerns that person and family. Does the person not wish to be a burden to his or her family members? Or does that person wish to die only because of physical pain that is not being (and potentially could be) relieved? What, for example, might be influencing Helene's weariness of life?

Understanding ethical choices in context suggests turning back to other forms of inquiry. How are autonomy and self-determination being lived in relation to the dominant ideologies that you are exploring through sociopolitical inquiry (as we will describe, the ideology of compliance serves as a good example here) and/or in relation to the empirical inquiry you are undertaking? So, following the lead of people and families and asking, "What do these people want?" and "What are this person's worries?" (aesthetic inquiry) requires taking other forms of inquiry into account. For example, what does this individual or family want within what is known and what is considered possible? For example, Hclene was eligible for another transplant due to her age and "proven medical compliance;" my (Colleen's) mother was not eligible for a bone marrow transplant due to her age; each situation set different possibilities for "choice."

Ethical inquiry provides significant direction for action. The questions "How am I being?" "What is the effect of how I am being?" and "How do I want to be?" reflect both analysis of your own values and of the relational context. These questions also suggest the possibility of being more intentional in your practice based on an analysis of your values in relation to the values of the people and families with whom you work and the values operating within the context of practice. These questions directly lead to the question "How shall we be together?" Given this knowledge and analysis, you can determine the "best" actions you can take and how you might best support capacity, equity, and justice.

BOX 6.3

Key Questions for Ethical Inquiry

What knowledge is valued or devalued?

- Whose knowledge is valued or devalued?
- What values, commitments, and obligations are being upheld?
- Whose values, commitments, and obligations are being upheld?
- What values, commitments, and obligations inform the knowledge that is being used and how knowledge is being applied?
- Intrapersonal: How are your values affecting this situation and being affected by this situation?
- Interpersonal: What values are you imposing, upholding, or undermining? How do your values match with the people, family, and communities to whom you are providing care?
- Contextual: What wider values are influencing this situation? What wider values can be influenced (health care organization, wider society)?
- HP lens: How are values arising from the worlds in which people are situated? How are people constituted by those values?
- Critical lens: How are power dynamics shaping what and whose values are upheld?

Aesthetic Inquiry

Aesthetics matter in nursing. Rachelle Lautischer, a nurse who works in a maternal/child unit and who recently took a relational inquiry course, offers a great example of how she has started to bring different modes of inquiry together and approach her work more aesthetically. She describes how the normative practice within maternal/child care is often disease-oriented and focused on risk assessment and disease management. Rachelle describes how relational inquiry reoriented her practice to be more "multidimensional" to consider how all things are interwoven and are meaningful to care. *"The omission of this consideration from my practice was not intentional. It was due to decreased awareness and understanding of the power dynamics in my practice. So now that I understand the powers that live within me, I deliberately ask my patients and families what matters to them during their labor and delivery experience and which family member they would like to have present in the room during the birth of their child."*

This inquiry into "what matters" is a wonderful example of aesthetic inquiry and the art of aesthetically meaningful nursing care. In a similar vein, Godfrey, Cloete, Dymond, and Long (2012) provide a concrete example in their study of hydration for elderly people. Given the importance of hydration, the diminished desire to drink among older people, fear of incontinence or frequent urination, and the high risk of dehydration, they explored the perceptions of elderly residents in care homes and elderly patients in hospitals and the perceptions of their caregivers. The role of the aesthetics of drinking was fundamental to problems with hydration. The emphasis was on fluid intake as a functional rather than a pleasurable activity. Taste, temperature, and appearance of drinks; the

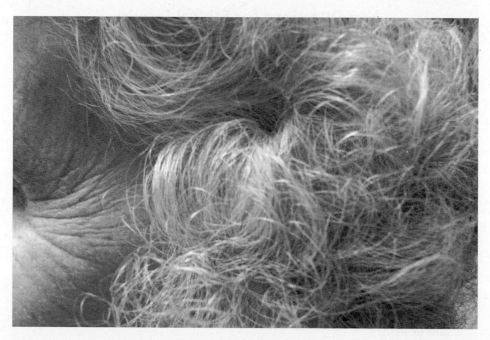

Aesthetics and beauty. (Photograph by Gweneth Doane.)

timing, availability, and presentation of drinks; and the utility of drinking aids impaired the quality of their drinking experience. Lack of attention to personal preference, independence in drinking, and the social aspects of drinking all contributed to the older people's lack of pleasure in drinking and hence contributed to dehydration. Drinking was perceived as a task or burden rather than as pleasurable. The study pointed clearly to the importance of aesthetics as key to supporting older people's well-being through drinking.

But what is aesthetic inquiry in nursing? To what does "aesthetics" refer? Chinn and Kramer (2011) say that aesthetic inquiry asks: What does this mean? How is it significant? Aesthetics are linked to art, beauty, taste, and sensory-emotional experiences. Aesthetics are also linked to suffering, because art and suffering are seen in many traditions as inseparable and because aesthetics are thought to be one way to counter suffering. To take a simple example, when I (Colleen) was being prepared for labor in anticipation of the birth of my son, my midwives told me to bring with me the most beautiful picture or object I could find that had meaning for me. I chose a picture I had taken of a canoe pulled up on the shore of a remote lake where I and my partner had portaged. Throughout my labor, I focused on the beauty of that picture and the peaceful memories with which I associated it. According to Chinn and Kramer (2011), aesthetic knowing involves establishing a meaningful connection with the person being cared for, appreciation, envisioning, improvising, creating and recreating storylines, and creating and developing embodied synchronous movement. To follow my example, meeting my midwife at the door of the hospital when I was in full labor was one of the most meaningful moments of my life; she opened her arms and gave me a hug. I felt known, safe, secure, and cared for, and consequently I was confident in myself and those who would be caring for me during the birth of my son.

Aesthetics in nursing has received some limited attention. Most recently, Archibald (2012) took issue with Carper's assertion that aesthetic knowing comprises the art of nursing, arguing that there is an important difference between knowledge development (i.e., aesthetic knowing) and the application of knowledge in practice (i.e., the art of nursing). She offers an alternative conceptualization of aesthetics in nursing, highlighting the distinction between artistry, which comprises the technical and deliberate skill that constitutes an art (e.g., skilled nursing practice), and aesthetics (e.g., the science of sensory perception), which is integral to exploring aesthetic knowing in nursing. Archibald draws on Dewey (1934/1995) to define aesthetics as the branch of philosophy concerned with sentiments of taste and judgment pertaining to sensory–emotional values. Importantly, in line with a pragmatist orientation (which also underlies a relational approach to nursing), Archibald also draws on Dewey to argue that the aesthetic pattern of knowing is the knowing of a unique particular experience rather than an exemplary class. So, for example, a "good death" cannot be known or described as a general experience exemplary of "good death" but must be known in its particulars. The aesthetics of a good death for one person may not be so for another. Similarly, for some people, the aesthetics of a hospital that give them a sense of control and safety would be preferred when birthing a baby while others may prefer a home environment.

She distinguishes an aesthetic experience from general experience according to its noteworthiness and the degree to which it is memorable (Dewey, 1934/1995). To return to my example of the birth of my son, I (Colleen) judge that I, my partner, my son, and my mother had a beautiful aesthetic experience. Despite the fact that my son had the umbilical cord around his neck and had to be resuscitated briefly, the nursing care, the labor room, the presence of my family—indeed all aspects—were beautiful and in line with my hopes and dreams.

We agree with Archibald and Dewey who both argue that aesthetic experience is integrative, wherein individual elements are synthesized into a meaningful and cohesive whole. In some ways, aesthetic knowing can be seen as the beauty in the whole of nursing practice.

TO ILLUSTRATE
A Cup of Tea

I (Gweneth) was reminded of the "beauty" of nursing care when Colleen told me the following story about making a cup of tea.

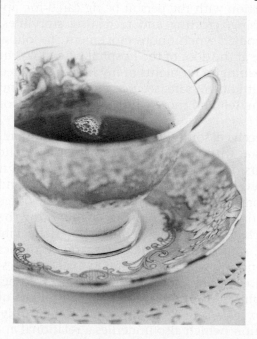

Aesthetic knowing.

I was working at a weekly drop-in for women at a primary health care organization in an inner city serving people marginalized by extreme poverty, racism, and/or stigma related to mental health illness and/or substance use. The drop-in typically provides lunch and activities. Sometimes we give the women manicures and hand massages, sometimes there is a craft to do, sometimes there are donated clothes to share, and

continued on page 267

TO ILLUSTRATE *continued*

A Cup of Tea

often there is someone playing piano or guitar with impromptu sing-alongs on occasion. If the women would like to see a health care provider, they can do so, and they can participate in the drop-in while waiting to see the health care provider rather than waiting in the (not very welcoming or safe) waiting room that is often dominated by men. Most of the women who attend are living on the street or in "single-room occupancy hotel" rooms in the neighborhood, and all have experienced significant violence of multiple forms.

Those of us who are care providers (staff from the organization, volunteers, students, and researchers) try to make the drop-in a welcoming, enjoyable break from life on the street, which is constantly dangerous and stressful. We serve the women food, invite them to sit, and invite them to be involved in whatever is going on or whatever we have to offer. In the routine course of participating in the drop-in, I invited a woman in as she stood tentatively at the door. I introduced myself and asked her if she would like to take a seat (indicating either the big table strewn with craft materials and snacks or the couches). She looked to be about 50 years old but hobbled painfully (people who live on the street or in shelters have to walk on concrete many hours per day and therefore often have terrible foot problems, especially given that they usually wear donated shoes that do not fit). She had many scars visible on her arms and face; the scars looked like the consequences of various injuries, knife wounds, and burns. She smiled appreciatively. I said, "The food isn't here yet, but could I make you a cup of tea?"

She paused thoughtfully and looked up at me saying, "No one has ever offered to make me a cup of tea before."

All my life, people have been making me cups of tea to socialize, to comfort, and just for fun. One of my earliest memories is my grandmother and mother making me "tea" (mostly milk). Putting on the kettle has been such an integral part of my social life that I found myself wondering what it would be like to live so long without having experienced such a simple caring gesture ever.

When Colleen told me this story, I (Gweneth) was struck by how this gesture of offering to make tea for someone was a profoundly meaningful one in terms of understanding aesthetic nursing practice. While tea may not hold the same meaning for the woman as it does for Colleen— it may not be associated with warm family memories, social interaction, and so forth— given the woman's background and life situation, the action of showing interest in and inquiring into the woman's comfort was one of aesthetic beauty. The meaningful connection described by Chinn and Kramer (2011) as a hallmark of aesthetic nursing was clearly created. Chinn and Kramer assert that aesthetic action involves appreciating what is of significance, envisioning and/or reimagining storylines, and improvising nursing care accordingly. As Colleen extended herself to promote the woman's comfort by offering to make her a cup of tea, she communicated that the woman was of value and that her comfort mattered—that *she* was significant. Regardless of what her life had been like, by offering to make her a cup of tea, in that moment, the woman's life was "re-storied"; she was a person of worth and dignity. While that same action may not have been relevant to another person, it was the "correspondence" (remember Chapter 3) that made it aesthetically meaningful. It was Colleen's improvisation in the relational moment that made the simple act of offering tea a health-promoting form of aesthetic care and beauty.

As you consider Helene and Dana, what would you imagine "beautiful care" to be? Karen Mahoney, one of the nurses who cared for Helene and Dana over many years, recently reflected on that question.

> *The first time I met Helene and Dana, I was working in the hospital as a casual in the renal unit, and we were going through the noon rush (patients coming off [dialysis], the next shift of patients being put on). Helene and Dana were standing rather prominently at the nursing station looking like they wanted someone to notice them, but they were being ignored. I was flying by but stopped to ask if they needed something. Helene told me she had taken her noon insulin but had no lunch. I phoned the kitchen and had a tray sent up, and it seemed that started what became a good working relationship over several years. I'm not saying I did anything "beautiful," but I knew how much they valued that seemingly small thing. What I remember about Helene was that she wanted to be "seen" (in the best sense) and not slotted into a category or role.*

We think that the bringing together of empirical, ethical, sociopolitical, and perhaps other forms of knowing into a coherent whole constitutes the aesthetics of practice. Clearly, as Archibald following Dewey (1934/1995) asserts, aesthetics and aesthetic experience cannot exist outside of the realm of values. What one values and finds beautiful in human experience will set the criteria for what one finds aesthetically pleasing. For example, as a nurse, I (Gweneth) found it aesthetically pleasing doing morning care for patients—assisting them with their grooming, refreshing their bed with clean linens, tidying up their bedside tables, and so forth. However, I quickly learned that while I valued having an orderly and tidy space, not all patients shared that value and aesthetic preference. Thus, it was important for me to ask what *their* preferences were before I just barged in and started doing "care." Similarly, aesthetic inquiry cannot be separated from the empirical or the sociopolitical. To return to the example of hydration care, Godfrey and colleagues (2012) found that the dominance of empirical knowledge about dehydration contributed to drinking being seen as a technical and functional task. They found that the context of practice, inadequate time, inadequate resources such as drinking aids, and the ethos that supported dependency in drinking for older people (helping them drink, rather than helping them independently drink) all mitigated against the aesthetics of drinking.

As with other modes of inquiry, aesthetic inquiry is conducted at all levels simultaneously (see Box 6.4). At the intrapersonal level, have you thought about nursing as an aesthetic experience? Nurses are with patients during some of their most meaningful moments—birth, illness, tragedy, grief, relief, healing, and death. If you think about it, these aspects of human experience are the stuff of art, so nurses are integral to the art of human experience. How do you work artfully? What aesthetic values do you hold? What, for example, is your sense of suffering well? And interpersonally, how do your aesthetic values align with the people to whom you are providing care? Contextually, what shapes the possibilities for an aesthetic experience in any situation?

TRY IT OUT 6.3

Washing the Dishes: An Aesthetic Inquiry

Thich Nhat Hanh is a Zen Buddhist monk, scholar, poet, and a political figure from Vietnam who has written extensively on the practice of mindfulness. His description of washing the dishes is illustrative of an aesthetic approach.

"I usually wash the dishes after we've finished the evening meal, before sitting down and drinking tea with everyone else. One night, Jim asked if he might do the dishes. I said, 'Go ahead, but if you wash the dishes, you must know the way to wash them.' Jim replied, 'Come on, you think I don't know how to wash the dishes?' I answered, 'There are two ways to wash the dishes. The first is to wash the dishes in order to have clean dishes and the second is to wash the dishes in order to wash the dishes.' Jim was delighted and said, 'I choose the second way—to wash the dishes to wash the dishes.' From then on, Jim knew how to wash the dishes. I transferred the 'responsibility' to him for an entire week.

"If while washing dishes, we think only of the cup of tea that awaits us, thus hurrying to get the dishes out of the way as if they were a nuisance, then we are not 'washing the dishes to wash the dishes.' What's more, we are not alive during the time we are washing the dishes. In fact we are completely incapable of realizing the miracle of life while standing at the sink. If we can't wash the dishes, the chances are we won't be able to drink our tea either. While drinking the tea we will be thinking of another thing, barely aware of the cup in our hands. Thus, we are sucked away into the future—and we are incapable of actually living one minute of life." (Nhat Hanh, 2013).

How we approach nursing can be likened to how we wash the dishes. Are we nursing to get our tasks done (treating and fixing patients to discharge them out the door), or are we nursing to nurse? The next time you are in clinical practice, do a "mindful inquiry" into your own aesthetic practice using the questions in Box 6.4. Ask yourself whether you are practicing to practice, or whether you are practicing only to finish your shift.

BOX 6.4

Key Questions for Aesthetic Inquiry

- How am I establishing a meaningful connection in this situation?
- What would constitute a meaningful and "beautiful" experience in this situation?
- Intrapersonal: Where is my attention? What am I appreciating and/or not appreciating? Am I being artful?
- Interpersonal: What matters and is of preference to the individuals and family members in this situation? How might I aesthetically correspond and reimagine my nursing care?
- Contextual: What wider influences are shaping the aesthetic possibilities in this situation? What wider influences can be changed (e.g., health care organization, wider society)?
- HP lens: What is of meaning to the people and the living experience of the moment?
- Critical lens: How are power dynamics shaping what aesthetic is valued, made possible, and upheld in any given situation?

Sociopolitical Inquiry

Sociopolitical inquiry directs attention to power and its relationship to knowledge, to structural conditions, and to language and ideologies. Although it seems logical that the context would be central in sociopolitical inquiry, as with all inquiry in relational practice, inquiry is conducted at the intrapersonal, interpersonal, and contextual levels simultaneously.

Beginning with the intrapersonal, your understanding of power and how it operates is crucial to sociopolitical knowing. If you see yourself as practicing within an immutable power hierarchy where your choices are constrained by that hierarchy, you will take a different approach than if you understand that every moment and every interaction is imbued with power. When nurses feel helpless and powerless, they can turn to enacting power in destructive ways. In reflecting on my mother's experience prior to her death, I (Colleen) have wondered if the nurses who were impatient and unkind perhaps were enacting power in the only way they could see to do so in a context in which they otherwise felt powerless. How you enact your power as a nurse should align with promoting the health and well-being of the patients and family members in your care. Thus, in each situation, sociopolitical inquiry involves asking whose interests you are serving. Finally the contexts of practice are a central focus in sociopolitical knowing—attending to structural conditions, language, and ideologies as they play out in context.

Sociopolitical inquiry invites paying particular attention to the context of health care as it affects particular people's and families' lives and experiences, and the wider sociopolitical context of particular people's and

BOX 6.5
Key Questions for Sociopolitical Inquiry

- What power relations are at play in this situation?
- Who dominates? Whose interests are being privileged?
- What structural conditions are influential? What ideologies?
- Who is advantaged or disadvantaged?
- How is domination being resisted?
- What might be done differently?
- Intrapersonal: How do I understand power, and how am I enacting my own power? How does my power position affect my approach? What do I get out of this arrangement? What do I see as my role in this situation? What advantages do I have that might blind me to the experiences of others? What experiences of disadvantage might sensitize me to others' experiences? To whom do I owe allegiance? What knowledge am I privileging through my enactment of power?
- Interpersonal: How am I enacting my own power in relation to individuals, family members, and colleagues in this situation? How is my enactment of power affecting the situation? How is my enactment of power aligning with my values? My aesthetic values? Whose interests am I serving?
- Contextual: What wider influences are shaping the power dynamics in this situation? What wider influences can be changed (health care organization, wider society)? How are dominant relations of power being reproduced and sustained?
- HP lens: How are all knowers (including myself) situated within, constituted by, and participating in multiple networks of power relations?
- Critical lens: How are power dynamics shaping every aspect of each situation in every moment?

families' lives and experiences. It involves examining how power plays out to support or thwart health and well-being. A beginning question might be, "What are the circumstances of this person or family?" In Helene's situation, the circumstances of being a person with a chronic condition (several, actually) on an acute medical unit might push her concerns to the side. Other acute priorities on the unit at a particular time might overshadow Helene's and Dana's chronic illness concerns.

Sociopolitical inquiry leads you to listen for the circumstances that are shaping people's and families' experiences. In Helene's situation, most salient to her circumstances at the time was the fact that Dana (an accountant) had a contract that required long hours of work, making visiting difficult. What ultimately concerns them? How do they enter into life with each other, with family and friends, and with other forms of power?

What are the patterns of capacity or adversity within their current life context? Such inquiry might turn attention to the obvious strength and power Helene and Dana must have within them to have lived through the many health challenges they have faced. Similarly, it might highlight the wealth of knowledge they bring having lived with both diabetes and renal failure for so long. For example, Helene has developed capacity in terms of knowing herself well enough to know what symptoms she needs to attend to and how to attend effectively. Dana has developed capacity in knowing how best to support Helene, and together they know how to keep their relationship and their relationships with their friends intact through repeated "life and death" experiences. Recognition of this family capacity turns attention to how contextual factors are enhancing and/or constraining such capacity. For example, how well does an acute care hospital setting facilitate nurses drawing on patients' knowledge of their own health when they have been living with chronic conditions? Similarly, you might pay attention to the adversities that seem to have particular significance and meaning. What is it that seems to be the most difficult part of their health experience? How might you collaboratively tap other contextual resources and capacities to enhance their already existing capacity? From the story, it is evident that Helene and Dana have a supportive and loving relationship and that as a couple, they also have the support of friends and community.

Structural conditions from wider social structures such as poverty/wealth, racial stratification, and so on, to more local structural conditions, such as nurse/patient ratios, shape your possibilities and your thinking. Consciously inquiring as to how particular structural conditions are shaping your practice provides you with opportunities to be more deliberate in your choices. For example, if you were to encounter Helene in emergency prior to her admission to the medical unit, how do you think your focus would be shaped differently than if you encountered her after admission? If the medical unit was overrun by a virulent infection, would you see Helene somewhat differently (e.g., thinking both of the fact that she is immunosuppressed and what such an infection might mean for your workload with other patients)? If you imagine yourself as Helene's nurse, how would the circumstances differ if you were a student new to the medical unit or if you were a nurse with 10 years of experience on that unit? What would be different if you had an elderly mother who had been refused a kidney transplant because of age-related eligibility criteria? What would be different if you were a home care nurse meeting Dana and Helene in their home rather than in a hospital setting? Imagine how the power dynamics shift in each of these situations as the structural conditions shift.

Finally, sociopolitical inquiry involves paying attention to ideologies. Allen and Hardin (2001) demonstrate how "social organization is not produced by external structures operating upon or causing people to adopt certain behaviors. Rather, social structure is an *effect* of taking up practices and reproducing and modifying them" (p. 163). For example, patients *become* "difficult" when you see them that way or label them as such. However, such patients *can* be seen differently, for example, as an opportunity to extend your nursing skills. Similarly, through my teaching career, I (Colleen) have tried to help teachers reframe "difficult" students as students who require the teacher's special skills; anyone can teach a "good" student, anyone can nurse a "good" patient, but difficulty can bring out the teacher's or nurse's best skills.

Throughout this book, we have pointed out how taken-for-granted ideas can shape thinking and practices, and we have encouraged the uncovering and challenging of such ideas. We now illustrate how this ideologic inquiry is an explicit part of your approach to nursing practice. Examining ideologies is particularly important in advancing knowledge toward social change. Rodney (1998) contends that "ideological inquiry can provide us with the theoretical and empirical tools necessary to challenge what is taken for granted in health care delivery and social policy" (p. 5). So, for example, Aasen and colleagues' (2012) study of nurses' perceptions of patient participation in their hemodialysis care showed that the nurses used power and control within an ideology of paternalism (the idea that those in greater positions of power know what is best and can exert control over others "for their own good"). They used biomedical explanations and the ethical principle of beneficence to justify their actions. They used their power to "sell" the idea that patients should have a fistula, which the nurses preferred, implying that the patients did not have a choice. However, the study also showed alternative practices, including sharing power with the patient. This sort of sociopolitical inquiry could help nurses question the value base of their practice, how they are using power, how they are using evidence in concert with their power positions, and what aesthetic they consequently uphold. In other words, sociopolitical inquiry can be a frame through which to examine how all forms of knowledge are brought together and can serve as a basis for change. For example, if hemodialysis nurses wanted to bring their practice more into line with values for respecting autonomy, they could shift their policies and practices to better enhance power-sharing.

In a relational inquiry approach, ideologies are also examined at the intrapersonal, interpersonal, and contextual levels, considering how certain practices are being taken up, reproduced, and modified. Examining ideologies can be guided broadly by four questions:

1. What ideologies do I subscribe to and how am I taking them up?
2. What ideologies is the person or family living?
3. What ideologies dominate this context?
4. How are we living these ideologies together in relation?

Analysis of your own ideologies relevant to nursing practice began at least as soon as you started reading this book. Examining your ideas about individuals, families, health, and health promotion automatically required you to consider the ways in which you take up, enact, and modify dominant ideologies. Similarly, your own spiritual and/or religious beliefs are a form of ideology. Considering what ideologies you might be living draws on the process of self-observation to consider what assumptions and biases you are living in your practice. The most telling place where ideology shows itself is in your actions.

TO ILLUSTRATE
The Ideology of Compliance

When you consider what ideologies you might be living in relation to Helene, your particular understandings, for example, about people who have diabetes, come into play. A popular ideology in use with people with diabetes (and renal and cardiac disease for that matter) is the ideology of compliance. Murphy and Canales (2001) analyzed the nursing literature and found that most nursing authors accepted the idea of compliance without apparent awareness of the long history of controversy in both medicine and nursing. Although nurse authors used various definitions and often did not define the term, usually they used compliance to mean the extent to which the patients and families followed the wishes, orders, or advice of health care providers. In other words, a nurse governed by the ideology of compliance assumes that "good patients" should follow the treatment protocols and regimens provided by expert health care providers. Other authors offered some critique but used the term despite the implications of paternalism, coercion, and acquiescence. Murphy and Canales thought this contradiction was ironic because the authors who rationalized use of the term wrote as though their critiques somehow distanced them from the associated assumptions and issues.

The term compliance has been widely critiqued because of its inherent assumption of patients and families yielding to more powerful health care providers and because through its use, nurses participate in disempowering patients and families and keeping them in line with the biomedical model. The use of the term "compliance" functions to perpetuate current systems of domination. For example, in my (Gweneth's) research with people living with diabetes, participants described how often health care providers' efforts to get them to comply with diabetic regimens (Matthews, Peden, & Rowles, 2009) seemed to take precedence over all other aspects of care (Hartrick, 1998). Moreover, they reported that when their blood sugars were "out of whack," the nurses would often assume they had not been following the regimen and would respond negatively toward them. They found it particularly frustrating that even when as "good diabetic patients" they had been "complying," the nurses would "not believe" them. What was particularly frustrating about this was that it was during these times of uncontrolled blood sugars that they, as patients, needed the most support and help from nurses. Yet because the nurses placed such emphasis on compliance and assumed uncontrolled blood sugars were a result of non-compliance, the nurses would become distant, less responsive, and at times even finger-wagging toward them (Atkin, Stapley, & Easton, 2010).

An important question to consider when examining the ideologies you are living is the extent to which they shape your approach to people. For example, if you think of a family as "noncompliant," are you able to approach that family as positively as if you think of that family as acting responsibly in terms of their own health? Similarly, if patients are making choices that are in opposition to your own particular religious beliefs, how

continued on page 275

TO ILLUSTRATE *continued*

The Ideology of Compliance

does that shape your ability to be with them in ways that honor *their* ultimate "spiritual" concerns? If you have strong opinions against same-sex couples, how will this affect your approach to Helene?

Considering what ideologies people and families are living requires actively listening for how dominant ideas are shaping their understandings and experiences, including their health care experiences and experiences of you. For example, in Helene's case, dominant ideas about medical units (as nonspecialized with less technology and less educated staff in comparison with other types of units) shaped Helene's and Dana's perceptions of the unit and its nurses. It is important to keep in mind that the goal is not to achieve some "right" way of thinking. We all live multiple, contradictory, taken-for-granted ideas. We can, for example, critique the ideologies of a youth-oriented society at the same time as working to look youthful. I (Colleen) feel pleasure at compliments that I don't look my age while at the same time being perturbed that aging women are not seen as attractive and recognizing that such compliments arise from that youth-oriented preoccupation. Rather than aim for a "right" way of thinking, the goal is to have a greater critical awareness so that we may more consciously and intentionally choose and act within and around the ideologies.

Such a critical awareness requires that we inquire into the ideologies that are available and operating in the wider sociopolitical context. For example, Simmington (2004) contends that Western society's practice of religion and models of helping often focus more on maintaining the particular system of religion or helping practice than addressing the needs of the human soul. The strength of the ideologic structures may lead us to lose sight of the human being and of human wholeness. Similarly, returning to the idea of compliance, different practice settings will take this idea up differently and to greater or lesser extents. When I (Colleen) was practicing in coronary care units, the idea of compliance was pervasive. Patient and family teaching was geared toward optimizing compliance with lifestyle changes prescribed by health care providers. However, there was a recognition that such changes were still within the control of the individual or family. When I began working with nurses in nephrology units, I was taken aback not only at how pervasive the idea of compliance was but also how patients and families were "punished" for noncompliance. For example, both nurses and patients told me that patients who came into hemodialysis "overloaded" (with too much fluid, sometimes from drinking too much or eating the wrong things) were punished in various ways—being made to wait, being verbally chastised, or by having the fluid removed rapidly in ways that caused discomfort. Compliance was a dominating ideology in those nephrology settings and was so normalized that it was difficult for the nurses to see the harmful impact of that ideology, never mind to think differently. Karen Mahoney, a clinical nurse specialist in nephrology says that this perspective persists today, despite ongoing efforts by leaders, educators, patients, and other concerned people.

Ideologic inquiry identifies directions for action. Critical analysis of how taken-for-granted ideas are shaping thinking and experience for both yourself and people and families opens up possibilities for understanding things differently and for helping others understand things differently. Ideologic inquiry identifies patterns in the ways practices are taken up and the possibility of naming and supporting the capacity of redefining situations and experiences. Our colleague Helen Brown's son Tanner was placed on life support at birth (Brown, 1997). Helen refused the taken-for-granted idea that physicians should not give their opinion in end-of-life decisions and invited her physician to speculate on what he would do. In doing so, she interpreted his willingness to share what he thought he would do as highly supportive.

It is important to emphasize that the goal of ideologic inquiry is not "consciousness raising" with people and families. In relational inquiry practice, the goal of ideologic inquiry is *not* to help families see things "right." Rather, as Banks-Wallace says, drawing on Collins' (1990) notion of womanist thought, the goal is "to affirm and rearticulate a conscious-ness that already exists" (Banks-Wallace, 2000, p. 36). As a nurse, your goal is not to shape how people think but rather to listen, help people consider and surface what they think, and tap into what they "already know." For example, when Helene was on hemodialysis, she did not need me (Colleen) to point out the ideology of compliance; she was living the consequences of an entire system of care organized around efforts to make her comply with medical advice. However, she found it affirming that I, too, could see the dynamics operating. Indeed, Helene helped me see how even in my critiques I was still using the idea, giving it "currency."

TRY IT OUT 6.4
Catch a Popular Ideology at Play

The next time you are in a clinical setting, see if you can identify a popular ideology operating. Think of ideologies of sets of ideas that are taken for granted and that imply the "way things are" or "the way things should be." We have used the example of compliance as an ideology in this chapter, and in previous chapters, we have suggested that ideas such as liberal individualism, choice, and responsibility operate ideologically (i.e., they operate to reinforce existing relations of domination). See if you can identify an ideology that is dominating—an ideology that might be obscuring other possibilities. Looking for people's frustrations, annoyances, or difficulties often points to ideologic

continued on page 277

TRY IT OUT 6.4 *continued*

Catch a Popular Ideology at Play

dynamics. Conduct an ideologic inquiry within the intrapersonal, interpersonal, and contextual domains. Ask:

■ What is the ideology?

■ Whose interests does it serve?

■ How is it operating?

■ Who participates in maintaining it?

■ What effects does it have?

■ What other "truths" does it obscure?

■ How do you want to relate to it?

Bringing It All Together

As we have shown, the various forms of inquiry are interrelated. Further, as we also have illustrated, each form of inquiry is conducted within the intrapersonal, interpersonal, and contextual levels. Table 6.3 offers some key questions using different modes of inquiry in concert with others.

Table 6.3: Key Questions Using Different Modes of Inquiry Together

	Empirical Inquiry	Ethical Inquiry	Aesthetic Inquiry	Sociopolitical Inquiry
Empirical Inquiry	What evidence?	What values shape what evidence is produced, valued, and used?	What aesthetic supports what evidence is produced, valued, and used?	What power dynamics support what evidence is produced, valued, and used?
Ethical Inquiry	What evidence is used to support selected moral choices?	What values?	What aesthetic shapes what values are upheld?	What power dynamics support what values?
Aesthetic Inquiry	What evidence is used to support selected aesthetics?	What values shape what aesthetic is upheld?	What beauty in human existence?	What power dynamics support what aesthetic?
Sociopolitical Inquiry	How is evidence selectively used to support certain interests?	What values support what power dynamics?	What aesthetic supports what interests?	What power dynamics?

THIS WEEK IN PRACTICE
Enlisting the Modes of Inquiry

This week, think about the first person or family you encounter as a "patient." Take a copy of Table 6.3 with you, and read the questions in relation to that person's or family's situation. It is possible to answer these questions in relation to any situation, so give it a try. What do you notice? What is "easy" to answer, and why? What is most difficult? If you have a colleague or fellow student doing the same exercise, compare notes.

YOUR RELATIONAL INQUIRY TOOLBOX

Add the following tools to your relational inquiry toolbox.
- Analyze your own allegiances and reference points in relation to particular situations, people, and phenomena.
- Appreciate the value of not knowing as a complement to knowing.
- Analyze the role of personal knowledge in your own nursing practice.
- Use empirical, ethical, aesthetic, and sociopolitical inquiry in an integrated way.

REFERENCES

Aasen, E. M., Kvangarsnes, M., & Heggen, K. (2012). Nurses' perceptions of patient participation in hemodialysis treatment. *Nursing Ethics, 19*(3), 419–430.

Abma, T. A., Baur, V. E., Molewijk, B., & Widdershoven, G. A. M. (2010). Inter-ethics: Toward an interactive and interdependent bioethics. *Bioethics, 24*(5), 242–255.

Allen, D., & Hardin, P. K. (2001). Discourse analysis and the epidemiology of meaning. *Nursing Philosophy, 2*(2), 163–176.

Allmark, P. (2013). Virtue and austerity. *Nursing Philosophy, 14*(1), 45–52.

Andorno, R. (2012). Do our moral judgments need to be guided by principles? *Cambridge Quarterly of Health care Ethics, 21*(4), 457–465.

Archibald, M. M. (2012). The holism of aesthetic knowing in nursing. *Nursing Philosophy: An International Journal For Health care Professionals, 13*(3), 179–188.

Atkin, K., Stapley, S., & Easton, A. (2010). No one listens to me, nobody believes me: Self management and the experience of living with encephalitis. *Social Science & Medicine, 71*(2), 386–393.

Austin, W., Goble, E., & Kelecevic, J. (2009). The ethics of forensic psychiatry: Moving beyond principles to a relational ethics approach. *Journal of Forensic Psychiatry & Psychology, 20*(6), 835–850.

Banks-Wallace, J. (2000). Womanist ways of knowing: Theoretical considerations for research with African American women. *Advances in Nursing Science, 22*(3), 33–47.

Benner, P. (1984). *From novice to expert: Excellence and power in clinical nursing practice.* Menlo Park, CA: Addison-Wesley.

Benner, P., Tanner, C. A., & Chesla, C. A. (1996). The social embeddedness of knowledge. In P. Benner, C. A. Tanner, & C. A. Chesla (Eds.), *Expertise in nursing practice* (pp. 193–231). New York: Springer.

Bergum, V. (2013). Relational ethics for health care. In J. Storch, P. Rodney, & R. Starzomski (Eds.), *Toward a moral horizon: Nursing ethics for leadership and practice* (2nd ed., pp. 127–142). Toronto, Ontario, Canada: Pearson.

Boockvar, K. S., & Lachs, M. S. (2003). Predictive value of nonspecific symptoms for acute illness in nursing home residents. *Journal of the American Geriatrics Society, 51*(8), 1111–1115.

Bourque Bearskin, R. L. (2011). A critical lens on culture in nursing practice. *Nursing Ethics, 18*(4), 548–559.

Brown, H. (1997). Tanner's story: A phenomenologic stance towards newborn death. *The Canadian Journal of Nursing Research - Revue Canadienne De Recherche En Sciences Infirmières, 29*(4), 21–31.

Brown, H., Rodney, P., Pauly, B., Varcoe, C., & Smye, V. (2004). Working the landscape: Nursing ethics. In J. Storch, P. Rodney, & R. Starzomski (Eds.), *Toward a moral horizon: Nursing ethics for leadership and practice* (pp. 154–177). Toronto, Ontario, Canada: Pearson.

Carper, B. A. (1978). Fundamental patterns of knowing in nursing. *Advances in Nursing Science, 1*(1), 13–23.

Checton, M. G., Greene, K., Magsamen-Conrad, K., & Venetis, M. K. (2012). Patients' and partners' perspectives of chronic illness and its management. *Families, Systems & Health: The Journal of Collaborative Family Health Care, 30*(2), 114–129.

Chinn, P. L., & Jacobs-Kramer, M. (1988). Perspectives on knowing: A model of nursing knowledge. *Scholarly Inquiry for Nursing Practice: An International Journal, 2*(2), 129–139.

Chinn, P. L., & Kramer, M. K. (2008). *Integrated theory & knowledge development in nursing* (7th ed.). St. Louis, MO: Elsevier.

Chinn, P. L., & Kramer, M. K. (2011). *Integrated theory & knowledge development in nursing* (8th ed.). St. Louis, MO: Elsevier Mosby.

Collins, P. H. (1990). *Black feminist thought: Knowledge, consciousness, and the politics of empowerment* (2nd ed). New York: Routledge.

Dewey, J. (1934/1995). Having an experience. In A. Neill & A. Ridley (Eds.), *The philosophy of art: Readings ancient and modern* (pp. 59–74). New York: McGraw-Hill.

Doane, G. H., Storch, J., & Pauly, B. (2009). Ethical nursing practice: Inquiry-in-action. *Nursing Inquiry, 16*(3), 1–9.

Ells, C., Hunt, M., & Chambers-Evans, J. (2011). Relational autonomy as an essential component to patient-centered care. *International Journal of Feminist Approaches to Bioethics, 4*(2), 79–101.

Eriksson, I., Gustafson, Y., Fagerström, L., & Olofsson, B. (2011). Urinary tract infection in very old women is associated with delirium. *International Psychogeriatrics / IPA, 23*(3), 496–502.

Evans, J. H. (2000). A sociological account of the growth of principlism. *Hastings Center Report, 30*(95), 31–38.

Falk-Rafael, A., & Betker, C. (2012). Relational ethics in public health nursing practice. *International Journal for Human Caring, 16*(3), 63–63.

Fox, R. C., & Swazey, J. P. (2010). Guest editorial: Ignoring the social and cultural context of bioethics is unacceptable. *Cambridge Quarterly Health care Ethics, 19*(3), 278–281.

Gill, P. (2012). Stressors and coping mechanisms in live-related renal transplantation. *Journal of Clinical Nursing, 21*(11/12), 1622–1631.

Gill, P., & Lowes, L. (2008). Gift exchange and organ donation: Donor and recipient experiences of live related kidney transplantation. *International Journal of Nursing Studies, 45*(11), 1607–1617.

Godfrey, H., Cloete, J., Dymond, E., & Long, A. (2012). An exploration of the hydration care of older people: A qualitative study. *International Journal of Nursing Studies, 49*(10), 1200–1211.

Goethals, S., Dierckx de Casterlé, B., & Gastmans, C. (2012). Nurses' decision-making in cases of physical restraint: A synthesis of qualitative evidence. *Journal of Advanced Nursing, 68*(6), 1198–1210.

Grant, A. (2001). Knowing me knowing you: Towards a new relational politics in 21st century mental health nursing. *Journal of Psychiatric & Mental Health Nursing, 8*(3), 269–276.

Hague, W. J. (1995). *Evolving spirituality.* University of Alberta, Edmonton.

Hartrick, G. A. (1998). The meaning of diabetes: Significance for holistic nursing practice. *Journal of Holistic Nursing, 16*(1), 76–87.

Hartrick Doane, G. A., Storch, J., & Pauly, B. (2009). Ethical nursing practice: Inquiry-in-action. *Nursing Inquiry, 16*(3), 232–240.

Hartrick Doane, G. A., & Varcoe, C. (2007). Relational practice and nursing obligations. *Advances in Nursing Science, 30*(3), 192–205.

Hoffmaster, B. (2001). *Bioethics in social context*. Philadelphia: Temple University Press.

Hufschmidt, A., Shabarin, V., Rauer, S., & Zimmer, T. (2010). Neurological symptoms accompanying urinary tract infections. *European Neurology, 63*(3), 180–183.

James, S. M. (1907). *Pragmatism. A new name for some old ways of thinking*. New York: Longmans, Green & Company.

Jowett, A., & Peel, E. (2009). Chronic illness in non-heterosexual contexts: an online survey of experiences. *Feminism & Psychology, 19*(4), 454–474.

Kneck, Å., Klang, B., & Fagerberg, I. (2012). Learning to live with diabetes – Integrating an illness or objectifying a disease. *Journal of Advanced Nursing, 68*(11), 2486–2495.

Kvåle, K., & Bondevik, M. (2010). Patients' perceptions of the importance of nurses' knowledge about cancer and its treatment for quality nursing care. *Oncology Nursing Forum, 37*(4), 436–442.

Lawler, J. (1991). *Behind the screens: Nursing, somology and the problem of the body*. Sydney, Australia: Sydney University Press.

Liaschenko, J. (1997). Knowing the patient? In S. E. Thorne & V. E. Hayes (Eds.), *Nursing praxis: Knowledge and action* (pp. 23–53). Thousand Oaks, CA: Sage.

Liaschenko, J., & Fisher, A. (1999). Theorizing the knowledge that nurses use in the conduct of their work. *Scholarly Inquiry for Nursing Practice: An International Journal, 13*(1), 29–41.

Malone, R. E. (1996). Almost 'like family:' Emergency nurses and 'frequent flyers.' *Journal of Emergency Nursing, 22*(3), 176–183.

Matthews, S. M., Peden, A. R., & Rowles, G. D. (2009). Patient–provider communication: Understanding diabetes management among adult females. *Patient Education and Counseling, 76*(1), 31–37.

McGrath, P., Pun, P., & Holewa, H. (2012). Decision-making for living kidney donors: An instinctual response to suffering and death. *Mortality, 17*(3), 201–220.

Murphy, N., & Canales, M. K. (2001). A critical analysis of compliance. *Nursing Inquiry, 8*(3), 173–181.

Nhat Hanh, T. (2013). *Washing the dishes*. ABuddhistLibrary.com.

Niebuhr, R. (1972). *Experiential religion*. New York: Harper Row.

Pergert, P., & Lützén, K. (2012). Balancing truth-telling in the preservation of hope: A relational ethics approach. *Nursing Ethics, 19*(1), 21–29.

Polanyi, M. (1962). *Personal knowledge*. Chicago: University of Chicago.

Rodney, P. (1998). Towards ideological inquiry. *Canadian Association for Nursing Research/Association Canadienne pour la Recherche Infirmière, 9*(1), 5–6.

Rodney, P., Brown, H., & Liaschenko, J. (2004). Moral agency: Relational connections and trust. In J. Storch, P. Rodney, & R. Starzomski (Eds), *Toward a moral horizon: Nursing ethics for leadership and practice* (pp. 154–171). Toronto, Ontario, Canada: Pearson.

Rodney, P., Burgess, M., Phillips, J. C., McPherson, G., & Brown, H. (2013). Our theoretical landscape: A brief history of health care ethics. In J. Storch, P. Rodney, & R. Starzomski (Eds.), *Toward a moral horizon: Nursing ethics for leadership and practice* (2nd ed., pp. 59–83). Toronto, Ontario, Canada: Pearson.

Rodney, P., Kadyschuk, S., Liaschenko, J., Brown, H., Musto, L., & Snyder, N. (2013). Moral agency: Relational connections and support. In J. Storch, P. Rodney, & R. Starzomski (Eds.), *Toward a moral horizon: Nursing ethics for leadership and practice* (2nd ed., pp. 160–187). Toronto, Ontario, Canada: Pearson.

Schaefer, K. M. (2002). Reflections on caring narratives: Enhancing patterns of knowing. *Nursing Education Perspectives, 23*(6), 286–294.

Shaha, M. (1998). Racism and its implications in ethical-moral reasoning in nursing practice: A tentative approach to a largely unexplored topic. *Nursing Ethics, 5*(2), 139–146.

Sherwin, S. (1998). A relational approach to autonomy in health care. In S. Sherwin (Ed.), *The politics of women's health: Exploring agency and autonomy* (pp. 19–47). Philadelphia: Temple University Press.

Sherwin, S. (2011). Looking backwards, looking forward: Hopes for bioethics' next twenty-five years. *Bioethics, 25*(2), 75–82.

Shorr, R. I., Guillen, M. K., Rosenblatt, L. C., Walker, K., Caudle, C. E., & Kritchevsky, S. B. (2002). Restraint use, restraint orders, and the risk of falls in hospitalized patients. *Journal of the American Geriatrics Society* (Vol. 50, pp. 526–529): Blackwell.

Simmington, J. (2004). Ethics for an evolving spirituality. In J. Storch, P. Rodney, & R. Starzomski (Eds.), *Toward a moral horizon: Nursing ethics for leadership and practice* (pp. 465–484). Toronto, Ontario, Canada: Pearson.

Smith, M. C. (1992). Is all knowing personal knowing? *Nursing Science Quarterly, 5*(1), 2-3.

Snellman, I., & Gedda, K. M. (2012). The value ground of nursing. *Nursing Ethics, 19*(6), 714–726.

Storch, J., Hartrick Doane, G. A., Rodney, P., Varcoe, C., & Starzomski, R. (1999-2001). The ethics of practice: Context and curricular implications for nursing: Funded by Associated Medical Services.

Sweeney, N. M. (1994). A concept analysis of personal knowledge: Application to nursing education. *Journal of Advanced Nursing, 20*, 917–924.

Thaler, R. H., & Sunstein, C. R. (2009). *Nudge*. New York: Penguin books.

Thayer-Bacon, B. (2003). *Relational (e) pistemologies*. New York: Peter Lang.

Van der Elst, E., Dierckx de Casterlé, B., & Gastmans, C. (2012). Elderly patients' and residents' perceptions of 'the good nurse:' A literature review. *Journal of Medical Ethics, 38*(2), 93–97.

Varcoe, C., Browne, A. J., Wong, S., & Smye, V. (2009). Harms and benefits: Collecting ethnicity data in a clinical context. *Social Science & Medicine, 68*(9), 1659–1666.

Varcoe, C., Doane, G., Pauly, B., Rodney, P., Storch, J. L., Mahoney, K., et al. (2004). Ethical practice in nursing: Working the in-betweens. *Journal of Advanced Nursing, 45*(3), 316–325.

Varcoe, C., Pauly, B., Storch, J., Newton, L., & Makaroff, K. (2012). Nurses' perceptions of and responses to morally distressing situations. *Nursing Ethics, 19*(4), 488–500.

Varcoe, C., Pauly, B., Webster, G., & Storch, J. (2012). Moral distress: tensions as springboards for action. *HEC Forum: An Interdisciplinary Journal on Hospitals' Ethical And Legal Issues, 24*(1), 51–62.

Varcoe, C., Rodney, P., & McCormick, J. (2003). Health care relationships in context: An analysis of three ethnographies. *Qualitative Health Research, 13*(6), 957–973.

Wainwright, P. (2000). Towards an aesthetics of nursing. *Journal of Advanced Nursing, 32*(3), 750–756.

White, J. (1995). Patterns of knowing: Review, critique, and update. *Advances in Nursing Science, 17*(4), 73–86.

Widdershoven, G., Molewijk, B., & Abma, T. (2009). Improving care and ethics: A plea for interactive empirical ethics. *The American Journal of Bioethics, 9*(6–7), 99–101.

Winkler, E. (1993). From Kantianism to contextualism: The rise and fall of the paradigm theory in bioethics. In E. Winkler & F. A. Coombs (Eds.), *Applied ethics: A reader* (pp. 343–365). Cambridge, MA: Blackwell.

Wolf, S. (1994). Shifting paradigms in bioethics and health law: The rise of new pragmatism. *American Journal of Law and Medicine, 20*(4), 395–415.

Woods, M. (2012). Exploring the relevance of social justice within a relational nursing ethic. *Nursing Philosophy, 13*(1), 56–65.

World Health Organization. (1984). *Health promotion: A discussion document on the concept and principles*. Geneva, Switzerland: World Health Organization.

Yen, L., Gillespie, J., Rn, Y.-H. J., Kljakovic, M., Brien, J., Jan, S., et al. (2011). Health professionals, patients and chronic illness policy: A qualitative study. *Health Expectations, 14*(1), 10–20.

7 All Nursing Is Theoretically Informed

LEARNING OBJECTIVES

By engaging with the material in this chapter, you will be able to:

1. Understand how theories support the enactment of effective nursing practice.

2. Understand how relational inquiry is a theorizing process.

3. Understand the value of theorizing at point-of-care.

4. Begin to articulate your own theoretical perspective.

5. Practice conscious theorizing to inform your nursing practice.

In previous chapters, we have described a relational consciousness and the ontologic capacities (the five Cs) inherent to relational inquiry. We have also explored the key role of knowledge and knowing in a relational inquiry process. Here, we continue to build on these ideas by turning our attention to the role of theory in nursing and how relational inquiry supports a conscious, intentional, theorizing approach to nursing practice.

THE VALUE OF PRACTICING WITH THEORETICAL INTENT

Do you know what theories guide your practice as a nurse? We begin with that question because, if you're like many nurses, you may not. As a result, you may be unintentionally working from a theoretical perspective that is not congruent with your nursing values, goals, and commitments. For example, without recognizing how they are theorizing health, many nurses slip into a biomedical approach to care because they are practicing in a context that privileges biomedical conceptualizations of health (e.g., as the absence of disease). Thus, their way of caring for people is often disease-oriented.

This chapter provides an opportunity for you to identify and reflect on the theories that currently guide your nursing practice. You'll also explore how theory can provide a foundation from which to act more consciously and effectively. This is important because how you practice is dependent upon how you *theorize* the purposes, goals, and processes of nursing.

Theory is often viewed as an abstract body of knowledge that is learned outside of the practice arena. This separation of theory from practice has

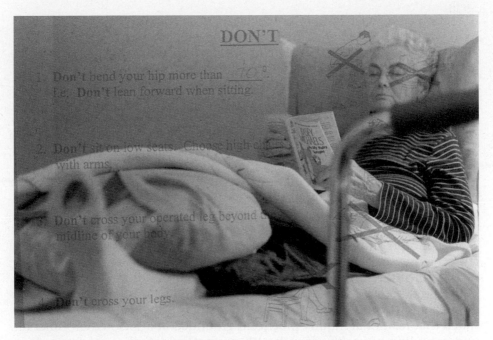

Don't. (Photograph by Gayle Alison.)

caused many nurses to devalue theory as having no relevance in the "real world" of nursing work. This is unfortunate. Intentional, theoretically informed practice is not only critical but also central to every nursing action.

Stop for a moment and try to think of a time when you are *not* acting from a theoretical base. For example, when you set off down the corridor to respond to two patient call bells, your decision about which of the two patients requires the most urgent attention is grounded in theory. When you make a bed with clean linen, your action is informed theoretically. Similarly, changing a dressing using sterile technique is a theoretically based action. Although you might not be conscious of the theories grounding your everyday work, you bring beliefs, assumptions, understandings, and hypotheses to each moment of your practice, and those ingredients constitute a theoretical base for action.

Although the theories that inform your action may not be formal or intentionally enlisted, they highly influence your actions and set parameters on how you provide nursing care. By more intentionally theorizing your nursing practice, you can strengthen the knowledge base for making clinical decisions. Sometimes, it can also expand the number of options you see open to you. It can also help you clarify your nursing goals and commitments, enabling you to feel more confident when you find yourself in complex and uncertain situations. Thus, practicing with a clear *theoretical intent* is vital.

Practicing without a conscious theoretical intent is comparable to setting off on a trip into unknown terrain without a roadmap or compass. Although you might eventually get somewhere and you might see interesting things along the way, it is far more difficult to make your way randomly and/or know if you are heading in a direction that is worthwhile—and one that is aligned with the direction in which you wish to go. Without theoretical tools, your knowledge of the terrain may be lessened, the choices of routes you see will likely be fewer, and you might not realize when you have stepped off the road you wish to take. That is, you are less likely to realize when you have lost your way or know how to get back on track when you *feel* lost.

So how do *you* theorize your nursing practice? For example, how do you theorize the purpose of nursing? If you read the nursing literature, you will see that different nursing theorists propose and emphasize somewhat different perspectives on that. However, Chinn and Kramer (2011) describe how most theories include four common concepts that give direction to nursing work: person, health (illness), society/environment, and nursing, the metaparadigm concepts articulated by Fawcett (1978, 2005). For example, consider how we have theorized nursing as a practice of relational inquiry. If you look back over preceding chapters you will see how we have outlined these concepts. Informed by the hermeneutic phenomenologic (HP) and critical lenses, we have theorized *people* as relational beings who are situated in and constituted by their sociohistorical backgrounds and locations. We understand people as interpretive and concerned beings who give particular meaning to any living experience (remember Chapter 2). We have also stated that relational inquiry practice is grounded in a socio-environmental understanding of *health* where health promotion activities are focused on enabling people/families to live meaningful lives and have the ability and resources to make choices and realize their aspirations. Since people inhabit and embody *environments*, we have said that context needs to be understood in its breadth and depth and in its embodied form. Substantively, we have theorized *nursing* as a responsive, compassionate process of relational inquiry and action that is oriented toward well-being and health in its broadest sense. These understandings serve as the roadmap for our nursing practice.

THE HUMAN SCIENCE OF NURSING

Different theories resonate with different nurses. Here, we have chosen three theories as examples that could support your relational inquiry nursing practice. All three are from the "human science" tradition, which has been shaped by the philosophies of existentialism and phenomenology. Human science nursing theories offer valuable insights into human caring and interpersonal relations (Roach, 2002; Watson, 1988). Beginning with Martha Rogers's (1970) theory of unitary human beings, human science nurse theorists have developed a range of theories to inform nursing practice. Watson (1988) summarizes the human science paradigm in nursing as being based upon:

- A philosophy of human freedom, choice, and responsibility
- A biology and psychology of *holism*, which recognizes nonreducible persons interconnected with their world
- A knowledge development process that includes not only empirical science but also aesthetics, ethics, values, intuition, and process discovery
- A way-of-being that is relational and process-oriented
- A scientific worldview that is open and ever-changing

Within each of the human science theories, nursing is theorized somewhat differently. For our theorizing purposes (which mostly are to illustrate the value of nursing theory for relational inquiry practice), we have chosen three nursing theories as examples of how nursing theories might inform your action as a nurse. Although the three theories we describe are grounded in the valuing of people, human relating, and expanded well-being, they define the four elements (people, health, society/environment, and nursing) in different ways. We are not suggesting that the theories we present below are the best theories or the only ones congruent with relational inquiry practice. In fact, there are many more that could inform your practice, and we suggest that you read Reed and Crawford Shearer (2012) or Parker and Smith (2010) to consider other theories that could inform your practice.

As you read the theories ahead, we invite you to read *pragmatically*. As we discussed in Chapter 1, pragmatists approach any knowledge or theory as a tool. Its value lies in its practical contribution—how it can enable us to be more effective in the world. Thus, we are inviting you to scrutinize the theories according to how useful they might be in clarifying your own theoretical perspective and enhancing your capacity to respond and practice nursing in ways that promote health and well-being. Consider the following questions:

■ What values are embedded within the theory?
■ How does this theory conceptualize relating?
■ How does this theory conceptualize people?
■ How does this theory conceptualize health?
■ How is environment conceptualized and incorporated?
■ How does this theory define the focus and purpose of nursing?
■ To what does the theory itself, as well as the ideas and concepts within the theory, draw attention?
■ What does it take for granted or assume about people, health, environments, and/or nursing?
■ What does it fail to address?
■ How might it inform your nursing practice?

As you consider the theories in terms of these questions, try to think of people and families with whom you've worked as a nurse or with whom you might currently be working. Consider what you see of value in the theories and what you see as limitations.

Paterson and Zderad's Humanistic Nursing Theory

Hildegard Peplau (1952) was one of the first nurse theorists to draw attention to interpersonal experiences between nurses and patients. Building on Peplau's work, in 1976, Josephine Paterson and Loretta Zderad published their classic book *Humanistic Nursing*. Describing nursing as "an experience lived between human beings" (Paterson & Zderad, 1988, p. 3), these nurse theorists inspire us to move beyond the technical "doing" of nursing and open ourselves up to the feeling and "being" of nursing. Believing that nursing theory should be rooted in practice, they contended that *knowing was cultivated from within nursing experience* and that it was the responsibility of each nurse to contribute to the evolution of nursing theory by paying close attention to their everyday practice experiences. Borrowing from R.D. Laing, they defined theory as "the articulated vision of experience" (Paterson, 1978, p. 45). To develop and evolve their theoretical practice, therefore, these theorists suggest that when engaged in everyday work, nurses needed to ask questions of their practice such as what, why, how, how better, ought, and ought not? According to these theorists, *theoretically sound practice requires that nurses tune into themselves as knowing places and reflect on new possibilities within their everyday work.*

Humanistic Nursing Is a Happening between People

O'Connor (1993) suggests that perhaps the major contribution Paterson and Zderad's humanistic nursing theory offers is the view of nursing as a particular kind of human relating. At the center of their theory is an understanding of nursing as a "happening between people." The theory emphasizes a particular way of being that involves presence and awareness to support a "withness" between nurse and patient. They emphasize the importance of this way of being within the "doing" of nursing. Said another way, their theory gives direction to "how" nursing should be practiced as well as the "what" of nursing.

Moreover, Paterson and Zderad take nursing practice beyond subjective/objective dualism to emphasize an approach that is trifold, recognizing the *objective, subjective,* and *intersubjective all at once.* Objective reality is what occurs "out there" and can be observed, pointed at, and examined. Subjective reality is what is known from the inside out or a reality that is the awareness of one's own experience. Intersubjective reality is what is experienced in the between space when two or more people come together. Humanistic nursing dwells primarily in the intersubjective realm, while simultaneously recognizing the trifold reality of the nursing world (O'Connor, 1993).

As you read the description of the central concepts below, notice the ways in which Paterson and Zderad's humanistic nursing theory informs relational inquiry nursing practice.

Humanistic Nursing Promotes the More-Being of People

A central premise of humanistic nursing theory is that nursing concerns go beyond the well-being of patients to the "more-being" of both patients and nurses. From the simplest greeting to the most advanced resuscitation, nurses act to call forth the potential in people (Paterson, 1978). Involving both assessment and intervention, this calling forth of "more-being" is accomplished by presencing (being attentively present) with people—by joining people in their situations, sharing knowledge and experience, and nurturing "responsible choosing."

Closely tied to the concept of more-being is the emphasis on the patient and nurse working together to search for the meaning of the health and illness situation. For example, one particular process these theorists suggest is listening to people and living past events with them (O'Connor, 1993). An example might be when a child is admitted to hospital with an episode of acute asthma. Instead of telling the parents what they need to do to prevent another attack, the nurse would begin by asking about their experience, including how it seemed to transpire and their own experiences (what was meaningful) during the situation and then use that knowledge and understanding to collaboratively consider options for future management of the child's asthma (more-being).

Characteristics of Humanistic Nursing

In articulating how nurses proceed in practice, Paterson and Zderad (1976) offer the following characteristics of humanistic nursing as

- Being with and doing with
- Dialogue
- Here and now
- Occurring in situations
- All-at-once
- Complementary synthesis

Nursing as Being with and Doing with

Paterson and Zderad (1976) highlight the inextricable link between nursing doing and being. Moving beyond the level of nurses "doing to" and/ or "doing for" people, these theorists call for nurses to focus on "being with and doing with" (p. 13). Being with involves "turning one's attention toward the patient, being aware of and open to the here and now shared situation, and communicating one's availability" (Paterson & Zderad, 1988, p. 14).

Nursing as Dialogue

Paterson and Zderad (1988) contend that nursing is a dialogue, not merely communication through words but a mutual, two-way process that happens in the "between" space. It involves "a purposeful call and response" (p. 24) to particular people and particular situations or needs. Nursing as dialogue involves meeting, relating, and presence. For dialogue to occur, there must be an openness that is revealed directly and indirectly "in a glance, a touch, a tone of voice" (p. 28).

Nursing as Here and Now

Paterson and Zderad (1976) highlight the connectedness between one's past, present, and future. Subsequently, they contend that humanistic nursing is always inclusive of both nurses' and patients' histories, meanings, hopes, fears, and possibilities (O'Connor, 1993). From a here-and-now perspective, each moment is significant, irreplaceable, and imbued with potential.

Nursing in Situations

Humanistic nursing theory points out that all nursing occurs against the backdrop of a situation; that is, the intersubjective "dialogue" of patient and nurse is always subjected to "all the chaotic forces of life," (p. 29) including the complex and conflicted realms of the health care world

(O'Connor, 1993). The situational nature of nursing practice means that both patients and nurses are affected by the network of relationships and social structures within which they exist.

Nursing All-at-Once

All-at-once is the way Paterson and Zderad (1976) convey the paradoxical, complex, and multifaceted nature of nursing practice. Patients are simultaneously strong and vulnerable, nurses are simultaneously being with and doing with, and when patient and nurse meet, they are simultaneously alone and in the world. Paterson and Zderad assert that a central skill of nurses is the ability to balance these multiple forces and situational elements to be present in the nursing act.

Nursing as Complementary Synthesis

Closely related to the concept of all-at-once, nursing as complementary synthesis highlights how nurses traverse both the objective world of biomedicine and the subjective and intersubjective realms of people and situations (O'Connor, 1993). Paterson and Zderad contend that the tensions between these realms are lived out in the moment of the nursing act (O'Connor, 1993).

TRY IT OUT 7.1
Translating Theory into Action

Stop for a minute and look back over the description of Paterson and Zderad's theory. What parallels can you see between humanistic nursing and relational inquiry? How are people conceptualized similarly and/or differently? How is health defined?

For example, these authors emphasize "more-being." What do you think they mean by that? Recently, I (Gweneth) was reading Mehl-Madrona's (2007) description of how people living through major illnesses often ask themselves "big questions" such as, "Who am I?" "Why am I here?" and "Where are we going?" I immediately thought of Paterson and Zderad's description of more-being—how illness can lead people to deeper places within themselves and in their lives and how they may widen their views of life to be and live more intentionally. I am also struck by how they point to the intrapersonal (e.g., "being a knowing place"), the interpersonal (nursing as a happening between people), and contextual (nursing occurs in situations).

As you think about the way Paterson and Zderad describe nursing, what resonates for you? How might their theory inform and reform your own practice and how you relate as a nurse? Finally, choose one concept or process described above to take into practice this week.

TO ILLUSTRATE
Another Turning Point

I (Colleen) was new to the bone marrow transplant unit and was feeling overwhelmed by all I had to learn: hematology, chemotherapy, a whole new set of unfamiliar lab results, and medications. My first patient was a 27-year-old woman with an acute disorder. She was having yet another bone marrow biopsy today, and I was quite concerned about knowing the preparation and setup required. As I entered the woman's room (gowned, gloved, masked, and a bit distracted by the fact that I had to get back to another patient whose chemo was just about finished), I noticed by her bed a photo of a toddler about the same age as my son. I also noticed that she had written a cute message on a white board letting people know that because of her immunosuppression, she was on strict isolation protocol and could not have physical contact.

I introduced myself and began chatting with her as I quickly set up for the biopsy scheduled for a few minutes later. She was composed and gave me some hints as to how to position the overbed table in the rather crowded room. I asked about the toddler, whom she identified as her 2-year-old son. At that moment, I thought of my own son and put myself in what I thought were "her shoes." With tears welling up, I said, "You mean you can't kiss your little boy?" She burst into tears, her composure gone. In that moment, I realized that I had NOT put myself in her shoes; I had put her in MY shoes. While she was composing herself for a painful procedure, in my less composed state, I had drawn her attention to other painful concerns.

The woman recovered quickly and told me how her illness and uncertain prognosis made her cherish each moment with her son in a new way that she had never thought possible. I apologized, admitting, "That wasn't very helpful of me." However, she objected, saying that she appreciated my reaction in contrast to how stoic most staff had been in the face of her grief. Although she tried to make me feel better, I knew that I had not served her well by not really attending to what her concerns were in that particular moment.

Colleen's story illustrates the way in which effective and responsive relating practice involves far more than a nurse compassionately talking with a patient. As Paterson and Zderad (1976) observe, nursing is a happening between people. Both nurses' and patients' histories, meanings, hopes, fears, and possibilities come into play in any nursing moment. For example, the context of Colleen's own life (having a son who was a similar age) triggered a particular intrapersonal response within her and ultimately shaped the way she related in the situation. In considering the situation in light of Paterson and Zderad's theory, would Colleen's action constitute effective relating practice (did it promote well-being and more-being)?

To consider that question, one needs to look beyond the behavioral words to the here-and-now of that nursing moment. Informed by Paterson and Zderad's theory, we are called to look at what is happening in the situation to determine effective relating practice. Given that the woman was in the midst of preparing for a painful medical procedure, it was probably not the most effective time to invite her emotions out into the room. The woman wanted and needed to focus on getting through the biopsy; thus, a more "complementary synthesis" (responsive action) might have been to join her in that here-and-now—to relate by supporting her to muster her strength and composure to get through the biopsy. That focus and goal was evident in the way the woman was composing herself and offering direction to Colleen in preparing the physical space for the procedure. By *corresponding* with the woman's here-and-now situation, I (Colleen) might have related more effectively at that moment.

Paterson and Zderad (1988) describe the challenge of actualizing humanistic nursing in the face of the hectic demands of everyday nursing practice. Thus, they contend that although no nurse may be able to live humanistic nursing in every moment of practice, it is "a goal worth striving for; an attitude that strengthens one's perseverance toward attaining the difficult goal; or fundamentally, a major value shaping one's nursing practice" (p. 15). Their theory offers direction to support you as a nurse in discerning effective relational comportment in particular situations. It is not a matter of finding the "right" response but "being a knowing place" by theorizing your practice to continually be more responsive in particular nursing moments.

Newman's Theory of Health as Expanding Consciousness

> (O)ne does not practice nursing *using* theory, but rather the theory becomes a way of being with the client—a way of offering clients an opportunity to know and be known and to find their way. (Newman, 2005, p. xiv)

In *Health as Expanding Consciousness*, author Margaret Newman (1994) describes what she came to learn as she cared for her mother during the 5 years she lived with amyotrophic lateral sclerosis.

> I learned that my mother, though physically incapacitated, was a whole person, just like anybody else. I came to know her and to love her in a way I probably never would have taken the time to experience had she not been physically dependent. The five years I spent with her before she died were difficult, tiring, restrictive in some ways, but intense, loving, and expanding in other ways. (p. xxii)

This personal experience informed Newman's subsequent work as a nurse theorist. Her work focused on articulating an understanding of disease as a meaningful aspect of health. For Newman, health and illness are not at two different ends of a continuum but are integrally related aspects of the unitary process of life. From this theoretical orientation, health is conceptualized as a process of expanding consciousness, and the ultimate goal of nursing is to foster higher levels of consciousness.

Consciousness in this sense is defined as information—how and what people know of themselves in the world. As people gain more knowledge and information (expand their consciousness), they are better able to identify and transform their life patterns. Let's take a closer look at this aspect of Newman's theory.

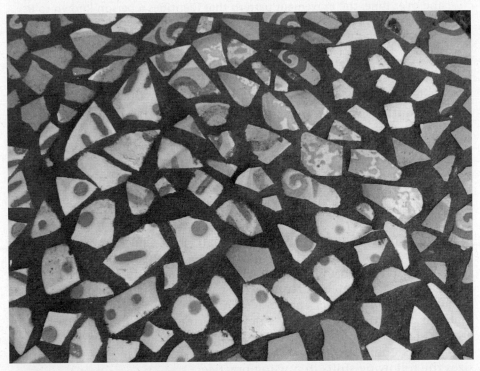

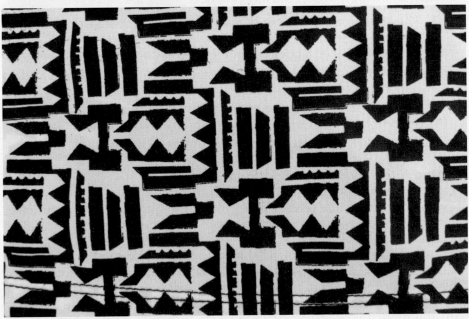

Identifying patterns. (Photographs by Gweneth Doane.)

Identifying Patterns

> From the moment we are conceived to the moment we die, in spite of changes that accompany aging, we manifest a pattern that identifies us as a particular person: the genetic pattern that contains the information that directs our becoming; the voice pattern that is recognizable across distances and over time; the movement pattern that identifies a person known to us a long way off even though no other features can be seen. These patterns are among the many explicate manifestations of the underlying (whole) pattern. It is the pattern of our lives that identifies us. (Newman, 1994, p. 71)

Newman (1994) contends that the task of nursing is not to try to change another person's pattern but to recognize it as information that depicts the whole of the person's life. Because all individuals and families have their own unique patterns, nursing action cannot be generalized. It must occur in response to particular people in particular situations. For example, we do not give the same information about asthma in the same way to all families.

Shifting Nursing Practice

Borrowing from Vaill (1984–1985), Newman (1994) emphasizes the importance of *process wisdom* and *response-ability*—of nursing being open, relational, and in synchrony with people and families. A nurse practicing from this theoretical orientation requires the capacity to be conscious of his/her involvement with others and to act from a knowing that transcends the material and intellectual level. Knowledge must also include the moral/ethical knowing that "what you are doing is somehow right" (p. 77).

Understanding health as expanding consciousness, Newman emphasizes the following shifts in nursing practice:

1. The shift from treatment of symptoms and disease to a search for patterns
2. The shift from viewing pain and disease as wholly negative to a view that pain and disease are information about the life pattern and an opportunity for growth
3. The shift from seeing the body/family/community as a machine in good or bad repair to seeing the body as a dynamic field of energy
4. The shift from seeing disease as an entity to seeing it as a process

Nursing Intervention as a Relational Process

A central premise within Newman's (1994) theory is that intervention aimed at producing a particular result is problematic. "To intervene with a particular solution in mind is to say we know what form the pattern of expanding consciousness will take, and we don't" (p. 97). Interestingly, if you stop and think about this quotation, you will likely recognize how it resonates with the goals of relational inquiry. The theory of health as expanding consciousness articulates with the view of nursing as a relational process in which the nurse enters into partnership with the person or family, often at a time of chaos, with the mutual goal of participating in an authentic relationship through which they all may emerge at a higher level of consciousness.

Moving beyond Problems

The theory of expanding consciousness also informs us that nursing practice must move beyond the deficit approach, which focuses on identifying what is wrong with a person or family and the reasons why it is wrong and then taking steps to fix the problem. Newman (1994) suggests that people often begin to interact with a nurse when they are in a situation that is new and disruptive. They don't know how to handle the situation because they are at a place where their old rules and patterns do not work or are not relevant. Rather than viewing such situations as problems to be fixed, Newman emphasizes that they are opportunities for promoting health—for expanding consciousness and evolving new patterns. For example, illness can provide "a kind of shock" that reorganizes the relationships and patterns of a person's or family's life in more harmonious ways.

> Consider the function of a high fever, or an emotional crisis, or the accident that occurs at a particularly crucial time. These, and other critical incidents, may provide the shock that facilitates a jump from one pattern to another . . . if we view disease as something . . . to be avoided, diminished, or eliminated altogether, we may be ruling out the very factor that can bring about the unfolding of the life process that the person is naturally seeking. (Newman, 1994, p. 11)

In this way, disease and illness provide the opportunity for people and families to expand their consciousness (gain information about their life patterns). Such experiences may lead them to "transcend a situation that seems impossible, to find a new way of relating to things, and to discover the freedom that comes with transcending the old limitations" (Newman, 1994, p. 99).

Entering into the Difficulty

By emphasizing *not* fixing and *not* reducing life situations and experiences to problems, this theory instructs nurses to enter into the difficulty of families' health and healing experiences and "hang in there" with them as they live the uncertainty and chaos in their lives. "The task . . . is to stop trying to change the world in accordance with our own image of what is healthy . . . to give up the old agenda to fix things" (Newman, 1994, p. 103). According to Newman, focusing on change and "doing to" people leads nurses into a pattern of diminished sensitivity. Change is unpredictable and transformational. Therefore, the intention guiding practice is for nurses to be in relation with people as they are, view their behaviors and experiences as indications of their current life patterns, and relate to that information (to their expanding consciousness) as it unfolds. As people expand their consciousness and gain information about their life patterns, their power and choice of action is enhanced.

Responding to Patterns

Again, this theory informs us that nursing actions must be offered in appropriate response to the patterns of the people and families involved. Newman (1994) contends that such patterns have a profound bearing on how people respond to other people and to therapeutic interventions. She explains that, just as a drug may have a fatal effect at one point of the circadian cycle and a therapeutic effect at another point, nurses must orchestrate the timing of their interactions in response to people's readiness and need. That is, "sensitivity to knowing when the need is there to connect with the client and when 'there is enough,' is an important skill for nurses to acquire" (Newman, 1994, p. 56). She calls this skill *interactional synchrony*. In the following example, nursing instructor Michelle Spadoni describes how Margaret Newman's theory of health as expanding consciousness informs her work as she teaches undergraduate nursing students.

TO ILLUSTRATE

"I Wish It Were This Clean!"

Late in the afternoon, a student came to my door, voicing her experience of a *troubling* clinical event—adequate pain control for someone who had a history of drug abuse. To help her discern an ethically informed intervention, her clinical teacher instructed her to reflect upon the experience utilizing an ethical decision-making tool. The student dug through her shoulder bag and pulled out the tool. She had written notes on the paper and crossed out and written over different points. Smoothing out the crinkled paper on my desk, she continued to explain how she had tried to identify the people involved in the event and their various positions. At some point, she sat back and said, "It just doesn't make sense to me. I can't find myself or my patient in this tool. I wish it were this clean, but it isn't!"

I asked the student to set aside the tool and reflect back on her experience. At first, she tried to create a detailed recollection of the event, what happened first and second, and who said what and when. She pointed out her own values and beliefs and what she thought were the values and beliefs of those involved, attempting to answer all the questions listed within the ethical framework. But then she said it wasn't a single event but a *pattern of things said, done, and sensed throughout her care of the patient that troubled her*. She said that she was especially troubled by the thought that she had at different times participated in her patient's suffering. "I didn't know what to do. My patient was suffering, and I felt hopeless. I couldn't get the nurses to see what I saw. They told me, 'You have to be careful with pain medication. The patient's system is failing because of years of abuse.'" At the same time, the student wondered if the staff felt helpless too. "Some nurses avoid the room. They don't answer the call bell right away, and they don't stay long; they don't really talk much to the patient or the family."

Nursing students often collide head-on into the underlying norms of the practice setting, the unspoken understandings and rules, beliefs, and values of practitioners and institutions that are intertwined and surface in moments of uncertainty. The student in my narrative found herself alone in the "in-between" of steps and rules and the norms of practice and the contextual realities of the living world. My challenge, as a nursing teacher informed by Newman's theory, is to embrace these moments of students standing in the doorway and crinkled paper conversations and see them as a space for transformational learning—for expanding consciousness, where a student's self-formation to being and becoming a nurse can be embraced. I have

continued on page 295

TO ILLUSTRATE *continued*

"I Wish It Were This Clean!"

learned that a student standing in the doorway is on the edge of something and requires of me intentionality, presence, and "being with" rather than "doing for." My focus as a teacher is to stay with the student in the tension that the student is experiencing as he or she comes up against the visible and invisible norms embedded in the social, political, historical, cultural, and economic context of nursing practice. As a teacher, I embody health as expanding consciousness (HEC) when I intentionally choose to know the student, be with the student, and recognize my own biases, beliefs, and values, to understand that I am interpreting my world through these views. It means letting go of certainty (e.g., offering an answer to "fix" her confusion) and giving way to ambiguity—when I intentionally am with a student, I give up fixed agendas and the urge to predict and control. HEC as nursing praxis is *"a place where we require one another"* and where we develop insights into self, meaningful relationships, and action. Having been a student of Margaret Dexheimer Pharris (2002), I have grown to appreciate that as human beings, we "must seek to understand rather than simply explain . . . because human beings are not just body, but also spirit" (p. 26).

TRY IT OUT 7.2

Trying out Newman's Theory

Look back over the description of Newman's theory and Michelle's story. What parallels can you see between her theory and relational inquiry as we have described it in this book? How are people conceptualized similarly and/or differently? How is health defined? For example, Newman discusses "expanding consciousness." How might that be similar to and different from Paterson and Zderad's "more-being?"

One of the elements that I (Gweneth) find particularly helpful in Newman's theory is the way she brings energy, pattern, and timing together. This expands my way of seeing and relating—it directs me to look and listen beyond words, to relate with all of my senses, and feel my way in and through the experience. It resonates with the example in Chapter 3 of how one needs to enter a patient's room—how important it is to be attuned to the rhythm and energy and join people as they are in that moment.

As *you* think about the way Newman describes nursing, what resonates for *you* as a nurse? How might it inform and reform your own practice and how you relate as a nurse? Choose one specific idea or concept from Newman's theory, and try it out in practice to see how it shifts your way of relating as a nurse.

Parse's Theory of Human Becoming

Rosemarie Rizzo Parse (1999) has created her nursing theory of human becoming by synthesizing ideas from Rogers's (1970) science of unitary human beings and existential phenomenology. Some of Parse's ideas and the language in which she expresses them are quite abstract and complex, and this abstractness poses a challenge to us as writers—how to present her theory in a way that is understandable in terms of your everyday practice while not losing its depth and complexity. We therefore decided to use her original words accompanied by descriptions of how *we* have found her theory to be relevant to our work in nursing. Because this is only our interpretation, you might find it helpful to explore Parse's ideas further with your colleagues or classmates and instructors.

Parse begins with nine philosophical assumptions (Parse, 1999, pp. 5–6). As you read the assumptions below, pay attention to three core themes that are running throughout them—meaning, rhythmicity, and transcendence. Also pay attention to the phenomenologic (remember the HP lens in Chapter 2) underpinnings that are obviously embedded in the assumptions.

1. The human is coexisting while co-constituting rhythmical patterns with the universe.
2. The human is open, freely choosing meaning in situations and bearing responsibility for decisions.
3. The human is unitary, continuously co-constituting patterns of relating.
4. The human is transcending multidimensionally with the possibles.
5. Becoming is unitary human living health.
6. Becoming is a rhythmically co-constituting human-universe process.
7. Becoming is the human's patterns of relating value priorities.
8. Becoming is an intersubjective process of transcendence with the possibles.
9. Becoming is unitary human evolving.

As you can glean from the above assumptions, Parse (1999) views people and the world as inseparable. The HP notions of constituted and situated experience that we discussed in Chapter 2 also run through Parse's assumptions.

In addition, we see a similarity between Newman's (1994) and Parse's (1999) assumptions of rhythmical patterns. For Parse, people are living patterns in the world. We also see correspondence between Newman's concept of health as expanding consciousness and Parse's concept of health as a process of human becoming. This human becoming is evolved in and through living experience. Health is the quality of life from the perspective of the person. Regardless of whether nurses are working with individuals or with families, the goal of nursing practice is to participate in co-creating quality of life. Parse believes that humans are free agents with an innate capacity to make intentional choices. Through this capacity, people are able to change moment to moment as they are in relation with the world, to invent new ways to actualize their dreams. In this capacity for choice lie possibilities for transcendence.

Looking beyond the Words

When I (Gweneth) first read Parse's theory several years ago, I remember struggling with the language and abstractness. Yet, at the same time the ideas within her theory resonated with what I "knew" about nursing. In reading about "health as a process of human becoming," I found myself thinking back to particular nursing moments that had affected me deeply, and I could see that at the center of those moments was the human becoming process that Parse was describing. I found myself remembering people and families for whom I had cared in the emergency department, in adult and neonatal intensive care unit, in psychiatry, and in my community work as a nurse. Regardless of the context of my practice, even in the briefest of moments, the lives of the people and families with whom I worked and my own life had changed and "become" something more. Whether it was a child with acute otitis media who was brought to the emergency room (ER) by an exhausted mother or a family who was living with a diagnosis of schizophrenia for one of its members, health as a process of human becoming was central.

As I thought about the significance of those human-becoming moments, I recognized the importance of my own nursing actions and, in particular, how I was "with" people in those moments. I resonated with Parse's contention that nurses should take the role of "nurturing gardeners" (as opposed to "fix-it mechanics") and could see how that description was in keeping with how I had intuitively found myself responding. At the same time, the distinctions she drew between biomedically based approaches and a human science approach to nursing echoed the limitations that I had experienced in the service delivery model of health care that seemed to dominate and limit my nursing potential.

Looking beneath the Words

When reading Parse's work, I (Colleen), too, struggled with the language. However, I was drawn to what I understood to be Parse's (1999) view that nurses are not experts engaged in doing "to" and "for" people. It seemed to me that Parse advocated more egalitarian relationships than those I regularly witnessed in my critical care practice. However, I wondered how nursing and non-nursing knowledge was to be drawn upon. Parse emphasizes "co-constituting," but I could not discern how a nurse contributes differently from any person being with another. I do value "bearing witness," whether during birth, death, illness, or any of the health experiences nurses are likely to share with people, but I see the role of nursing as being more than bearing witness. I could not see in Parse's theory direction for how nurses might bring their knowledge into practice.

In addition, I saw in my daily practice that the ability of people and families to freely choose meaning and bear responsibility for their decisions was severely constrained by the resources and discourse available. To me, these constrained possibilities often seemed to overwhelm the ability of people and families to freely choose. I continue to question the relative importance of the role of nurses in expanding the possibilities and co-creating quality of life, given the complexity of peoples' lives and the multitude of influences shaping them.

Practicing from True Presence

Nurses who practice from Parse's theoretical perspective live and practice nursing in "true presence . . . [Nursing from this perspective] is an unconditional loving, non-routinized way of being with, in which the nurse bears witness to changing health patterns of persons and families" (Parse, 1997, p. 34). The nurse enters people's worlds as a not-knowing stranger (Parse, 1996), is open to what people are experiencing, and is willing to share in particular moments. Parse emphasizes that all nurse-person processes are led by the person. Parse (1996, 1997, 1999) articulates particular ways of relating, including face-to-face discussions (dialogue and conversation), silent immersion (a deep place of no words), and lingering presence (being still to reflect and abide with).

THEORIZING YOUR OWN NURSING PRACTICE

As you pragmatically consider the theories we have described above in light of your own nursing practice, what stands out? Bringing a pragmatic attitude to theorizing your nursing action enables you to clarify the meaning and relevance of any conceptual idea or thought. It directs you to unpack any theory or concept to look for the practical consequences. For example, pragmatically, you might ask what a particular concept or theory leads you to focus on, to attend to, and to do in your nursing practice. Looking at theory pragmatically, we are called to ask what concrete difference this theory makes in actual practice:

- How would I enter nursing situations differently?
- How would I see and relate to people differently?
- What matters most?
- How would I relate to myself and the contexts in which I work differently?
- What is the value of the theory in experiential terms?

For example, if you look at the three nursing theories we have described, you will see that they have a particular focus on the interpersonal domain of relational comportment. That is, the theories emphasize what transpires between a nurse and a patient. Paterson and Zderad (1976) describe nursing as an experience lived between people. Similarly, Newman (1994) describes nursing as a practice focused on expanding consciousness, and Parse (1999) emphasizes the fostering of human becoming. Thus, the theories help us see beyond "the absence of disease" and beyond "the aortic repair in room 2" to pay closer attention to the relational interaction. Students have also told me (Gweneth) that one of the most helpful aspects of nursing theories is how they help orient and ground their practice in *nursing*; the theories extend the nursing view to see commitments and goals beyond disease treatment.

As you read more theory, you will probably find that some resonate more than others, and that you and a colleague might interpret the same theory differently. For example, in considering the theories within the human science paradigm, Kleffel (1996) has proposed that the theories are congruent with an ecologic approach to nursing practice. However, Browne (2001) has argued that the assumption of individual free will and choice that underpins these theories is problematic since the theories do not attend to the way in which the interpersonal process is contextually shaped. The difference in how the theories have been interpreted by these different nurses points to the importance of *your* own theorizing process.

Theorizing Extends Your Own Practice

Similar to Kleffel and Browne, as nurses, we have considered the human science theories in light of our own nursing interests and concerns. In bringing a pragmatic lens to our own nursing practice, we have found ourselves compelled to go further in our theorizing of nursing in two particular ways.

First, as we have scrutinized our own practice, we have found it necessary to extend our view of nursing beyond the interpersonal domain. We have found that nursing practice is shaped not just by what transpires between a nurse and a patient. Rather, our nursing actions are greatly affected by what occurs within and between the intrapersonal, interpersonal, and contextual domains. *Subsequently, we believe we need to extend our actions toward the well-being of not just patients and families but also health care providers and the health care system. Thus, in theorizing our nursing action we have extended our view to consider all three domains, how those domains are influencing and informing each other, and what actions might be necessary to affect well-being at all three levels.*

The second aspect we have intentionally included in our theorizing process is an emphasis on how one relates and acts within those three domains. Our pragmatic orientation pushes us to go beyond descriptive theorizing to engage in situation-producing theorizing. For example, while there are many nursing theories that give direction by *describing* nursing and what effective, responsive relating should look like, as Dickoff and James (1968) have suggested, theorizing in nursing has the potential to go beyond description to actually *produce* situations. Situation-producing theory is practice-minded theory, the purpose of which is "to allow the production of situations of a desired kind" (p. 105).

Relational inquiry focuses specifically on how our theorizing action can produce situations of a desired kind—specifically, situations that promote health and well-being. Dickoff and James (1968) contend that situation-producing theory is the highest level of theory, since it exists and is produced for practice. They have argued (and we concur) that "theory for a profession of practice discipline must provide for more than mere understanding or 'describing' or even predicting reality and must provide conceptualizations specially intended to guide the shaping of reality to that profession's professional purpose" (p. 102). Thus, in our own practice we have found ourselves compelled to extend our theorizing to the action level within the intrapersonal, interpersonal, and contextual domains.

Describing nursing as a practice of relational inquiry, we have intentionally included a focus on how our ways of theorizing/relating/acting may serve to produce particular kinds of situations. My (Gweneth's) description in Chapter 5 of how I re-theorized family as a relational living experience is an example of action-oriented theorizing. My goal as a nurse was to relate and act in such a way that all people and families, regardless of their life circumstances, might have relational experiences of being cared for and about. Thus, by theorizing family as a relational living experience, I began paying more attention to each moment of my nursing actions as a potential relational, health-promoting experience. Looking beyond the individual in the bed or the family unit, my focus of attention became more consciously and intentionally relating to who was and was not in the room so I could respond to the meaningful experience of people with and/or without actual families.

Theorizing to Produce Situations

By *engaging in a process of relational inquiry to consciously theorize your practice*, you are positioned to produce health-promoting nursing situations by fine-tuning your understandings and your nursing action. By engaging in a continual inquiry and tracking the consequences of your actions and of the way you're theorizing, you'll have the opportunity to recreate your understandings, actions, and the situation. That is, you'll be able to consciously try out, evaluate, and revise your ways of thinking/acting/relating and become more effective in promoting the well-being of people, the health care system, and yourself and other nurses. Regardless of the context of your practice or the patient population with whom you work, the way you theorize makes a profound difference to what transpires. How might nursing theory enhance the care *you* give? How might consciously theorizing your actions enhance your effectiveness as a nurse?

THIS WEEK IN PRACTICE
Being Informed by Nursing Theory

Choose one nursing theory from the list provided to research and try out in practice this week:

Pamela Reed's theory of self-transcendence

Marlaine Smith's theory of unitary caring

Barbara Dossey's theory of integral nursing

Katherine Kolcaba's comfort theory

Read about one of these theories in Reed and Crawford Shearer (2012) or Parker and Smith (2010) or online. As you read the theory, begin by identifying how it conceptualizes people, health, environment, and nursing. Reflect on the following questions:

■ Does the theory offer a different perspective of nursing than you currently hold?

■ To what does the theory draw your attention?

■ What does it take for granted about people, health, and/or nursing?

In your practice, try looking through this theoretical lens as you go about your work. Consider the following:

■ How does the theory change your view?

■ How does it extend your capacity and effectiveness as a nurse?

continued on page 301

THIS WEEK IN PRACTICE *continued*

Being Informed by Nursing Theory

- What does the theory lead you to question about yourself and your own nursing practice?
- What do the theoretical understandings lead you to do differently?
- What actions compelled you to take to practice in accordance with the theory?

 # YOUR RELATIONAL INQUIRY TOOLBOX

Add the following tools to your relational inquiry toolbox.
- Scrutinize what theories are informing your current nursing practice.
- Enlist nursing theories to help you orient and ground your day-to-day work.
- Engage in more conscious and intentional theorizing (how might you theorize health, people, nursing, and environment).

REFERENCES

Browne, A. J. (2001). The influence of liberal political ideology on nursing science. *Nursing Inquiry, 8*(2), 118–129.

Chinn, P. L., & Kramer, M. K. (2011). *Integrated theory & knowledge development in nursing* (8th ed.). St. Louis, MO: Elsevier Mosby.

Dickoff, J., & James, P. (1968). Symposium on theory development in nursing. A theory of theories: A position paper. *Nursing Research, 17*(3), 197–203.

Fawcett, J. (1978). The "what" of theory development. In *Theory development: What, why, how* (pp. 17–33). New York: National League for Nursing.

Fawcett, J. (2005). *Contemporary nursing knowledge: Analysis and evaluation of nursing models and theories* (2nd ed.). Philadelphia: F. A. Davis.

Kleffel, D. (1996). Environmental paradigms: Moving toward an ecocentric perspective. *Advances in Nursing Science, 18*(4), 1–10.

Mehl-Madrona, L. (2007). *Narrative medicine: The use of history and story in the healing process.* Rochester, VT: Bear and Co.

Newman, M. A. (1994). *Health as expanding consciousness* (2nd ed.). New York: National League for Nursing.

Newman, M. A. (2005). Preface. In C. Picard & D. Jones (Eds.), *Giving voice to what we know: Margaret Newman's theory of health as expanding consciousness in research, theory, and practice* (pp. xxiii–xxvi). Sudbury, MA: Jones and Bartlett.

O'Connor, N. (1993). *Paterson and Zderad humanistic nursing theory. Notes on nursing theory.* Newbury Park: Sage.

Parker, M. E., & Smith, M. C. (2010). *Nursing theories & nursing practice* (3rd ed.). Philadelphia: Davis Plus.

Parse, R. (1996). The human becoming theory: Challenges in practice and research. *Nursing Science Quarterly, 9,* 55–60.

Parse, R. (1997). The human becoming theory: The was, is, and will be. *Nursing Science Quarterly, 10*(1), 32–38.

Parse, R. (1999). *Illuminations: Human becoming theory in practice and research.* New York: National League for Nursing.

Paterson, J. G. (1978). *The tortuous way toward nursing theory. In theory development: What, why, and how?* New York: National League for Nursing.

Paterson, J. G., & Zderad, L. T. (1976). *Humanistic nursing.* New York: John Wiley.

Paterson, J. G., & Zderad, L. T. (1988). *Humanistic nursing* (2nd ed.). New York: National League for Nursing.

Peplau, H. E. (1952). *Interpersonal relations in nursing.* New York: G. P. Putnam's Sons.

Pharris, D. M. (2002). Coming to know ourselves as community through a nursing partnership with adolescents convicted of murder. *Advances in Nursing Science, 24*(3), 21–42.

Reed, P. G., & Crawford Shearer, N. B. (2012). *Perspectives on nursing theory* (6th ed.). Philadelphia: Lippincott Williams & Wilkins.

Roach, S. (2002). *Caring, the human mode of being: A blueprint for the health professions* (2nd rev. ed.). Ottawa: Canadian Health care Association Press.

Rogers, M. E. (1970). *An introduction to the theoretical basis of nursing.* Philadelphia: F. A. Davis.

Vaill, P. G. (1984–1985). Process wisdom for a new age. *Revision, 7*(2), 39–49.

Watson, J. (1988). *Nursing: human science and human care. A theory of nursing.* New York: National League for Nursing.

8 All Nursing Is Relational Practice

LEARNING OBJECTIVES

By engaging with the material in this chapter, you will be able to:

1. Understand how nursing is a relational practice.

2. Understand how values shape relational practice.

3. Identify the five Ws of relating.

4. Identify the relational reference points shaping your nursing action.

In this chapter, we explore how nursing is a relational process shaped by personal values, dominant values in health care settings, and broader social values. We also identify the drawbacks of a service-provision way of relating and further consider how taking a relational inquiry approach can support more effective nursing action.

RE-THEORIZING RELATIONAL NURSING PRACTICE

Paterson and Higgs (2008) contend that, given the breadth of knowledge and evidence available to inform health care practice, one of the most significant challenges we face is that of making visible and credible "the many invisible, tacit, and as yet unexplored aspects of professional practice that are vital" (p. 181) to high-quality care. We believe that one of the tacit aspects of nursing that needs further clarification is the way in which nursing *is* at its core a relational practice.

Relational Practice Is More than Interpersonal Communication Skills

Decades ago, nurses began attempting to articulate a conceptual foundation for relational practice in nursing by borrowing concepts and strategies from the social sciences—in particular, psychology (Hartrick Doane, 2002a, 2002b). This borrowing occurred during a time when mainstream psychology was governed by behaviorism, an orientation that focuses on observable behaviors. As a result, specific emphasis was given to interpersonal communication skills and the behavioral performance of those skills as nurses interacted with patients (Hartrick Doane, 2002a, 2002b). This behavioral conceptualization has been appealing because it has identified concrete behaviors for nurses to enact; namely, to engage in effective communication skills such as active listening, open-ended questioning, paraphrasing, summarizing, and so forth (Hartrick Doane, 2002a, 2002b; Hartrick, 1997).

While there is no question that communication skills are helpful, they offer an incomplete picture of what is entailed in relational nursing practice. In particular, they do not reveal the complexities and/or the "how to" of effective relational practice in nursing (Hartrick Doane, 2002a, 2002b; Hartrick, 1997). Worse, this incomplete picture has limited effective action, at times actually serving to direct nurses in such a way that they fail to respond appropriately to what is happening in the moment (Hartrick Doane, 2002a, 2002b; Hartrick Doane & Varcoe, 2005; Hartrick, 1997). For example, when I (Colleen) was first taught communication, I was taught phrases such as "I hear what you're saying," but I was not taught how to figure out when they might be useful. Similarly, in teaching relational practice, I (Gweneth) find the majority of nurses begin with the assumption that relational nursing practice is about "saying the right thing" or about the "touchy feely stuff of nursing."

While borrowed theories and strategies such as those from psychology can be enlisted to inform our nursing action, as Chinn and Kramer (2011) contend, to determine the value of any borrowed knowledge, it needs to be examined from the perspective of nursing itself. In particular, the knowledge needs to be considered in light of the purpose and nature of nursing work and the realities of everyday nursing practice.

In presenting a relational inquiry approach to nursing practice, we are proposing that relational practice extends far deeper into human "being" and "relating" than interpersonal communication skills (Hartrick Doane, 2002a, 2002b; Hartrick, 1997, 1999). Relational practice is a process that involves nursing values, intent, knowledge, commitment, decision making, and actions (Watson, 1988) and is shaped by intrapersonal and contextual elements as well as interpersonal ones. Skillful relational practice includes how nurses orient and focus their attention in health care situations, how they use knowledge, and how they make clinical decisions. It also includes their way of being with (remember the five Cs) and relating to patients, colleagues, and the contexts in which they are working.

Having studied communication and interpersonal practice in both nursing and psychology, and more importantly having practiced as both a registered nurse and a registered psychologist, it is clear to me (Gweneth) that nursing is its own unique relational practice. My relational practice as a nurse is distinctly different from practice as a psychologist. For example, even if I enlist communication skills, the nature of how I do so differs. Nursing is a practice that is most often done "on the move." While I might occasionally have time to sit and talk with a patient, most of my "relating" is done while I am doing other forms of care—while I am doing a physical assessment, changing a dressing, measuring vital signs, and so forth. Thus, while communication skills might be helpful to nursing, they are not sufficient for effective practice. Moreover, to determine what *is* useful for effective relational practice in nursing, the starting point needs to be nursing itself. Specifically, we need to start by considering the nature, goals, and challenges of everyday nursing situations.

Complexity Theory Can Help Us Re-Theorize Relational Nursing Practice

Pause for a moment, and try to think of a time when you are *not* relating. Although you might start to think about solitary activities, if you think carefully, you will see that in each of the activities, you are still in relation with something or someone. During a walk in the forest, you are in relation with nature. While reading a book, you are in relation with the text. Even during meditation, people are in relation with larger forces of energy.

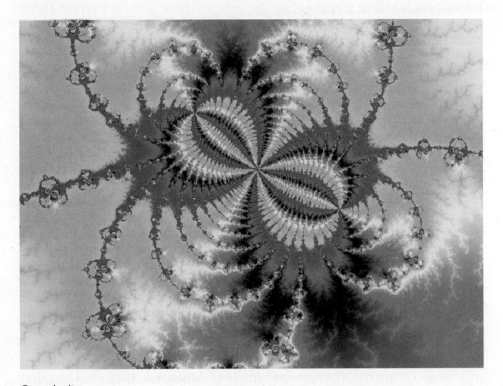

Complexity.

This relational nature of life is one of the foundational principles of complexity theory, a fundamental theory within the field of quantum physics. Complexity theory proposes that all things in nature are inter-related. The universe is interdependent and relational, a realm where the observer cannot be separated from the observed. "In the quantum world, relationships are not just interesting; to many physicists, they are *all* there is to reality" (Wheatley, 1994, p. 32).

Complexity theory can help us understand that nursing practice is not a linear independent practice (Hartrick Doane, 2002b). Rather, your nursing actions and the impact of those actions are mediated by many intrapersonal, interpersonal, and contextual variables, including what is happening for and around the person with whom you are relating. Specifi-cally, complexity theory reveals that people always act in relation to some-thing or someone else (Zohar, 1990) and that multiple elements relate and converge to create any outcome. The result of this relational interaction may be subtle or profound.

A good example offered in discussions of complexity theory is the butterfly effect. The beat of a butterfly's wing could trigger a breath of a breeze that eventually, through a series of initially minute and unforeseeable changes to a complex set of variables, could become a tornado (Vicenzi, White, & Begun, 1977). The actual outcome of the beat of the butterfly's wing—the force and the path of the breeze it generates—is ultimately determined by an infinite number of variables and their relational interactions.

Take a minute and think about these ideas in the context of your own life. Do you find that you are different in different situations and with different people? Have you ever had the experience of getting a report about a patient or reading his or her medical chart and then finding when you meet that person he or she is quite different from what you thought based on what you had heard or read? Complexity theory contends this is due to the relational nature of matter. That is, subatomic particles change their behavior according to that with which they come into relation. So when we relate to a person, what we observe is the person presenting *in response to us* and the particular context within which we are relating. This means that we influence and in some way determine who we meet and what we observe in people just as they somewhat determine who and what they meet in us. For example, can you think of people or environments that "bring out the best" in you? This relational nature of being and observing underscores the influence that you have as a nurse in the relating process. It also highlights how every moment of nursing action is relational, and thus it is important to be mindful and intentional in how you relate.

Ray (1994) and other researchers have come to recognize that re-examination of nursing practice in light of complexity theory has the potential to revolutionize nursing science. For example, in observing that a biomedical lifestyle approach to diabetes care is no longer adequate, Cooper and Geyer (2009) contend that complexity theory offers a way of knowing and understanding diabetes that accommodates what patients and health practitioners actually experience—"that living, caring, and working with diabetes is not separate from the real world but embedded within it in a series of interrelated systems" (p. 764). Moreover, they contend that complexity theory offers a practical application to chronic disease management and "'tools' for patients, caregivers, and practitioners that capture the reality of managing chronic disease" (Cooper & Geyer, 2009, p. 761). In a similar vein, health geographers Curtis and Riva (2010a) have offered examples of ways in which complexity theory is and can be used to understand health, emphasizing interconnectedness and the relationality of therapeutic care and care settings.

Overall, complexity theory illuminates how our lives are lived relationally—and how every moment of nursing involves some form of relating. To assume that we function independently (i.e., that we function separately from each other and from our world) is to miss all of the ways we are connected and relating. Thus, I (Gweneth) am continually perplexed when I hear nurses exclaim that they "don't have time to relate," as though *not* relating is even possible. What this thinking overlooks is that (a) it is impossible to *not* relate, and (b) *how* you relate is shaping everything you do and accomplish as a nurse. Simply put, you do not have a choice about whether you will relate. However, you do have a choice about *how* you relate—a choice that you need to consciously make since the choices you make about how you relate matter.

To illustrate the importance of conscious relational practice, we offer the following story of an experience I (Gweneth) had while in hospital a number of years ago following the birth of my daughter Teresa. The story illustrates that, whether nurses intentionally engage or disengage with people, they are always in relation and those relational moments are always affecting and shaping health and healing (Cooper & Geyer, 2009; Curtis & Riva, 2010a, 2010b; Geary & Schumacher, 2012; Hast, Digioia, Thompson, & Wolf, 2013; Hodges, 2011; Jayasinghe, 2012; Mitchell, Jonas-Simpson, & Cross, 2012; Rantz, Flesner, & Zwygart-Stauffacher, 2010; Ricca, 2012).

TO ILLUSTRATE
Two Relational Moments

The nurse knocked gently on my door and, thinking I was asleep, came quietly into my room. As I opened my eyes, she smiled, said hello, and began to check my IV. Silence seemed to fill the room. As I lay there in silence, I could feel the nurse's discomfort. I watched her busily checking tubes and dressings. Throughout her tasks, she did not look at my face; she seemed to be carefully avoiding my eyes. I was puzzled by the gentleness and concern I could sense she felt toward me despite her seeming desire to not engage with me. I asked if it would be possible for me to go and see my baby. (My daughter had been born by cesarean section the day before. She had stopped breathing in the delivery room, was on a ventilator, and was progressively becoming worse. No one could figure out what was causing her distress.) As I began to get myself up, I could feel the emotion rising within me and found myself swallowing hard to keep the tears in. The nurse busily got the wheelchair and helped me into it, all the while avoiding my eyes. Just as we were about to head out of the door, an old (medical) friend stepped into the room with a big smile on his face. He had seen my name on the patient list and had wanted to stop in to congratulate me. As I tried to speak, the emotion welled up. Looking into his eyes that showed such care and warmth, it was like the dam broke, and the tears began to pour out. Without saying a word, my friend took two steps across the room and reached out to hug me. It felt so good to express the emotion I felt! As the tears slowed and I reached for some Kleenex, I looked around for the nurse and realized she had left.

I have often thought about that nurse and wondered what her experience was that day. What led her to relate by maintaining such a distance between us? I remember that the ward was very quiet, so I don't think it was other demands that stopped her from engaging. Also, I could sense her caring and compassion, and yet she was giving a clear message that she was not willing to be with me in my pain. In response, I found myself desperately trying to keep my pain within me.

The response of that particular nurse is not unique. Many nurses choose such distance in their practice. It is not uncommon to hear nurses say things like, "I didn't know what to say," or "I didn't want to open that can of worms." Often, nurses believe they have to know how to handle a patient's discomfort; they have to do something with it. As a result of that belief, they relate by offering advice or choosing not to speak with people about difficult things. Their own discomfort with not being able to make things better and/or at the uncertainty of what might happen (e.g., "What if the person gets more upset or starts to cry?" or "What if I don't have an answer?") sometimes leads nurses to pull back. At times, nurses may also pull back because they themselves (as people) do not want to feel such deep emotion and pain.

Nurses may also relate by distancing themselves at least in part because of the messages they get about what is and is not of importance and value within the practice context and in order to deal with the way they are expected to practice within the business-driven context of health care. In my research on emergency nursing, I (Colleen) found that nurses criticized one another for being "too emotional" or "too involved" (Varcoe, 2001; Varcoe & Rodney, 2009). They called nurses who spent time with patients "bleeding hearts" and so on. Nurses modeled and promoted emotional distance, and although they talked about wanting more time to be with patients, meaningful engagement did not fit with an overall work pattern that was focused on "emptying the stretchers." Even when they had ample time, many nurses often chose to sit at the desk engaging with colleagues rather than with patients and families. With other colleagues who noted similar practices in other clinical settings, I concluded that nurses relationally disengaged to some extent in order to make the organization work (Varcoe, Rodney, & McCormick, 2003). They disengaged and kept emotional distance in order to more easily move people along and be ready for the next stretcher.

Whatever the underlying reasons, ignoring our relational impact reduces our capacity to respect, honor, and promote people's health and healing. It also restricts our knowledge about the people for whom we are caring, our ability to effect positive change, and our opportunity to experience one of the greatest sources of satisfaction from our nursing work.

RELATIONAL NURSING PRACTICE IS A VALUING PROCESS

The way you relate in your nursing practice is strongly shaped by your personal values and the health care and societal values that dominate your everyday world. Enlisting the hermeneutic phenomenologic (HP) and critical lenses (remember Chapter 2) can be helpful in illuminating this valuing process in action.

Personal Values Shape How Nurses Relate

Personal values shape how you relate. For example, having worked in the emergency room (ER) and adult intensive care unit (ICU) where I (Gweneth) saw a number of serious brain injuries from cycling accidents in which people were not wearing protective head gear, I have personally come to greatly value helmets. Specifically, I *relate* helmets to well-being. Thus, when my son Taylor was going to university in Germany and a friend gave him a bicycle to use as transportation, my first question was, "Do you have a helmet?" He laughed (since he knew I would be asking him that question) and told me how he had mentioned getting a helmet at a gathering the evening before, and everyone there had burst out laughing at the idea that someone would actually wear a helmet while cycling around town. They obviously did not see a value for helmets. Helmets held different meaning for them than they do for me. More importantly, because they did not invest helmets with the same meaning (and thus value them as I did), they did not relate to them in the same way and/or see their relevance (e.g., they did not relate helmets to well-being as I did).

Contextually, I do not know what the injury rate from cycling accidents is like in the city where Taylor lived, but when I visited, I did observe how the culture of cycling was quite different from the cycling culture where I live. The speed, look, and nature of the bikes and the way people used them were quite different. For example, the bikes were not built for speed; thus, the body position while on the bike was more vertical and upright. Everyone from children to elderly people could be seen cycling from place to place on the well-groomed bike paths and sidewalks where bicycles actually had the right of way (over pedestrians). Indeed, where we (Gweneth and Colleen) live, activists have pointed out that helmet laws (including tickets and the requirement for costly helmets) disproportionately disadvantage people with fewer material resources and that structural changes such as bike paths and lanes and subsidized helmets would be a more equitable public health approach.

We use this example to highlight how personal experiences shape our values, and these in turn shape how we interpret and subsequently relate to people and objects. Within health care, you only have to listen to nurses discuss a patient situation to hear their personal values: "His daughter hasn't shown up for 3 days," "That homeless guy I had to admit was filthy," or "I wish her family would just get out of the way and let me do my work." Statements such as these communicate personal values. Yet, the HP and critical lenses inform us that these personal values do not arise in isolation. As we discuss next, they are formed as we participate in particular contexts with particular value systems.

Health Care Values Shape How Nurses Relate

The systems and contexts within which you work are structured according to values, and those values determine what is given priority and worth. As you look at the normative practices (at the interpersonal level) and policies and structures (at the contextual level) that shape how health care and nursing is organized, it is possible to see particular values at play and how practice is strongly shaped by what the health care system accords value.

As we discussed in earlier chapters, the health care system in which we practice is structured according to a disease-treatment, service-oriented business model of care. This model of care shapes nursing actions. For example, many nurses approach their practice believing they are responsible for quickly making things better. As a result, they may relate more meaningfully to the disease than to the person living with that disease. Kelley Doucette, an ER nurse, describes her own experience of practicing in the value system of a busy ER and how through learning about relational inquiry she began to see the way in which her own values and her nursing practice had been shaped by that value system.

TO ILLUSTRATE

Enacting Values in the Emergency Room

Being able to practice with a relational inquiry approach has been such an influence in my practice, as it has shaped everything I do in every situation. I have to say it again because it is so ingrained in our hospital nursing culture of labeling patients. This occurs regularly in the ER, especially with patients who are being "overly dramatic," in our opinions. Previously when these patients presented, I would do the standard rolling of the eyes to my coworkers and take the patient in so we could assess them and find out the "asthma attack" was truly an anxiety attack. Now my practice has changed completely.

For example, recently, a woman came in with an asthmatic attack, and upon assessing her, I found no wheezing in her chest, her oxygen saturation was 95% to 100%, and she was sobbing uncontrollably while sounding stridorous with inspiration. A nebulizer of Ventolin was given as per the doctor's orders, and once she was able to speak again, I spoke to her about what was going on in her life at the moment. She started to tell me about the stresses she had been experiencing—trying to be the sole care provider for her special needs adult son, her sister was now dying of lung cancer, and she and her husband were struggling financially as he had been laid off a month ago. By relating more to her as a person, I was able to move beyond her "initial presentation" and seek the real reason she ended up in the emergency department; she needed more support and she was feeling overwhelmed. Subsequently, we were able to set her up with both our cancer care coordinator and social work program so she was able to find the respite resources she required to help her care for her son and sister. She had limited socioeconomic resources but was unaware of the resources that were available to assist her with her current situation. Had I given her a "placebo" Ventolin and a couple of Ativan for her anxiety without asking these questions, I wouldn't have given this woman the help she needed in a time when she needed it the most.

Societal Values Shape Nurses' Relational Practice

Societal norms and customs also shape how we relate as nurses. For example, in the Western world, feminism opened up the question of women's value in society. As people of all genders increasingly recognized women's equal value, gender relations began to change, and they continue to do so. The value of men in what traditionally had been women's terrain (e.g., the home, nursing, teaching) also shifted. A simple example of how this societal change has affected health care is how we relate to fathers in the delivery room when their children are being born. When I (Gweneth) was a student, having fathers in the delivery room was a relatively new practice and a controversial one. In fact, at the hospital where I did my delivery room rotation, the attending doctor was the one to decide whether a father was "allowed" in the room, with progressive doctors "accommodating" fathers' requests while conventional doctors barred their entries. Today, in most settings in North America, fathers are expected not only to be present at but also to participate in the birth. In turn, these expectations shape interpersonal action. For example, my (Colleen's) son-in-law, whose background includes a patriarchal family structure within a male-dominated logging community, found the nurses' expectations that he participate fully in child care (e.g., diapering) contrary to his values and norms. Social norms related to gender continue to shift and affect health care. For example, many health care contexts are seeking ways to be gender inclusive beyond the male/female binary, an inclusivity fueled in part by activism by transgendered people and their allies.

These examples highlight another feature of valuing—that values set the expectations and parameters for our judgments, and those judgments shape how we relate and respond in action. For example, we now expect "good" fathers to participate in the birth and make negative judgments when they don't. When particular individuals and families do not align with the norms and values dominant in your community or society, how do *you* respond?

Values Inform Our Relating Practices

Personal values, dominant health care values, and societal values all converge to "in-form" our action. By "in-form," we mean that we actually come to embody the values in concrete ways. For example, Elias (1978, 1982) has described how value systems and ways of thinking become so deeply integrated that they influence how we conduct ourselves bodily. People learn to discipline and control their own bodies according to the social groups within which they live and work. Thus, by watching the way people relate, we can often discern their values and the value systems at play in the particular situation. How people greet one another, their body language as they turn toward or away from one another, and so on, convey values. As Brown (2008) has observed, "It all shows up in the face-to-face" (p. 110). That is, values are revealed in how people relate to one another in face-to-face encounters.

TO ILLUSTRATE
Inconsistent Value Messages

As a student, I (Gweneth) found myself greatly confused by the contradictory messages I was receiving about practicing as a nurse. On one hand, I learned in class that as a nurse I should treat all people equally and with

continued on page 312

TO ILLUSTRATE *continued*

Inconsistent Value Messages

respect and dignity. On the other hand, while out in clinical, I saw very inequitable relational practices. This inconsistency was particularly evident during my rotation on pediatrics where I noticed that nurses racialized some of the families and made judgments about them according to those distinctions. Moreover, the nurses acted in ways disrespectful to these families. For example, they would refer to a particular racialized group, saying "those women who don't look after their kids properly, and then when the kids get sick they dump them at the hospital." These nurses, who were serving as my mentors, informed me in frustrated voices that "you can never get a hold of the mothers to come and get their kids because they're off drinking somewhere." At the same time, I watched how the nurses' interpretations and judgments (and their own value systems) led them to use derogatory tones with these families and to speak with frustration in their voices and coldness in their eyes. I found myself thinking that if I were one of these mothers, it would be difficult for me to show up and face such harshness.

My confusion about the mixed messages led me to feel uncertain about how to be "a good nurse." It was when I first read postcolonial theory (Chapter 2) that I started to gain some clarity and also began to see how the nurses' personal values were shaping their relational actions on pediatrics and how both had been contextually influenced. Moreover, I saw how important it was for me to enlist the postcolonial lens to examine my actions to see how my own values, interpretations, and judgments might have been "colonized."

My grandparents had emigrated from the United Kingdom, and I grew up in Saskatchewan, a province in Canada that had been colonized by European settlers who took over the land and displaced the indigenous people. Thus, my world was strongly shaped by colonial values, beliefs, and assumptions, including norms that were communicated to me both explicitly and implicitly. I grew up with the privilege of speaking English (with an "accent" of the dominant group) and being a white, British descendent in a country where British dominance shaped everyday life. Being in this white, English-speaking, privileged position and assuming a liberal individualist ideology, I took the colonial values, structures, and ways of being that dominated my world as normal. And as I did so, they became invisible to me. That is, I was colonized. Perhaps one of the most detrimental effects of this normalizing/colonizing process was that, in HP terms, I became constituted by them. I did not see that I had embodied norms that I had not chosen consciously and would realize later (thanks to my exposure to postcolonial theory) that I did not believe.

This experience is not unique. As constituted/situated beings, we are all shaped by the value systems in which we live—and those values serve to shape our interpretations, judgments, and ultimately how we relate and act. However, undertaking such a self analysis requires courage. It is not only difficult to see our own ideologies (fish don't see the water they swim in) but it is also challenging to name and take into account our own privileges and biases.

TRY IT OUT 8.1
Take a Snapshot of Yourself in Practice

To help you consider the knowledge, values, assumptions, and normative practices that are shaping your own relational practice, we invite you to do an inquiry. Next time you are in your clinical practice area, observe yourself for 1 hour, and take a careful look at your practice and how you relate.

■ What patterns do you see?

■ Can you identify any particular values (personal, health care, and/or societal) that are shaping your actions? If so, how?

■ Are your actions in line with the values and nursing ideals you espouse?

■ What knowledge informs your relational practice?

■ How does all of this influence your nursing action?

PRACTICING IN RELATIONALLY RESPONSIVE WAYS

Given that our nursing action is shaped by so many factors, practicing in relationally responsive and effective ways is supported through a process of inquiry and conscious choice. The story earlier in the chapter about how Kelley's practice in the ER shifted after she began practicing relational inquiry illustrates the profound difference conscious inquiry and choice can make.

The Five Ws of Conscious Inquiry

Focusing your attention on the "who, what, why, when, and where" of your relational action—what we will refer to as the five Ws (see Box 8.1)—is an important part of relational inquiry practice. As exemplified by Kelley, it involves having the courage and commitment to take an honest and sincere look at *how* you are relating. Are you conscious of *what* and *who*, *why*, *when*, and *where* you are relating and whether your actions are aligned to your nursing values and commitments?

What are you relating to? *What* are you focusing your attention on? *What* are you prioritizing and privileging? *What* are you valuing and not valuing? To use Kelley's example above, are you relating by unconsciously privileging the value system that prioritizes asthma over an anxiety attack—moreover that stigmatizes an anxiety attack and labels it "overly dramatic?" *Who* are you relating to? Do you find yourself joining colleagues in disrespectful and judgmental actions (e.g., rolling your eyes in response to a woman who is clearly in distress)?

BOX 8.1

The Five Ws of Relating: Choosing *How* You Will Relate

- *What* are you relating to? On what are you focusing your attention? What are you prioritizing and privileging? What are you valuing and not valuing?
- *Who* are you relating to? Who are you privileging? From whom are you distancing?
- *Why* are you relating? Identify the purpose and goals that are directing you.
- When are you relating? When do you extend or distance yourself? How do time and timing shape your relating practices?
- Where are you relating? How is context shaping your relating practice?

Do you look beyond the "initial presentation" to extend and widen your view so you can relate to the "whole" of a person and her living experience?

Third, do you consciously look to consider *why* you are relating? What purpose and goals are directing you? Is your attention focused on fixing the body in the bed or emptying the stretcher? Do you consider how you might work in concert with your nursing goals and also with what is meaningful to the person in the bed? Or, do you practice as the "burly nurse" (remember Nepo's example in Chapter 3) and just do what needs to be done?

Do you consider the fourth W and consciously pay attention to *when* you relate? Of course, as we described earlier, you are always relating, so really, this question of *when* directs your attention to the circumstances in which you relationally extend yourself and those in which you do not extend yourself—for example, when you relate by distancing, ignoring, or leaving. The *when* of relating draws particular attention to "timing" and the temporal aspects of practice. For example, Kelley first related to the "what" of the asthma symptoms by addressing the woman's breathing distress. Once that was reduced and the woman was able to speak, Kelley related by focusing her attention on the woman's living experience (her experience of being an overwhelmed caregiver with limited financial resources).

The fifth W of conscious relating is the *where*. This contextual aspect is vital since the way we relate and the choices we have are highly influenced by the contexts in which we work. For example, working in a busy ER shapes Kelley's relational practice by setting parameters on how her time is structured and the number of patients that need her attention. However, as she so eloquently described, once she began more consciously examining the who, what, why, and when of her actions and made the choice to revise her practice to better align with her nursing values and commitments, she was able to work more effectively within that context.

Kelley's action illustrates that in relational inquiry, we don't choose to focus on only one aspect of a situation. That is, it is not about whether you relate by addressing the physical symptoms *or* relate to the woman's socioeconomic experience. You relate to both because they are intricately connected—to promote well-being requires a "both/and" approach (as opposed to an "either/or").

To be clear, when we say that you are consciously choosing the five Ws, we are not saying you have complete choice in terms of the who, what, why, when, and where of any situation. Rather, we are saying that the more you pay attention to the relational choices you are making, the more you can ensure your actions are aligned with your nursing obligations and commitments. In addition, once you have identified these factors, you can then more consciously choose *how* you will relate. This distinction is an important one. As complexity theory suggests, we are always relating; thus, we don't have a choice about whether to relate. However, as we said earlier, we *do* have a choice about *how* we will relate in and to the five Ws.

TRY IT OUT 8.2

Inquiring into the Five Ws of Relating

Watch another nurse in practice for 5 minutes. Take a snapshot in your mind, and walk through the five Ws using the questions above.

- What does this tell you about values?
- What does it tell you about relating—what is the purpose, what goals are being pursued, and whose interests are in the foreground?
- What is happening simultaneously? For example, is the nurse relating effectively while also doing care tasks?
- Does this serve as a model for your own relational practice? In what ways?
- In what ways would you have acted differently to promote health and well-being?

Choosing to Relate to Uncertainty

Realizing the relational, nonlinear nature of human life and experience highlights how there is no linear cause–effect of "if I am compassionate, the patient will respond." Rather, what actually happens in an interaction, and the outcomes of that interaction are determined by many factors. As the butterfly effect in complexity theory highlights, one small relational variation can dramatically change the outcome of a situation. Thus, while consciously choosing how you will relate is vital, that is where your choice (and control) ends. That is, there are so many variables, and the complexity of interactions among those variables is so great that the actual outcome of your particular action can never be fully known or predicted. It is always uncertain.

If you think about this idea—that relational practice is uncertain—you will probably be able to see how you have experienced this feature of nursing work. For example, as nurses we have found that there have been times when our deeply concerted efforts have had little impact on the people with whom we are working. No matter how we have related and/or what we have done, we have not been able to produce the outcomes for which we are striving. At the same time, we have had experiences where a seemingly brief connection or minor effort on our part has had a profound effect on a person or family.

For example, I (Colleen) remember the first thank you card I received as a nurse (I can still see the yellow roses on the card in my mind's eye). When I received the card, I was shocked because I didn't think I had done anything special, and I barely remembered the situation. I had been looking after an elderly woman with Parkinson's disease. I do remember how I felt watching her try to brush her own hair with great difficulty, and I do remember saying how difficult I imagined her life must be. Somehow, something I did or said led her to write on the card that I had "given her hope to go on living."

This nonlinear, uncertain nature of people's experience and of relational nursing practice heightens the importance of your relational action; it means that you are always impacting the situation in some way. Thus, the question arises: What are you perpetuating through the way you relate or act? Moreover, (as we discussed in Chapter 7) how might you focus your relational actions toward your nursing commitments and toward "situation-producing" goals? That is, how might you relate or act in ways that might foster desirable situations?

TO ILLUSTRATE

An Uncertain Situation

Mr. Gray's body was swollen beyond recognition. He was septic following a bone marrow transplant and was critically unstable. I (Colleen) had been expecting his wife to return to the unit with their daughter who was flying in from California, not having seen her dad since he had become ill. Mr. Gray was semiconscious, and although I could not be sure he heard and understood me, I talked to him continuously as I suctioned his endotracheal tube, completed my routine vital sign checks, and titrated his drugs, trying to maintain some sort of blood pressure.

As I was completing these actions, Mr. Gray's wife and daughter arrived, the senior resident immediately behind them. He urgently told me to take a new set of cardiac output and hemodynamic parameters and gave me

continued on page 317

> ### TO ILLUSTRATE *continued*
> ### An Uncertain Situation
>
> several new drug orders. The resident was not the sort of physician who appreciated being contradicted, and my habit was to follow orders. However, the look in his daughter's eyes as she took in the alien sight of her father amidst the multiple lines, monitors, tubes, lights, and sounds led me to say, "I think it is more important for his daughter to have some time right now." I was shocked at myself (this marked a turning point for me in my practice in terms of my clarity and convictions regarding my allegiances within the health care power hierarchy) and at the resident's response. He nodded and quietly left.

Colleen's decision about how to respond in the situation arose through a combination of clinical judgment, a sense of empathy for Mr. Gray's daughter, and an obligation to care for Mr. Gray's family as well as Mr. Gray. Although it would have been within her purview to privilege the doctor's orders and the biomedical imperatives of the situation, Colleen extended her modes of inquiry to encompass the particularities of the moment, then consciously chose her action from a number of competing options.

This story illustrates how being clear in your nursing commitment and consciously choosing your relational response can serve as the anchor for your nursing action in the midst of "uncertain" nursing situations. Being clear in your nursing commitments enables you to make conscious choices and intentionally look to see the choices you might have within the very real constraints of a situation. Thus, effective relational practice entails developing the disciplined habit of really looking to see more clearly and more critically what is happening for you, for the patients and families you care about, and what is happening within your context so you can consciously choose your own response to and in those realities. While we cannot predict or determine the impact of our actions, we can choose to direct our actions in particular ways.

Choosing to Promote Well-Being

One of the reasons it is important to scrutinize how you are relating within situations and more consciously choose your relational action is that any relational experience in itself has the ability to promote well-being or potentiate harm. If you listen to anyone who has had a "bad" health care experience, you can hear the remnants of that experience and how people continue to carry the wounds from those experiences. Similarly, if you listen to anyone who has had a particularly positive experience, you can hear the impact that experience had and continues to have. This points to how relational experiences are in themselves a health intervention. Through relational presence, people have the opportunity to experience the power of human connection in the healing process (Anderson, 2007; Segrin & Domschke, 2011; Turpin, McWilliam, & Ward-Griffin, 2012; Wilson, 2008). For example, Anderson (2007) describes the central role of nurse presencing in a community-based cardiac rehabilitation program, emphasizing how the relational connection with nurses led patients to become more invested in the program. Similarly, Wilson (2008) describes the significance of relational presence for people living with chronic illness, while Turpin and colleagues (2012) examine the impact in the context of older adults in home care and long-term care.

My (Gweneth's) work as a nurse/psychologist with families experiencing loss and grief also exemplified this health-promoting quality of relational presence and connection. When I was with families in their grief and we entered into the realm of deep relational connection, it was common for one or more of the family members to afterward question how it was possible to feel so out of control and in such incredible pain and yet simultaneously feel they were okay. I have come to understand that, at least in part, what promotes this feeling of being okay is the human connection of being cared about and sharing a compassionate space. Although our togetherness did not lessen their grief or pain, it provided the space and opportunity for them to live what they were experiencing—to open up to their grief and express it. Moreover, it helped them to experience their own capacity to handle the adversity they were facing. That is, having experienced that they could be in their pain *and* be okay, they discovered aspects of themselves they had never before experienced and began to see the strength and capacity they had within them. It also provided the opportunity to see what they didn't have and what they might need to support them as they lived through the challenging circumstances. In essence, the relational experience promoted their reconnection with themselves and a feeling of choice and centeredness amidst their grief.

Purposeful relational presence enables people and families to more deeply connect with themselves as they go through adversity. When their life circumstances feel out of control, supporting people to be in their experiences and connect with their capacities is not only empowering but also healing. Rushing in to "fix" or "do for" may actually impede their own capacities to live these experiences *and* heal. This process of being with and supporting people to deepen their connection with themselves resonates with the nursing theories you read in Chapter 7 (Paterson and Zderad's "more-being," Newman's "expanding consciousness," and Parse's "human becoming").

As nurses, we do not have the power to fix or change people and families or control the outcomes of situations (e.g., biomedical intervention may "fix" disease processes, but people still have to live in and through the illness experiences). Any change or healing that occurs will be the result of a multitude of relational factors. However, because our actions *always* impact the outcome in some way, we must be very thoughtful as we relate. If a breath of a butterfly wing can spark a tornado, we must tread lightly and "care-fully" as we act and be deeply mindful of how we may be impacting the situation we are entering because our smallest actions can promote hurting or healing (Hartrick Doane, 2002a).

A Question of Time

Practicing in relationally responsive ways is not about having more time. As we mentioned earlier, we commonly hear nurses explain that they do not have time to relate or be with patients in meaningful ways. Yet, every nursing action is relational and meaningful in some way. Thus, the question becomes: "How might you use the time you have to practice in the most relationally responsive way?" *Core to relational inquiry is the assumption that meaningful, health-promoting nursing action can occur in any amount of time.* Thus, your nursing attention needs to focus on effective and efficient use of your time and energy to make the time you have count.

Della Roberts, an advanced practice nurse who teaches workshops on care of people with dementia, asserts that even if you have only a moment to make eye contact with or smile at a person, that action can be significant.

TO ILLUSTRATE
Making Moments Meaningful

An example of how a small shift in relating can have an impact happened in a workshop with interprofessional staff in residential care for people with advancing dementia. Participants expressed frustration and distress as they had so little time to be with the person with dementia. Gina Gaspard, a skilled clinical nurse specialist in geriatric care, shared a powerful video clip of a social worker making a connection with a woman in the advanced stage of dementia (Memory Bridge: The Foundation for Alzheimer's and Cultural Memory, 2007). The video clip demonstrates how a person never loses his or her ability and longing for connection, even when they have lost their ability to speak. Gina emphasized that the person with dementia lives in the moment, so staff members need to "make moments meaningful" by entering into the reality of the person with dementia and make connections. At the end of the session, participants were asked to write down one thing they would do differently tomorrow in their practice. Many of the participants wrote down "make moments meaningful." Their comments demonstrated a shift in understanding and the realization that the few moments they had to connect with the person with dementia could promote well-being. Rather than seeing a few moments as insignificant and feeling badly about not doing enough, they decided to begin using the few moments they had in purposeful ways.

Since the impact of your action is not just a matter of whether you have time to form relationships or how much time you spend, it comes down to a question of *how to invest the time you have* (even if that time is a minute or two as you pass someone in a hallway, take vital signs, dispense a medication, or complete a home care evaluation). Relational nursing practice, then, is a matter of intentionally choosing what and how you will invest your time, energy, and attention. If you cultivated only one relational practice to enhance your nursing effectiveness and that practice was to more consciously and compassionately choose how you relate in particular situations at particular moments, that practice alone would stand you in good stead to be a more effective and competent nurse.

SHIFTING YOUR INTERPERSONAL REFERENCE POINTS

By inviting you to examine your relational practice, we are attempting, in Thaler and Sunstein's (2009) words, to "nudge" you toward more effective reference points for making decisions about nursing action. Influenced by contextual values and normative practices, many nurses have developed reference points that constrain their relational responsiveness. Thus, we need to scrutinize our choice-making reference points to ensure that they meet the needs and desires of our patients, families, and communities. For example, because nursing practice is often anchored in a biomedical model, nurses often make choices from that model; in other words, their practice is anchored in a biomedical reference point. But what happens when nurses add new points of reference?

For example, when the nurses with whom I (Colleen) currently work initially began providing care to people living with HIV/AIDS, they anchored their care to viral load counts. However, as they become more skilled, while viral load counts remain important, the nurses increasingly anchor their care to what is meaningful to the patient.

Doreen Littlejohn, an expert nurse who has been overseeing a program for people who are HIV-positive for many years, recently gave an example of the effect this shift in reference point is having. By inviting women to a support circle and encouraging the women to "lead" according to what is important to them, new possibilities are emerging.

TO ILLUSTRATE
The Power of Group Support

A woman who attended brought her antiretroviral (ARV) meds to the group today. She was quite defensive in earlier groups, but through the one-on-one with the nurses and the group support, she is actually committing to take her meds and is using the group support to walk her healing journey. She requested I have her meds bubble-packed for 1 week at a time and said she would bring the empty package to the group next week. This is a huge step for her as the (clinic) staff had tried (unsuccessfully) for the past 2 years to devise a strategy to support her "medication compliance."

Thinking about this anchoring process in terms of how you relate as a nurse highlights the importance of consciously considering and perhaps shifting the reference points you are using as you make choices about who, what, why, when, and where you relate (the five Ws). In what are you anchoring your practice? If you think you don't have time to relate to patients, what reference points for "efficiency" are you using in determining that? For example, consider the earlier story about the woman who presented to the ER with an asthmatic/anxiety attack. If your reference point for efficiency was "quick treatment of acute symptoms and speedy discharge," you could have achieved that goal by giving the patient Ativan. However, if your reference point for efficiency was decreased visits to the ER, that approach probably would not have been the most efficient since the woman likely would have returned to the ER when her anxiety and stress level rose again. Moreover, if your reference point was the promotion of health, giving Ativan would not have been an efficient use of time regardless of whether you define health according to the biomedical, behavioral, or socio-environmental perspectives (as we discussed in Chapter 1). That is, even from a biomedical perspective (health as the absence of disease), it becomes clear that although the symptoms would have been lessened, the condition would still have been present. To treat a situation-triggered anxiety attack by merely addressing momentary symptoms would be comparable to treating someone who presented with a myocardial infarction with morphine and sending the person home because the chest pain or neck pain had lessened. Thus, Kelley's example is an interesting one even when you think about competence and what serves as a reference point for competent practice. Without her "relational intervention" (e.g., if she had just given Ativan and sent the woman on her way), would her nursing action have been competent?

TRY IT OUT 8.3

What Are Your Allegiances and Reference Points?

Think about your current or most recent practice setting. First, identify what reference points are encouraged. What is the one thing that "can't be missed?" What ideas are in the background guiding priority setting and the measurement of efficiency? If you are in community health practice, is it immunizations that "trump" everything else? If so, what drives that? See if you can articulate at least one "reference point" that dominates the setting in which you work.

Second, identify how you act as a result of that reference point. Do you always comply with that reference point as your guide? Does it shape your interpersonal action? Or do you sometimes "go against the grain?" If so, how? When, where, why, what, and with whom? If, for example, medication

continued on page 322

TRY IT OUT 8.3 *continued*

What Are Your Allegiances and Reference Points?

administration is the central reference point, do you ever go against that as guiding your priority setting, and if so, under what conditions? Do you ever try to work in concert with different reference points to do both/and? For example, do you look to see how you can give priority to both immunizations and a parent's distress?

Shifting Your Reference Point from Service Provision

Often, developing skillful relational practice involves some unlearning (Hartrick Doane, 2002a, 2002b; Hartrick Doane & Brown, 2011). Varela, Thompson, and Rosch (1993) provide a helpful analogy for this unlearning, asserting that we are born "already knowing how to play the violin and practicing with great exertion only to remove the habits that prevented one from displaying that virtuosity" (p. 251). This captures the way in which we develop relational skillfulness (Hartrick Doane, 2002b). Becoming a skillful relational nurse requires us to identify and step out of the ways of relating that are hindering our effectiveness. One constraint that hinders many of us is a service-provision point of reference.

Over two decades ago, McKnight (1989) observed that health care systems are dominated by a service-provision model in which initiatives and activities (such as nursing) most often focus on providing a service. Specifically, relating to people as patients in need of servicing is the normative practice. As McKnight and Kretzmann (1992) explain, this model rests on the underlying premise that people with health problems require outsiders to meet their health and healing needs. This service-provision model still dominates today. That is, service provision is most often the central point of reference from which health care providers, including nurses, act.

What are the drawbacks of this model? First, as McKnight (1989) contends, it contradicts the principles of socio-environmental health promotion by focusing on pathology or deficiency. The more disadvantaged people are, the more problems can be found (by well-meaning nurses and others) and the more people can be pathologized. If my reference point and main job as a nurse is to provide a service, my attention will be focused on looking for what it is that needs servicing. If what needs to be serviced are problems, I will be focused on problematizing people and situations. Indeed, entire health care systems are structured to focus on servicing problems.

For example, two home care nurses with whom I (Colleen) work were recently told by their administration that they could no longer visit patients unless they needed a procedure (e.g., dressing change, medication administration). These nurses, who have worked for many years with impoverished people living in an inner city, routinely visited their patients, knowing that their health would often otherwise deteriorate without anyone knowing because

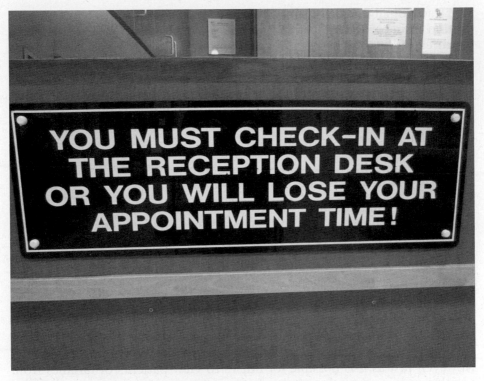

Welcome sign. (Photograph by Colleen Varcoe.)

they lived alone and had few social supports. Despite hundreds of examples of situations in which they had averted catastrophic health consequences through such visits, their practice was clawed back to a service model.

Although a person or family may have many strengths and resources, the servicing of deficiency may become the overriding emphasis of nursing assessment and intervention. For example, scan any admission form, intake form, or initial assessment form in the health care agency where you are doing your clinical work. How do these forms set you up as a nurse? To what do they draw your attention? How much focus is on deficiency or problems and on what service the client needs? If strengths and capacities are included in the forms, are they centrally located or are they add-ons? Do the forms direct you to consider the integral relationship between strengths or capacities and adversities or problems?

A second effect of the service-provision point of reference is that the power of the professional may push aside the expertise, technique, and capacity of people and families to address their own health and healing needs (Hartrick, 1997). A service model of health care rests upon the assumption that it is nurses (and other health professionals) who possess the knowledge, expertise, technique, and technology necessary to manage people's health and healing experiences, and these override the knowledge and experiences of people and families. According to McKnight (1989), as the power of the professional and service systems ascends, the legitimacy, authority, and capacity of people to increase control over and improve their health (in their own lives) descends.

Traditionally, the nursing literature has tended to link health promotion conceptually with this servicing approach to health problems (Hartrick, 1997). This service-provision, problem-oriented reference point is evident in the language used in many descriptions of nursing. For example, nurses speak of "treatment and outcomes," of "assessing, diagnosing, and intervening" to identify and address "problems." Often, the fundamental emphasis of nursing assessment and intervention is problem-focused service provision. Health promotion is seen as something an expert nurse does through the provision of health services.

Shifting Your Reference Point to What Is

Given the dominance of the service model of care, nurses are often well-schooled in being what Parse (1999) has termed "fix-it mechanics." In consequence, when entering any nursing situation, their focus (their central reference point) is what needs changing or servicing. This can have a limiting effect on the people and families for whom they are caring; for example, they are so focused on what concerns them as nurses that they often fail to ask what is important to the person or family. It can also have a detrimental impact on nurses themselves; for example, when they see themselves as ineffective because they have not achieved the health outcomes they wanted, such as getting someone with COPD to stop smoking. However, just as it is possible for nurses to view patients or families from a half-empty perspective, it is also possible to view them as half-full (Hartrick, 1997).

To practice from a socio-environmental perspective of health in line with the purposes and goals of nursing as outlined in the human science theories of nursing requires shifting your reference point to *what is*—relating to the particular situation as it is and responding to what is meaningful to the people in those situations (Hartrick Doane, in press). In contrast to a service-provision model that directs attention to problems, a socio-environmental perspective of health directs the nurse never to lose sight of what nursing assessment and intervention are fundamentally for and about—namely supporting people's and families' choices and capacities to live meaningful lives within their particular personal and social contexts. Although nurses may well attend to a problem and provide a service, at the center of nursing care are people and families and what is meaningful to them.

I (Gweneth) witnessed a basic yet exemplary illustration of a nurse who practices from the reference point of *what is* while doing a buddy shift with a nurse, Michelle, during an ethics research project (Rodney, Hartrick, Storch, Varcoe, & Starzomski, 2002). It was basic in that all Michelle was doing was greeting her patients at the beginning of her shift. What made it exemplary was *how* she did that. The first patient she greeted was a burly man who was self-employed as a logger and was anxious to get out of hospital and back to work. Before Michelle could say hello, he began asking when the doctor would be there to discharge him. Already dressed at 7:30 in the morning, the man who was pacing the floor declared that he was anxious to get on the road since he had a long drive home to his small rural community. Entering the second room, Michelle greeted an elderly woman with dementia who, confused and anxious, asked where her son and daughter had gone. As we rounded the corner into the third room, we heard a woman crying—the woman, a young mother who had just been given a terminal diagnosis, lay weeping in her bed. In each case, Michelle relationally attuned to where and how each person was in that moment, responding to each in a very simple and particular way (simple in that she merely met them where they were and particular in that she responded to their very particular concern at that moment). Each greeting lasted only a matter of a minute or two, during which time Michelle assessed needs and priorities and determined the order of things to be attended to. Telling the young mother she would return in a few minutes (and thereby letting her know she had seen her need and was going to respond), she returned to the nursing station to place a call to the first man's doctor to get the discharge rolling. Next, she settled the elderly woman into her breakfast. Completing her rounds to check that the rest of her patients were okay, she returned to spend a few minutes with the woman who was weeping.

As I watched Michelle, I found myself wishing that I could package her up and take her to class with me (and I actually told her that). She was a living example of what I try so hard to convey to students—that responsive relational practice is at the heart of all nursing care—and that it takes many different forms. Effective relating is not just about the "touchy feely stuff"; it is about effectively responding in and to each moment of nursing care! It is about orienting in living experience, relating to what is, and recognizing and responding to significant patterns.

For Michelle to practice as she did required focused intention and inquiry. Specifically, her focus was to know and relate to her patients as they were—to relate to "what was." As Thayer-Bacon (2003) contends, the first relational step toward understanding another is to notice them—to value them enough to notice and try to understand. It also involves taking the initiative to reach out and extend oneself toward people—listening and inquiring intently and suspending judgments long enough to make sure we have seen and heard what the other is relaying (Thayer-Bacon, 2003). This inquiry involves the desire and ability to move beyond reference points that block such connection and/or that hinder one's ability to see and hear what is meaningful and significant to particular people and families.

Once again, it can be helpful to use the analogy of looking through a camera and adjusting your lens. A nurse practicing from a socio-environmental understanding of health focuses the lens on people and families in context. The reference point becomes who this person or family is; what is meaningful and significant to them in their lives; what their particular health concern means to them at this moment; what capacities they have both personally and contextually; the adversities that might be constraining their power, choice, and ability to realize their aspirations; and the potential actions that might be taken (by the person or family and nurse) to simultaneously enhance capacity and address adversity. The following story was told to me by Sandi, a nurse I (Gweneth) taught last term. It is a story of Sandi practicing the strategy of joining a patient in a meaningful way to relate to "what is."

TO ILLUSTRATE
Sandi Relates to What Is

Anna has been in the ICU for 6 weeks following a double lung transplant. She remains in the ICU post lung transplant because she has barely tolerated any weaning from the ventilator. After 2 weeks, Anna was labeled as a needy patient by the nurses. My first questions were, "Why is she needy?" What is she looking for?" "What needs are perhaps not being met?" "What does she fear?" "What does she expect?" "Does she understand what we expect of her?" Luckily, I have spent several shifts with Anna and began asking her some of the questions I was asking myself. I know her rituals that comfort her in the ICU, yet I found myself pondering the double-edged sword of helping her feel comfortable and at home in the ICU. Does she really want to be that comfortable in the ICU? "Does she plan to live here?!"

During my shift, after talking with Anna, she tolerated a 35-minute weaning trial. This is a measurable progress from the 3-minute weaning trials that she began 2 weeks ago. She told me that the weaning trials were hard and long. I tried to reframe this for her. I asked her, "What if you were to go home and be independent of the ventilator?" I know she wanted to go home and eat Cheezies. For Anna to go home and eat Cheezies would require some degree of independence from the ventilator. I know this made her think. After 1 or 2 weeks, Anna was transferred to the step-down unit with her weaning trials lasting over 13 hours. I like to believe that the conversations I had with Anna helped her. I cannot be sure.

Sandi's story illustrates relating to what is by orienting to what is meaningful to the patient. Sandi did not simply abide by the label of "needy patient" and relate to Anna accordingly. She sought to understand and connect with Anna. She extended herself to inquire into what might be meaningful to Anna and joined her in that. While in the context of a high-tech biomedically oriented ICU, the desire to eat Cheezies could be interpreted as irrelevant or a somewhat superficial focus, what was important was how Sandi enlisted the Cheezies to help Anna reconnect with what mattered to her—namely, living a meaningful life. This example highlights that no matter the disease condition or illness situation, relating human being to human being and inquiring into and relating to people's living experience and what matters to them in a particular moment serves to promote health and simultaneously fosters competent, effective care.

Simply put, relational inquiry involves shifting our reference point from service provision to people and situations as they are. By purposefully relating to people and situations—to "what is"—the situation can be known and understood more fully and thus responded to more effectively. Kelley's example of how she approached the woman in the ER is a prime example of relating and responding to "what is." Looking beyond servicing an asthmatic/anxiety attack (beyond the symptoms and the administration of Ventolin and Ativan), Kelley inquired into what was happening for the woman. She related to "what was." She related by opening the relational space to know what was significant in the woman's life situation and how her symptoms were meaningful within that context and the particular moment in time.

As Newman (1994) explains, when life is received as it is, change can happen as it needs to. For that reason, relating to "what is" is perhaps the most powerful way in which change and well-being are promoted (Hartrick, 1997), and it is a central reference point for relational inquiry practice (Hartrick Doane, in press).

Relating to "what is" involves some fundamental shifts in terms of the rules you might currently be following. Thus, you might need to do some re-schooling and reforming of your practice. Specifically, some of the actions you might need to consider and cultivate include:

- Relating to "what is" without labeling
- Relating to "what is" without trying to fix it
- Relating to "what is" without decontextualizing
- Relating to "what is" by relating to complexity and difficulty
- Relating to "what is" by being a knower/not-knower
- Relating to "what is" by collaborating

Relating to What Is without Labeling It

In Chapter 2, we observed that labeling turns people into things (e.g., drug users, high-risk mothers, asthmatics), and then prompts us to relate to them accordingly. Given that we are assigned the responsibility to assess and discern patterns and make clinical judgments, of course we identify health problems that need treatment. However, any health or illness experience involves far more than a "thing" to treat. That is, there are always meanings, emotions, contextual elements, choices, and ambiguities. Shifting our point of reference to "what is" requires us to drop the labels and orient to these multiple and complex aspects of the patient's or family's experiences. What capacities do they have? What might impede their ability to cope with this situation and/or meet their aspirations?

Relating to What Is without Trying to Fix It

As we move beyond seeing people and situations as problems to be solved, we also begin to see another reference point that often underpins our interpersonal choices and actions—that of fixing. We are not suggesting that offering support for people to address problems in their lives is problematic—rather we want to open up the question of nursing action. Might we move beyond orienting our practice as expert "fixers" to become inquiring facilitators? Rather than taking up a professionally distant stance, treating people as objects we are observing or taking up our busy gait and "doing to" people in the name of efficiency, might we shift from an I-It to an I-Thou relation (Chapter 3) even in brief and transitory moments and respond to living experience as Kelley did in the ER?

Relating to What Is without Decontextualizing

Throughout this book, we have described how people and situations are often decontextualized in health care. Because decontextualizing is so common in the majority of health care contexts, we need to develop the relational practice of seeing decontextualizing as it is happening. For example, within the business model of health care and the trends of health care reform, efficiency is the overriding value, and the overriding assumption is that time and resources are simply "not there." While of course resources are always finite, what is often missing is the understanding of how existing resources are allocated and the contextual elements that determine allocation. That is, the discussion of limited resources is decontextualized. By paying attention to the contextual elements shaping this discussion, we shift our reference point and begin to ask the question of resources in another way: What values and priorities are directing the use of resources (e.g., as opposed to assuming that everyone—including patients—just has to learn to do with less)?

The public is encouraged to think that they need to make sacrifices in health care (Northcott, 1994). Nurses (along with the rest of the public) are encouraged to take these ideas for granted and focus on making the best of things, rather than recognizing that these "realities" are choices and relating to them as such (Abma, Baur, Molewijk, & Widdershoven, 2010; Jones, Pykett, & Whitehead, 2010; Lim, 2012; Williams & Maruthappu, 2013). When, for example, a hospital decides to lay off nurses at the same time as purchasing an expensive new computer system, this decision is not simply about limited resources; it is a series of *choices* driven by certain values. Nurses often have opportunities for input at a system level. To participate effectively, we need to see when "what is" is being discussed and viewed in a decontextualized manner. So, for example, nursing input is often sought when new bedside computers are introduced or a switch to a new model of equipment is being contemplated. Considering the context within which this new equipment will be used allows you to engage more effectively in system-level decisions. For example, as electronic patient record systems are developed, you might carefully look to see the kinds of information that are being privileged and/or ignored. Will they help you be more or less responsive to patients? Will they actually save time, or will they shift how you use it to more "screen" time and less "face" time?

Relating to What Is by Engaging with Complexity

Another habit or normative practice, given the fix-it reference point, is to try to reduce complexity. Effective relational practice requires that we actively shift that reference point to more intentionally engage with complexity. For example, rather than simplifying a situation by locating problems in people ("that woman is overly dramatic"), relational inquiry intentionally looks for the complexities beyond immediate people and families. Again, Kelley's example in the ER illustrates engaging with complexity. She did not reduce the woman's health situation by labeling her "overly dramatic" or foregrounding only her anxiety but invited the complexities into the room. She looked beyond the presenting symptoms to the complexities giving rise to her symptoms. Relating to complexity involves looking to see how health care situations are being shaped by language, structures, organizations, cultures, policies, and so on. Relating to complexity allows nurses to inquire about the influences shaping the patterns they see and to discern wider social patterns that shape experiences. Such understanding widens possibilities for intentional action beyond relationships with particular patients and families.

Relating to complexity involves developing the capacity to practice in ambiguity—to understand that any human experience is complex, ambiguous, and uncertain and needs to be related to accordingly. As one corresponds with the complexity (remember Chapter 3's discussion of corresponding), one simultaneously inquires, being curious and questioning the feelings, thoughts, and meanings within the situation and the multiple (and often conflicting) understandings. Engaging with complexity involves a concurrent process of inquiry to "know more" and discrimination to make connections among the different elements and meanings within the experience and, with the help of the patient or family, realize the relevance of the experience for subsequent action.

While on the surface it can seem as though engaging with complexity is unrealistic in today's health care environment where the dominant push is to simplify and streamline, if you observe carefully, you will see that it is in fact how all competent practitioners work. For example, when patients present in the ER with chest pain, they are not simply given analgesia. Rather, the first step is to look at the situation in all of its complexity by taking a full history and developing as much knowledge as possible through clinical investigations. In doing so, treatment can be targeted and much more effective.

Relating to What Is by Knowing/Not Knowing

We have already discussed the process of knowing/not knowing, emphasizing that not knowing is *not* a sign of incompetence. Given that human life and illness situations are complex and changeable, there is no possible way we can know for certain which is the best way to proceed or nail down in any final way "what is really going on" for people. While a physician might ascertain what is going on medically, nursing someone living with that medical condition involves looking beyond the diagnosis. Thus, as we described in earlier chapters, *competent, skillful practice does not rest on the certainty of a medical diagnosis but rather on inquiry; safe practice is grounded in a continual process of questioning how best to proceed with particular people and families in particular situations.* Yet, if you observe health practitioners in action, it is often possible to see how they are working toward control and certainty; there is an underlying assumption that they "should know." While they may consciously know and even say that the outcomes are unpredictable, they are invested in being more certain so they can control what happens.

Of course, trying to ascertain what is happening and to control the progress of a disease is a central reason people seek health care. Thus, we are not suggesting that knowing and/or such interventions are not relational. Rather, we are suggesting that practicing by investing and orienting one's practice primarily or exclusively around a control or certainty reference point is highly limiting for *nursing*. It is limiting because it serves to privilege certain things and ignore others. To reference Kelley's ER experience, it can narrow the focus to the disease process and direct attention away from other aspects that might be just as if not more significant to the patient or family and to the disease itself. Moreover, focusing on certainty, nurses can fail to respond to all of the uncertainties that are part and parcel of any illness experience. For example, while you can be certain that everything is being done from a biomedical perspective to treat a sick neonate in the neonatal intensive care unit, what is often overlooked are important *nursing* aspects. How do you care for parents living in uncertainty? What is it like for these specific parents to live in the uncertainty (whether their baby will live, whether there will be long-term disabilities, etc.), and what is the impact of that uncertainty on the family's health?

Not knowing is the first step to figuring out how to act. When we don't know, we are forced to look, inquire, and more carefully choose our actions. *Therefore, relating to what is by accepting "not knowing" as part of competent nursing practice actually enhances your nursing effectiveness.* "Not knowing" becomes merely a site for further inquiry and learning (it is not seen as a problem or something lacking in you). This relational practice of knowing/not knowing involves paying attention to how the expectation of certainty is shaping the contexts in which you are working. Often, we are pushed toward certainty by colleagues, patients, and managers who encourage us to be "knowers." By adjusting our reference point and working between knowing and not knowing, we can be more purposeful in our responses to such pressure. Moreover, we can resist the pressure to "fake" certainty and thus actually be more competent. We can be confident in what we both know and don't know and enlist relational inquiry as a way of responding to both further our knowledge and act effectively.

Relating to What Is by Collaborating

Given the individualist orientation and liberalist ideology that dominates most health care practice, health practitioners have been schooled to see themselves as autonomous agents who are expected to exercise their free choice in meeting the standards of professional practice. However, if you ask nurses about their actual experiences of providing care, you will undoubtedly hear them speak of interpersonal and contextual forces that shaped the care they provided and the choices that were possible. In other words, their range of choices is context-dependent; choices are not made in isolation. All nursing work is carried out in a relational matrix (Rodney, Brown, & Liaschenko, 2004). Whether we are aware or not and whether we consciously attend to the relational matrix or not, our nursing actions are shaped by our colleagues, patients/ families, and the structures organizing our nursing care. *Thus, we need to pay attention to when we are working in isolation and develop the practice of collaborative action.* Rather than unmindfully allowing the relational matrix to influence us, we can purposefully choose and act to make the most of these relations. While we discuss collaborative practice in more detail in Chapter 10, at this point we want to highlight how the strategies we outline in this book are collaborative in nature. That is, they are intended to be taken up to foster collaborative action *with* patient/ families and *colleagues.*

THIS WEEK IN PRACTICE
Relating to What Is:
Engaging with a "Challenge"

Pick your favorite clinical area to think about.

Identify the "challenging" people and families or "problem" situations in that area. List the people who are commonly seen as "difficult," "problematic," or "challenging." How are they commonly labeled or identified? In emergency nursing, patients who repeatedly return to the hospital are often labeled "frequent flyers" and seen as challenging. Sometimes patients who are angry are seen as challenging. Families who are demanding, particularly those who demand to be seen ahead of others, are considered challenging. Patients with substance abuse problems or serious mental illnesses are often considered challenging. In maternity, women who have not had prenatal care are seen as problematic and suspected as "unfit" mothers.

Select an example from your list of "challenging" people or situations.

Analyze the dynamics of your example, thinking at the intrapersonal, interpersonal, and contextual levels. What values and attitudes prevail in this example? What judgments? How do nurses tend to relate to people or situations deemed to be challenging or difficult? What contextual variables (e.g., stereotypes, workload priorities) might be at play? For example, in the case of women who do not access prenatal care, what judgments do nurses tend to hold? What attitudes are conveyed? How do they act toward them? To what extent are the barriers to prenatal care (such as racism, poverty, transportation, child care, violent and controlling partners who prevent access, etc.) understood?

Imagine how you might act with such a person or situation. What would be easy for you? What would be challenging?

Re-imagine the challenge. See if you can think relationally and locate the problem beyond people or contexts. If you look "relationally" and enlist the relational inquiry tools you have learned up to this point, do you see it differently? Might you act more effectively?

YOUR RELATIONAL INQUIRY TOOLBOX

Add the following tools to your relational inquiry toolbox.

- Look to see how every moment of nursing is occurring in a relational matrix.
- Pay attention to how personal, health care, and social values are shaping your nursing action.

continued on page 332

YOUR RELATIONAL INQUIRY TOOLBOX *continued*

- Enlist the five Ws to make conscious "relating" choices.
- Notice the reference points that are dominating your practice.
- Extend your reference points beyond a service model of health care.
- Consciously relate to uncertainty, complexity, and not knowing.
- Make conscious choices about how you will effectively and efficiently use the time you have with patients and families.
- Relate to what is without labeling, decontextualizing, or trying to fix things.

REFERENCES

Abma, T. A., Baur, V. E., Molewijk, B., & Widdershoven, G. A. M. (2010). Inter-ethics: Towards an interactive and interdependent bioethics. *Bioethics, 24*(5), 242–255.

Anderson, J. H. (2007). The impact of using nursing presence in a community heart failure program. *Journal of Cardiovascular Nursing, 22*(2), 89–98.

Brown, H. (2008). *The face to face is not so innocent: The relational construction of interpersonal spaces of maternal-infant care* (Doctoral dissertation). University of Victoria, Canada.

Chinn, P. L., & Kramer, M. K. (2011). *Integrated theory & knowledge development in nursing* (8th ed.). St. Louis, MO: Elsevier Mosby.

Cooper, H. C., & Geyer, R. (2009). What can complexity do for diabetes management? Linking theory to practice. *Journal of Evaluation in Clinical Practice, 15*(4), 761–765.

Curtis, S., & Riva, M. (2010a). Health geographies I: Complexity theory and human health. *Progress in Human Geography, 34*(2), 215–223.

Curtis, S., & Riva, M. (2010b). Health geographies II: Complexity and health care systems and policy. *Progress in Human Geography, 34*(4), 513–520.

Elias, N. J. (1978). *The history of manners: The civilizing process* (Vol. 1). Oxford, United Kingdom: Blackwell.

Elias, N. J. (1982). *State formation and civilization: The civilizing process* (Vol. 2). Oxford, United Kingdom: Blackwell.

Geary, C. R., & Schumacher, K. L. (2012). Care transitions: Integration transition theory and complexity science concepts. *Advances in Nursing Science, 35*(3), 236–248.

Hartrick, G. A. (1997). Relational capacity: The foundation for interpersonal nursing practice. *Journal of Advanced Nursing, 26*, 523–528.

Hartrick, G. A. (1999). Transcending behaviorism in communication education. *Journal of Nursing Education, 38*(1), 17–22.

Hartrick Doane, G. A. (2002a). Beyond behavioral skills to human-involved processes: Relational nursing practice and interpretive pedagogy. *Journal of Nursing Education, 41*(9), 100–404.

Hartrick Doane, G. A. (2002b). Beyond interpersonal communication: The significance of relationship in health promoting practice. In L. Young & V. Hayes (Eds.), *Transforming health promotion: Practice, concepts, issues, and applications* (pp. 49–58). Philadelphia: F. A. Davis.

Hartrick Doane, G. A. (in press). Cultivating relational consciousness in social justice practice. In P. Kagan, M. Smith, & P. Chinn (Eds.), *Philosophies and practices of emancipatory nursing: Social justice as praxis*. New York: Routledge.

Hartrick Doane, G. A., & Brown, H. (2011). Recontextualizing learning in nursing education: Taking an ontological turn. *Journal of Nursing Education, 50*(1), 21–26.

Hartrick Doane, G. A., & Varcoe, C. (2005). *Family nursing as relational inquiry: Developing health-promoting practice*. Philadelphia: Lippincott Williams & Wilkins.

Hast, A. S., Digioia, A. M., III, Thompson, D., & Wolf, G. (2013). Utilizing complexity science to drive practice change through patient- and family-centered care. *Journal of Nursing Administration, 43*(1), 44–49.

Hodges, H. F. (2011). Preparing new nurses with complexity science and problem-based learning. *Journal of Nursing Education, 50*(1), 7–13.

Jayasinghe, S. (2012). Complexity science to conceptualize health and disease: Is it relevant to clinical medicine? *Mayo Clinic Proceedings, 87*(4), 314–319.

Jones, R., Pykett, J., & Whitehead, M. (2010). Big society's little nudges: The changing politics of health care in an age of austerity. *Political Insight, 1*(3), 85–87.

Lim, M. K. (2012). Values and health care: The Confucian dimension in health care reform. *Journal of Medicine and Philosophy, 37*(6), 545–555.

McKnight, J. (1989). Do no harm: Policy options that meet human needs. *Social Policy, 20*(1), 5–15.

McKnight, J., & Kretzmann, J. (1992). Mapping community capacity. *New Designs for Youth Development, 10*, 9–15.

Memory Bridge: The Foundation for Alzheimer's and Cultural Memory (2007). *There is a bridge*. Retrieved August 12, 2013, from http:// www .memorybridge.org/videos/clip1.swf

Mitchell, G. J., Jonas-Simpson, C. M., & Cross, N. (2012). Innovating nursing education: Interrelating narrative, conceptual learning, reflection, and complexity science. *Journal of Nursing Education and Practice, 3*(4), 30–39.

Newman, M. A. (1994). *Health as expanding consciousness* (2nd ed.). New York: National League for Nursing.

Northcott, H. C. (1994). The politics of austerity and threats to Medicare. In B. S. Bolaria & R. Bolaria (Eds.), *Women, medicine and health* (pp. 7–24). Saskatoon, Saskatchewan, Canada: University of Saskatchewan.

Parse, R. (1999). *Illuminations: The human becoming theory in practice and research*. New York: National League for Nursing Press.

Paterson, M., & Higgs, J. (2008). Professional practice judgment artistry. In J. Higgs & A. Titchen (Eds.), *Professional practice in health, education and the creative arts* (pp. 181–189). Oxford, United Kingdom: Blackwell Science Ltd.

Rantz, M., Flesner, M., & Zwygart-Stauffacher, M. (2010). Improving care in nursing homes using quality measures/indicators and complexity science. *Journal of Nursing Care Quality, 25*(1), 5–12.

Ray, M. (1994). Complex caring dynamics: A unifying model of nursing inquiry. *Theoretic and Applied Chaos in Nursing, 1*(1), 7–14.

Ricca, B. (2012). Beyond teaching methods: A complexity approach. *Complicity: An International Journal of Complexity and Education, 9*(2), 31–51.

Rodney, P., Brown, H., & Liaschenko, J. (2004). Moral agency: Relational connection and trust. In J. Storch, P. Rodney, & R. Starzomski (Eds.), *Toward a moral horizon: Nursing ethics for leadership and practice* (pp. 154–177). Toronto, Ontario, Canada: Pearson Prentice Hall.

Rodney, P., Hartrick, G. A., Storch, J., Varcoe, C., & Starzomski, R. (2002). Ethics in action: *Strengthening nurses' enactment of their moral agency within the cultural context of health care delivery*. British Columbia, Canada: Social Sciences and Humanities Research Council, University of Victoria.

Segrin, C., & Domschke, T. (2011). Social support, loneliness, recuperative processes, and their direct and indirect effects on health. *Health Communication, 26*(3), 221–232.

Thaler, R. H., & Sunstein, C. R. (2009). *Nudge*. New York: Penguin.

Thayer-Bacon, B. (2003). *Relational (e) pistemologies*. New York: Peter Lang.

Turpin, L. J., McWilliam, C. L., & Ward-Griffin, C. (2012). The meaning of positive client-nurse relationship for senior home care clients with chronic disease. *Canadian Journal on Aging, 31*(4), 457–469.

Varcoe, C. (2001). Abuse obscured: An ethnographic account of emergency nursing in relation to violence against women. *The Canadian Journal of Nursing Research/Revue Canadienne De Recherche En Sciences Infirmières, 32*(4), 95–115.

Varcoe, C., & Rodney, P. (2009). Constrained agency: The social structure of nurses' work. In B. S. Bolaria & H. D. Dickinson (Eds.), *Health, illness and health care in Canada*

(4th ed., pp. 122–150). Toronto, Ontario, Canada: Nelson.

Varcoe, C., Rodney, P., & McCormick, J. (2003). Health care relationships in context: An analysis of three ethnographies. *Qualitative Health Research, 13*(7), 957–973.

Varela, F. J., Thompson, E., & Rosch, E. (1993). *The embodied mind. Cognitive science and human experience.* Cambridge, MA: The MIT Press.

Vicenzi, A., White, K., & Begun, J. (1977). Chaos in nursing: Making it work for you. *American Journal of Nursing, 97*(10), 26–32.

Watson, J. (1988). *Nursing: Human science and human care. A theory of nursing.* New York: National League for Nursing.

Wheatley, M. (1994). *Leadership and the new science.* San Francisco: Berrett-Koehler.

Williams, C., & Maruthappu, M. (2013). "Healthconomic crises:" Public health and neoliberal economic crises. *American Journal of Public Health, 103*(1), 7–9.

Wilson, M. H. (2008). "There's just something about Ron": One nurse's healing presence amidst failing hearts. *Journal of Holistic Nursing, 26*(4), 303–307.

Zohar, D. (1990). *The quantum self: Human nature and consciousness defined by the new physics.* New York: Williams.

9 Relational Inquiry Strategies

LEARNING OBJECTIVES

By engaging with the material in this chapter, you will be able to:

1. Identify several checkpoints for ensuring that you are orienting your practice as a relational inquiry.

2. Describe the checkpoints that support relating to and with "what is."

3. Explain the value of the strategy of collaborative knowing and not knowing, and identify specific inquiry checkpoints that can enhance this capacity.

4. Discuss the importance of recognizing and responding to patterns and the checkpoints that support this strategy.

In Chapter 1, we included a story that illustrated the gap between what the nurse telling the story wanted to do and what was realistically possible. That Chapter 1 story illustrates a common pattern that we have observed—the difference between responsibility and response-ability.

The strategies we outline in this chapter flow directly out of the ideas you have been reading about in the earlier chapters, as we show in Figure 9.1. We discussed in Chapter 1 that as a result of our pragmatic approach to knowledge, relational inquiry does not rest in one particular theoretical perspective. Relational inquiry is a way of relating to people, situations, and knowledge, and it is guided by the overriding goal of being as responsive and response-able as possible. *At its core, relational inquiry is a practice of attention—of focusing attention and acting in a more conscious and intentional manner.* The relational inquiry ideas and tools provide (a) a concrete orienting structure for your nursing attention, (b) a means of expanding your choices for action, and (c) an inquiry structure to guide and inform your knowledge and your actions. In this chapter, we offer four specific strategies to add to your relational inquiry toolbox. Each of these strategies includes a series of relational inquiry (RI) checkpoints to help you assess whether or not you're putting the strategy into action.

Table 9.1 identifies the checkpoints that support your implementation of each of the four strategies.

Orient Relationally

Choose How You Relate
- Who?
- What?
- Why?
- When?
- Where?

Use Lenses
HP lens
Critical lens

Use Modes of Inquiry
- Empirical
- Aesthetic
- Ethical
- Sociopolitical

Use Strategies
- Orient in living relational experience
- Relate to and with "what is"
- Collaborate through knowing/ not knowing
- Recognize and respond to patterns

Inquire at Three Levels
Intrapersonal
Interpersonal
Contextual

Develop Capacities
- Curiosity
- Compassion
- Commitment
- Competence
- Correspondence

Fig. 9.1 Relational Inquiry Tools

STRATEGY 1: ORIENTING *IN* LIVING RELATIONAL EXPERIENCE

As we have stated throughout this book, relational inquiry requires us to orient toward the relational complexities and interplay occurring in any situation in order to work intentionally and skillfully in response to them. Recall from Chapter 2 that you can enlist the HP and critical lenses to both expand your view of an experience and guide your actions. Looking through the HP and critical lenses is a way of orienting in living relational experience in all of its complexity. Five orienting checkpoints can help you implement this strategy.

Table 9.1: Relational Strategies and Checkpoints

Strategies	Relational Inquiry Checkpoints
Orienting in living relational experience	How am I orienting to health and well-being?
	How am I orienting in the five Cs?
	How am I orienting in the five Ws?
	Am I orienting at all levels?
	Am I orienting problems relationally?
Relating to and with "what is"	Am I "letting be" to know what is?
	Am I discerning the specifics?
	Am I in sync?
	Am I being *in* the complexity and difficulty?
Collaborative knowing/not knowing	Am I following the lead?
	Am I listening to and for?
	Am I looking beyond the surface?
	Am I enlisting multiple forms of knowledge?
	Am I willing to "backtrack?"
Recognizing and responding to patterns	Am I creating opportunities for choice-making?
	Am I creating opportunities for enhancing capacities and addressing adversities?

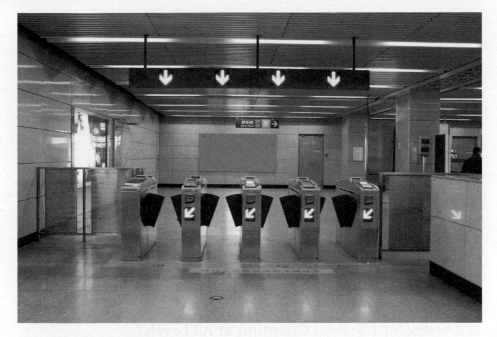

Checkpoints. (Media Bakery.)

RI Checkpoint 1.1: How Am I Orienting to Health and Well-Being?

The first orienting checkpoint is to identify the definitions of health and well-being from which you are working. Given that you are responsible for promoting well-being through your nursing action, the question becomes: How am I orienting to health and well-being? Whose well-being am I directing my actions toward (e.g., patient, nurse, system)? How is my working definition of health and well-being the same and/or different from the people or families for whom I am caring?

Revisit the opening story in Chapter 1. How would your own definition of health have focused your attention if you were the nurse in that situation? On whom and what would you focus your attention? For example, what would be particularly important in the immediate situation (your proximal view)? What more distal aspects might be important?

RI Checkpoint 1.2: How Am I Orienting in the Five Cs?

The second orienting checkpoint is to center yourself in the five Cs we discussed in Chapter 3. What attitudes and ways of being are you bringing to the situation?

- How are you being compassionate?
- Are you being curious, identifying what you know and don't know?
- What obligations and commitments are directing your actions?
- What would being competent mean within the complexities of this particular situation?
- How are you corresponding with the people and the situation?

Bringing these ways of being to the situation, are you valuing and opening to the living experience of the person or family for whom you are caring? Are you willing to be in the uncertainty of the situation and work between knowing and not knowing? Take a moment to think about how the answers to these questions would differ for the people involved in the story of Kelley's experience in the ER, told in Chapter 8. Recall the ER nurse who was rolling her eyes at the woman experiencing an anxiety attack. How would she answer these questions? What about Kelley, who decided to consciously practice relational inquiry?

RI Checkpoint 1.3: How Am I Orienting in the Five Ws?

The third orienting checkpoint is to tune into the five Ws of relating described in Chapter 8. This means you intentionally choose the who, what, why, when, and where of your actions. Tune into the five Ws throughout your day to orient your action before, during, and after any situation. For example, as Kelley more intentionally chose her way of relating (the five Ws), she reoriented her nursing assessment and greatly enhanced the effectiveness of her nursing action.

RI Checkpoint 1.4: Am I Orienting at All Levels?

As we have already described in relational inquiry practice, there are three levels or domains of inquiry, including the intrapersonal, interpersonal, and contextual. Thus, to act effectively as a nurse, you need to consider and act at all levels. The intrapersonal action may be as simple as noticing what is triggering you when you feel upset, annoyed, concerned, or unsure so you can exercise your choice and power in terms of how you are in the situation and how you respond. For example, as the nurse in Chapter 1 was able to do, your own emotional response can be used as a cue to look more carefully at what is happening interpersonally and contextually—to see and respond more fully at those levels. Acting interpersonally might involve extending your proximal view to see the wife of a dying man also as your patient. Acting contextually might be talking to your manager and colleagues about how patients might be better cared for by reworking transfer protocols.

Although in any particular moment you might focus the lens of the camera on a particular level, all three levels are always relevant to the picture. Moreover, each can and needs to inform the others. For example, intrapersonal inquiry enhances our view both inwardly and outwardly. Merleau-Ponty (1962) describes that our bodies are our first openings to the world. Our bodies do our living—they sense themselves in our physical, cultural, social, and human situations and environments. As such, our bodies offer a window into what is happening at all three levels and how we ourselves are relating. Take a minute and tune into your body. Try taking some slow deep breaths to help you begin to feel your bodily sensations. Pay attention to the air going into your lungs and to how it feels when you breathe out. As you breathe out, what bodily sensations do you feel? Are your shoulders up around your ears? Sitting at my computer and having done so for the past several hours, I (Gweneth) am aware of how tight my shoulders are from sitting over my computer so long. This simple example shows how if we listen and pay attention, we can physically sense our bodies implying the situation and the next steps we should take (Gendlin, 1992a). For example, my tight shoulders serve as cues to remind me that I should take a break and replenish myself if I want to continue thinking clearly and carry on writing. In this way, our bodies sense the intricacy of a situation and implicitly shape our next action (Gendlin, 1992a). Our bodies are the *site* of knowledge and decision making as well as the *medium* for action and knowledge development.

Although we may not tune into or be aware of it, this implicit, intricate "body-sense" functions in every situation, and according to Gendlin (1992b), we would be quite lost without it. Body-sense includes more than conscious awareness. Gendlin contends that body-sense is not merely perception or feeling but involves an intricate interaction of conscious and unconscious "knowing" that offers more than you can see, feel, or think. Our bodies are the sites where many forms of knowledge come together, are present simultaneously, and are weighed and interrelated as possible next moves (Gendlin, 1992a). It is this understanding of how knowledge comes together in the body that highlights the significance of bodily knowing for nursing practice. The body allows one to navigate and flourish in the ambiguity of everyday nursing practice (Benner, 2000) by offering a site where multiple forms of knowledge (e.g., personal, experiential, theoretical, contextual, cultural) come together and imply direction.

As human beings, we each are like one large relating organ—relating through our skin, eyes, touch, hearing, taste, energy, and so forth. Thus, body sensation offers a rich source of knowledge and a guiding foundation for nursing practice (Hartrick Doane, 2004). A simple example of bodily knowing in a nursing context is when I (Gweneth) worked in critical care. Often, my more experienced nursing colleagues would describe "having a gut feeling" that a particular patient wasn't doing well. As a new nurse, I quickly learned that more often than not, bodily sense—that gut feeling—was accurate. I also learned to rely on my bodily sensing during tasks such as starting an intravenous line. Once I started listening to my bodily sense and let my fingers *sense* the way, I became much more adept at successfully finding and entering a vein.

Sensory organs, the detailed structures of our living bodies, contextual forces and structures, and our interactions determine bodily knowing. Subsequently, embodied knowledge is not objective knowledge, nor is it merely subjective. Embodiment keeps it from being purely either (Lakoff & Johnson, 1999). Our bodily sense is shaped by our cultural, social, and corporeal worlds. As Merleau-Ponty claimed, the flesh of our bodies is inseparable from the "flesh of the world" (Gendlin, 1992a). Similarly, our bodies intimately shape what we touch, taste, smell, see, breathe, and move within. It is through sentient bodily interaction that we take up language, history, and culture and also exceed them (Gendlin, 1992a). In this way, the body conveys knowledge and information about ourselves, others, and the sociopolitical context that we may not be capable of yet articulating.

As we consciously access our body-sense and also tap the knowledge that may be gleaned through a more explicit process of inquiry and analysis (e.g., interpersonal and contextual inquiry), we can profoundly enhance our nursing practice. Attending to bodily sense offers the opportunity to step out of and possibly challenge habitual ways of practicing and/or the dominant sociocontextual norms that may be pressing in upon us and/or constraining our nursing effectiveness.

TO ILLUSTRATE

Practicing with a Gun at Your Head

During an ethics research project (Varcoe et al., 2004), we conducted a focus group with operating room nurses who talked about how their work environment was making it difficult for them to practice ethically. As they attempted to put the challenges they faced in their work environment into words, the following interaction occurred between them:

Nurse 1: The pressure is relentless. It is relentless . . . It's one of the most demarolizing environments you can ever imagine being in.

Nurse 2: I can speak of having to do 10 cataract extractions every day and feeling as though you're working with a gun at your head. Literally, that is the emotional feeling that I have.

Nurse 3: That's it, that describes the feeling perfectly. A very real and present revolver at your temples.

This interaction offers an excellent example of how our bodies sense, take up, and help us express knowing what we may not yet have put into thoughts or language. By becoming aware of the knowing living in our bodies at any moment (practicing with a gun at one's head), we are offered the opportunity not only to expand our understanding of ourselves and our reactions but also what might be happening for others in the situation and what contextual factors are pressing upon us. This bodily sensing can also enhance our ability to articulate aspects of our experience more clearly and serve as a compass to help us navigate through the complexities and ambiguities of any nursing situation.

TRY IT OUT 9.1

Addressing Well-Being at All Levels

Try to imagine yourself as the nurse in the Chapter 1 story. Picture the situation in your mind. Next, consider the intrapersonal, interpersonal, and contextual inquiry questions in Box 9.1. As you consider each set of questions, intentionally relate the different levels to each other. Look to see how your answers to the contextual questions might shape your answers to the intrapersonal and interpersonal questions and how the

continued on page 341

TRY IT OUT 9.1 *continued*

Addressing Well-Being at All Levels

answers to the questions at one level can offer insights into the other levels. For example, if the nurse had more consciously evaluated her interpersonal nursing actions in light of the contextual questions, might she have seen her actions differently? Might she have been better able to identify ways she was effectively impacting the situation in spite of the contextual limitations? Might that interpersonal and contextual knowledge have shaped her intrapersonal experience differently? Similarly, if she was better able to connect her intrapersonal experience to what was happening interpersonally and contextually, might she have had more confidence to address her nursing concerns (e.g., interpret her concerns as valid nursing issues that needed to be addressed at the system level)?

RI Checkpoint 1.5: Am I Orienting Problems Relationally?

Stop for a moment and consider the way we talk about problems and concerns in our nursing and health care world. A common practice of language, both in our everyday conversations in the health care world as well as in the professional literature, is to locate the problems or relational "hard spots" (areas of disagreement, conflict, uncertainty) *in* people and families (patients, ourselves, colleagues) or in the context (health care system). Examples include "This person is not complying with treatment," "This diabetic patient isn't eating like he should," "That colleague is difficult to work with," "These are at-risk youth," "She doesn't communicate openly," and "That is just the way the system works."

A *central working principle of relational inquiry is to see and locate problems relationally*—that is, one always looks to the relational space *between* people and *in* situations. By approaching difference relationally, we are able to look at and relate to differences and problems from multiple vantage points and extend our choice and action.

Difference implies more than one perspective and thus draws attention to the place *among* different perspectives and to the action of *"relating across difference."* For example, health care providers may blame a person with diabetes, heart disease, or kidney disease for dietary decisions. Often in this blaming process, contextual factors such as economic hardship, a controlling family member or partner, or a variety of other factors that constrain the person's choices may be overlooked. It also reinforces the focus on the health care providers' definition of the problem. For example, while nurses may expect patients to comply with dietary restrictions "for their own good," people consider pleasure, social aspects, and convenience when they make dietary decisions. Helene (in Chapter 6) always balanced restricting her fluid and salt intake against the extent to which she could tolerate feeling deprived. If she felt totally deprived of enjoyment, she became depressed, which she saw as also detrimental to her health.

BOX 9.1

Inquiry at All Levels

Intrapersonal Inquiry Questions

- What am I thinking, feeling, and how am I responding to myself?
- How are patients, families, and colleagues thinking, feeling, and responding?
- What interpersonal and contextual elements are influencing my interpretations, feelings, and actions?
- What values, commitments, and obligations are shaping my actions and those of others?
- What competing values, commitments, and obligations are at play?
- From what reference points and allegiances am I orienting?
- What and/or who am I privileging in my interpretations?
- How am I being compassionate to myself?

Interpersonal Inquiry Questions

- How might I meaningfully connect with this person or family?
- What reference points and allegiances are shaping my interpersonal practice?
- What is happening between us, and how am I participating in this interpersonal process?
- What normative practices are shaping the situation (labeling, categorizing, etc.)?
- What values, commitments, and obligations are being privileged?
- What competing concerns and/or obligations are at play in the situation?
- How is power being enacted by myself and by others?

Contextual Inquiry Questions

- What values, structures, and ideas dominate this context?
- How do these values, structures, and ideas tend to shape people's experiences and the health care situations?
- How does the way resources are being allocated and/or accessed support or constrain health-promoting practice?
- How does the way health care is organized support and/or limit health-promoting practice?
- What reference points are structuring policies and organizational directives?
- How are language practices, economics, sociocultural elements, politics, and historical factors shaping this particular health care situation and the way health care is occurring?

An important aspect of relational inquiry is the way it moves us beyond blame and criticism and helps us address any situation more effectively by locating hard spots and problems relationally.

TO ILLUSTRATE
Revisiting the Operating Room

Think back to the example of the OR nurses "practicing with a gun" at their heads. You know little about the situation, but what strikes you about what might be going on for them? What emotions can you hear or imagine from their words (intrapersonal)? How do you imagine this situation might influence them to relate (interpersonally) with one another, to patients, surgeons, the OR janitorial staff? What does their description suggest about the context in which they work? Change toward more health-promoting practices can't be achieved by simply changing individual staff attitudes; similarly, helping staff to relate to one another better is unlikely to improve the situation substantially. Policies and resource change are likely needed but would also require intrapersonal and interpersonal shifts; in other words, all levels need to be addressed at once. Yet, when one of the OR nurses went on stress leave, the problem was located in her—she was described by other staff as "just not cut out for the pace."

Locating problems *in* people and/or contexts can promote blaming people and families for their health problems and obscure other elements that are shaping their behaviors and the challenges they face. Moreover, it leads nurses to solutions that involve trying to force people to change themselves and their behaviors and fosters coercive relationships. Similarly, locating the problem with nurses blames nurses for whatever the hard spots are, which implies that nursing practice is entirely within the nurses' control.

Rather than abstracting and objictifying problems, relational inquiry highlights how problems arise out of a combination of complex multilevel factors. For example, rather than objectifying and abstracting problems that arise in interprofessional teams as "communication" problems or "time" constraints, relational inquiry extends the view to the complex relational interplay and in so doing extends possibilities for action (Hartrick Doane, Stajduhar, Bidgood, Causton, & Cox, 2012). Certainly, particular people do present challenges, and there can be communication problems. However, talking about problems abstractly and locating them only within the context of practice (as with communication and/or time) can overlook the capacity of the people involved and absolve both of responsibility for action and change. Similarly, it can set up simplified solutions and/or adversarial relationships that do not match the complexities of the situation. For example, I (Colleen) was told about a surgery that was conducted mistakenly on the wrong eye of a patient and how blame was placed on OR team communication. This resulted in better procedures being put in place; however, what was over-looked were the systemic problems such as work load, stress, and the hier-archical tensions in the team that contributed to the cause of the problem.

As responsibility and blame become intermingled, nurses' response-ability is hindered, and they feel powerless to change or affect the situation. Viewing and approaching difference relationally promotes taking respon-sibility rather than laying blame; inquiry to understand rather than en-trenchment in one's own position; connection rather than defensiveness and distancing; empathy rather than guilt or anger; and response-ability rather than a sense of powerlessness and frustration.

Orienting problems and hard spots relationally involves (a) bringing a compassionate attitude, (b) naming the interplay at all levels, and (c) posing helpful questions. So, for example, take the phrase "she doesn't communicate openly." One way of relationally reframing this would be to say, "I wonder how our unit culture and practices could foster more open communication with her?"

TRY IT OUT 9.2
Locate the Problem Relationally

For each of the following examples, try rewriting the problem by naming the interplay at all levels and posing a question.

"This person is not complying with treatment."	
"This diabetic patient isn't eating like he should."	
"That colleague is difficult to work with."	
"These are at-risk youth."	
"That is just the way the system works."	

STRATEGY 2: RELATING TO AND WITH "WHAT IS"

Although we have discussed the importance of relating to "what is" earlier, we discuss this strategy again here because in the midst of complex nursing situations, we often forget to practice it. Ironically, our relational efforts tend to be oriented more toward avoiding or changing what is than relating in and to it (Hartrick Doane, in press). This is particularly so when we run into relational hard spots—for example, when we find ourselves unsure, upset, frustrated, fearful, or even angry at particular people (patients and colleagues) and/or situations. Most often, we relate to those people or situations by trying to change or fix them.

For example, when a family member is angry over the care a loved one is receiving, nurses often respond to the anger by trying to deflect it, deny it, explain it away, or ignore it. Depending on how they view the situation, they may label the problem as a difficult family member, a demanding patient, or an overwhelming workload. Similarly, when patients are experiencing pain or suffering, we may try to make them feel better in a way that imposes a solution that may not align with what they actually need. For example, my (Colleen's) friend recently broke several cervical vertebrae and was temporarily partially paralyzed. Following, he could not get adequate relief of his shoulder and neck pain, despite the proffered solutions of multiple anti-inflammatory and pain medications. Once I tried listening to his explanation of "what is," I discovered that he was worried about addiction. To cultivate our ability to "relate to what is," the following checkpoints can be helpful.

RI Checkpoint 2.1: Am I Letting Be to Know What Is?

Because of the "fixing" tendency most nurses share, perhaps one of the most important skills of relational inquiry is developing the skill to "let be" (Hartrick, 2002). Situated in and constituted by powerful discourses of problem-solving, alleviation, change, management, intervention, and efficiency, nurses experience tremendous anguish at the thought of being with people and situations as they are—of letting be. The habit of striving to alleviate the problem is a difficult one to move beyond. Yet, as we discussed earlier, as nurses we do not actually have the power or ability to effect change in any predictable or linear (cause-and-effect) way. For example, even when we give pain medication, multiple influences affect whether or not pain will be relieved. Thus, in order to relate to and with what is, we must first let be. Rather than immediately striving to effect change, we must purposefully act to know and understand people and circumstances as they are.

The distinction between doing nothing and letting be is crucial. Many nurses interpret letting be to mean doing nothing; everything remains the same, and things are not changed. Yet, *letting be is active and purposeful*. Returning to the example of pain relief, when we routinely jump in to offer medication when a person is in pain, our action may well align with what is needed in that moment. However, it may miss the mark entirely, mask an underlying or different problem, and obscure other possibilities. This is not to say that we shouldn't offer pain medication; rather, our point is that we need to check ourselves continuously, especially when we are merely following common or routine practices. It's about not jumping to the quick fix. Letting be involves purposefully acting to more fully know what is. So although we may administer pain medication, we also want to know about the nature of the pain—when it is exacerbated, the thoughts, feelings, and worries that are part of the pain experience, and so forth so we can be more targeted in our intervention. Indeed, to follow this example, the act of inquiring and listening to a person describe his or her pain experience can in itself be pain-relieving. To be believed, not judged, and affirmed, and to experience being cared about can alleviate tension and fear and in turn alleviate pain. To develop the skill of letting be, it is helpful to move beyond the dualism of either doing nothing or changing (Hartrick, 2002). When we step out of dualistic thinking, we can begin to see the way in which "purposefully acting by letting be" is one of the most powerful ways in which we promote change. Box 9.2 offers an example of ideas for "letting be" from a patient perspective.

TRY IT OUT 9.3

Responding to Pain

The next time you encounter a person in pain (a patient, a friend with a headache, etc.), before you offer or recommend anything, extend your inquiry. Ask *one more* question than you would normally. Make your question appropriate to the situation, and draw on what you know about pain assessment. What is the pain like? Does it change when you move? Have you found anything that helps? What do you think is going on? What else are you doing to help it? Expand your inquiry by one more question.

BOX 9.2

Be with Me

If you are going to be with me:

1. Please be patient while I decide if I can trust you.
2. Let me tell my story. The whole story, in my own way.
3. Please accept that whatever I have done, whatever I may do, that this is the best I have to offer and seemed right at the time.
4. I am not a person. I am this person, *unique* and special.
5. Don't judge me as right or wrong. Bad or good. I am what I am, and that's all I've got.
6. Don't assume that your knowledge about me is more accurate than mine. You only know what I've told you. That's only part of me.
7. Don't ever think that you know what I should do—you don't. I may be confused, but I am still the expert about me.
8. Don't place me in a position of living up to your expectations. I have enough trouble with my own.
9. Please hear my feelings. Not just my words, and accept all of them. If you can't, how can I?
10. Don't save me! I can do it myself. I knew enough to ask for help, didn't I?

—Anonymous

RI Checkpoint 2.2: Am I Discerning the Specifics?

In relational inquiry, there is no linear laid out sequence or method since *it all depends on the particularities of specific nursing situations*. The same action may be responsive and health-promoting in one case and not in another case. Because the experiences of people and families and meanings of health are so varied, as are the realities within which health care occurs, nursing action needs to be both dynamic and specific. Thus, an important checkpoint is to discern the specifics of a situation to ensure you are focusing both broadly and specifically enough to determine the most significant elements. This checkpoint helps you look specifically at all levels (intrapersonal, interpersonal, and contextual) and consider the challenges, limitations, and possibilities to see even small ways that we can positively affect a situation.

If you think about it, you will probably see that this checkpoint is central to any good clinical decision-making process. Sound clinical decision making is by its nature specific to a particular patient and clinical situation yet broad enough to consider the wider picture. Yet, as we have said earlier, if you watch many nurses do assessment and intervene, they are not necessarily working in that specific way. They may be generalizing, and/or they may not be intentionally attuned to the particularities of the people and/or the specific factors and levels of experience to discern "best" action. For example, think back to Chapter 8 and Kelley, the nurse in the ER who cared for the woman with the asthmatic/anxiety attack. Consider on what the nurses who were rolling their eyes and labeling the woman as "overly dramatic" were basing their clinical decision making. Might they have been using generalized understandings of asthma and normative values of what counts as a valid health concern?

RI Checkpoint 2.3: Am I in Sync?

To be relationally responsive requires us to get in sync with both the situation and the people within that situation. As Newman (1994) articulates in her nursing theory, it also involves being in sync energetically. For example, often getting and being in sync involves paying attention to how you are moving as you work between the energy on the ward on a particular day (which might be frenzied) and an ill patient and anxious family. Do you absorb that frenzied energy, rush into the room to check the IV and rush out quickly? To get in sync and attune to the energy (and anxiety) of the patient or family, you might act by consciously taking a slow, deep calming breath and consciously exhaling the frenzied energy you have absorbed before you enter the patient's room. On the other hand, if you enter a room where people are relating to each other through humor and there is a lot of laughter happening, you might get in sync by joining in the laughter. Yet, if there are other patients in the room who are in need of quiet space, you might need to relate between the two competing elements. As you can see from these descriptions, getting in sync is about attuning and noticing what is happening and joining people and situations in relationally responsive ways.

Often getting in sync involves multilayered attention. For example, it involves attention to moments. As we have said earlier, a particular feature of nursing is that our work is often done on the move. That is, while there may be times when we sit down to talk with a patient or family, most often we relate as we do other things, like give a medication, change a dressing, check an IV or vital signs, take an admission history, and so forth. Thus, as we have described earlier, getting in sync involves paying attention to the possibilities and needs within a particular situation and making those moments count (remember Della's example in Chapter 8 about the impact of brief moments with people with dementia; or remember the example from Kelley committing to connect more fully at triage).

TO ILLUSTRATE

Getting in Sync by Multilayered Attention

Nepo (2005) tells a story of a friend who through aging experienced a gradual loss of hearing. "At first I would notice her straining to pick up pieces of conversation. As she accepted her loss of hearing, as she lived into it more and more . . . She didn't strain anymore." As the author asked her friend about this, she replied, "Yes, I've been forced to go beyond and listen below. One day I just got tired of straining so hard for all the words, and in my exhaustion, I settled on my sister's eyes as she was talking. It was then that I realized there are many things to listen to. When the words fell out of reach, I began to listen to eyes, to bodies, to gestures, to the face behind the face. I began to listen to the warmth coming from another." (Nepo, 2005, p. 260).

RI Checkpoint 2.4: Am I Being in the Complexity and Difficulty?

Because the health care system in the Western world is most often structured according to a service model of care, our attention most often focuses on narrowing our focus to "the problem." Thus it can seem contrary to nursing to *intentionally engage the complexities and be in difficulty*. Paradoxically, being willing to be in complexity and/or difficulty is essential if you are to be an effective nurse. For example, when we see someone upset and try to make them feel better before we really understand the situation and what it means for them specifically, our interventions are unlikely to correspond with their particular needs. Also, the more we try to control the outcome, the less likely people are to respond to our interventions.

Certainly all people need to feel a sense of power and control in their lives, and this need for their own control is heightened during illness or stress. It is only by joining them in their difficulty that you are able to understand what a particular person or family is experiencing and how you can best support them in their choice and power. Being in the difficulty is therefore the most effective way to promote health.

Unfortunately, it is not uncommon for nurses to be working in ways that are opposite to this strategy. For example, many students have told me (Gweneth) about situations in which patients with histories of addiction are not given pain medication when they request it. When the students try to advocate for the patients to receive medication, they are told by the attending nurses that, "You have to be careful and not just liberally give narcotics to people who have addiction issues." What troubles the students, however, is that the attending nurses often make these decrees without any kind of clinical assessment. In many cases, even though there is an order for pain medication, the nurse works from her or his own rule—don't perpetuate addiction. The nurse fails to enter into the complexities of the situation to discern how best to care for the particular person at that point in time.

Similarly, in Chapter 3, we described how a multidisciplinary group of practitioners in an asthma program changed their practices to be more health-promoting. If you reread that description, you will see that being in complexity and difficulty was a significant shift that occurred in their practice. For example, the nurses described that at the beginning of the project, they would go into a family's home as change agents armed with all kinds of information about asthma and launch into giving the information to the family (for the purpose of reducing the asthma "problem"). As they evolved their practice to be more health-promoting, they gradually found themselves asking the family about their asthma experience. They would listen carefully to learn about the complexities the family faced in managing the asthma. In doing so, the nurses could discern the specific target of their actions by looking for significant patterns. A central goal of that asthma program was to reduce the number of hospital admissions. By the end of the first year of the project, the nurses had managed to effect a significant decrease in admissions.

This checkpoint helps you keep people and families at the center of any action. It prompts you to address what matters to them and at the same time identify experiential, social, economic, environmental, and political complexities that are constraining the health of people and families. For example, as the nurses in the asthma program listened to families' experiences of living with asthma, they learned that limited economic resources made it difficult for some families to attend follow-up appointments. A lack of child care and poor accessibility to public transportation got in the way of families being able to access the support and resources the asthma program had to offer. Consequently, instead of trying to fix the families (such as by lecturing them on how important it was to attend the appointments), the nurses began looking for ways to increase the families' access to child care and transportation.

TRY IT OUT 9.4

Find a Complex, Difficult Moment

The next time you are in a clinical context, notice the first complex, difficult moment you encounter. What makes a difficult moment? Notice:

- Who is in sync with whom?
- How are people relating to the difficulty? What emotions arise? What strategies are used?

continued on page 350

TRY IT OUT 9.4 *continued*

Find a Complex, Difficult Moment

- Does anyone jump in to fix the difficulty? If so, is the situation well known first, or would a little more letting be make a difference?
- To what extent is health and well-being being promoted, and for whom?
- What can you learn from this moment?

STRATEGY 3: COLLABORATIVE KNOWING/ NOT KNOWING

By orienting relationally and relating to and with what is, you create space for collaborative knowledge development. A central tenet of the socio-environmental approach to health promotion (and relational inquiry practice) is collaborative working relationships between people/families and health care professionals. In many ways, collaboration has become a buzz word in health care. But what does it really mean to collaborate? As we have lived this question in our practice and worked with other nurses who are also attempting to collaborate, we have observed something interesting. Although many of us desire to be collaborative, our habit of being the one in charge of health care relationships and of health care leads us to take charge. If you listen carefully to nurses and other health care professionals speak and if you study the nursing literature, you will notice that discussions of collaboration are often phrased in such a way that puts the emphasis on *nurses* (e.g., nurses collaborate with families as opposed to families collaborate with nurses).

Although on the surface this distinction may appear to be merely semantics, we think it is quite telling about the power dynamics that dominate nursing practice. Specifically, it is evidence of the nursing habit to assume that care is about what *nurses* do (i.e., it communicates that care is only about nursing action and ignores the work and action of people and families). In truly collaborative relationships, the nurse is not in charge of the process. Rather, collaboration is a mutual process in which people with different forms of knowledge (such as family members and nurses) work together. There is a relation of shared power and decision making.

When you watch a nurse who is in collaborative relation, one of the first things you will notice is the way in which that person is being a knower. As we discussed in Chapter 6, the act of knowing *is* a way of relating. How we relate to knowledge and how we use knowledge shapes the way we relate to people and families, to colleagues, to the larger health care organization, and so forth. As nurses, we are often educated to relate primarily as expert knowers. This typically requires us to assume that we are the ones with knowledge and the ones in control of the knowing process.

Indeed expert knowledge is required, and of course as the nurse, you are the one doing a clinical assessment, exercising clinical judgment, and making clinical decisions about nursing intervention. However, to relate by collaboratively knowing draws attention to *how* you *do* that. That is, it is not a question of *whether* you enlist your expert knowledge, but how, why, when, and what kinds of knowledge you enlist. Recall from Chapter 1 that all knowledge is incomplete, fallible, and subjective. Thus, relational inquiry emphasizes not only knowing, but also not knowing, which in turn prompts inquiring and collaborating. This broad stance enables you to enlist multiple forms of knowledge simultaneously and ensures that your knowledge is as adequate as possible.

Remember the story in Chapter 6 about Mrs. Smith, the woman with undiagnosed congestive heart failure who was admitted to the psychiatric unit with a diagnosis of bipolar illness. That example illustrates the profound importance of collaborative knowing/not knowing. The reality is that as nurses, we are continually working in situations where we do not know what we do not know—and in situations in which other people (e.g., Mrs. Smith) may have knowledge that we need if we are to be as effective as possible. Again, effective nursing involves relating collaboratively as both a knower and an inquirer.

TO ILLUSTRATE
Collaborating in Chronic Illness

A prime example of the importance of collaborative knowing is nursing people with chronic health challenges. Chronic conditions are pervasive. The Centers for Disease Control and Prevention (2012) state that in 2005, 133 million Americans were living with at least one chronic condition. By 2020, that number is expected to grow to 157 million. The incidence of multiple chronic illnesses is also expected to grow from 63 million people to a high of 81 million by 2020. Given the incidence of chronic health challenges in the general population, as a nurse you will care for many people living with some kind of chronic condition. In examining effective chronic illness management, Thille and Russell (2010) highlight the importance of patient involvement and in particular the central role that patients need to play in the care process. Emphasizing collaborative relationships between patients and health care providers as crucial, these researchers conclude that ensuring patient concerns and goals are at the center of any decision making is a critical aspect of ensuring successful health outcomes.

The expert knowledge of health care providers is indisputably crucial. However, people with chronic health challenges manage their conditions on a daily basis and are the most knowledgeable about their own particular illness care. A palliative approach to chronic disease management provides an excellent example to consider collaborative knowing in nursing practice. Della Roberts describes a palliative approach to nursing care in Box 9.3 and offers some powerful illustrations of how she has put collaborative knowing and not knowing into practice. (*Della Roberts is an advanced practice nurse who specializes in the care of people living with life-limiting illness.*)

TO ILLUSTRATE

Della Shares a Story of Knowing/Not Knowing

Al was living in a residential care facility because his dementia had progressed, and his brain function no longer enabled him to feed himself, walk, or express himself in words. His wife, Ella, had come to the facility daily to be with him and give him his lunch and dinner ever since Al had been admitted. Al died during his sleep one night. When the nurse called her, Ella was very upset and expressed surprise that Al possibly could have died, saying, "If something as important as dying was likely, why didn't anyone tell me?" Although Ella had visited every day, she had not seen that Al was dying. Had the nurses? Or were they waiting until they saw death clearly on the horizon? If those nurses had been asked, "Would you be surprised if Al died in the next six months?" they would likely have said no, they would not be surprised. The framework of viewing palliative care as something that begins when death is clearly visible was not serving the nurses, Al, or his wife.

When I and my colleague Gina Gaspard tell this story and nurses have time to reflect, they quickly identify that almost all people moving into residential care need palliative dimensions of care from the time they are admitted. With similar stories, nurses on medical units can see that many patients they are caring for need the dimensions of a palliative approach during their hospitalization.

A palliative approach offers a wonderful example of collaborative knowing/not knowing. At the core of a palliative approach is the recognition of the uncertainty of the illness situation. It is in fact the uncertainty that makes the palliative approach so vital and that serves as the guide for action. For example, while as an advanced practice nurse Della brings a wealth of knowledge to her work with people and families living with life-limiting illnesses, the way she enacts care is to collaborate with them to determine the care they want. She begins her conversation with people and families by acknowledging the uncertainty of the situation. By opening the collaborative space to consider the uncertainty and simultaneously make some care decisions (e.g., about palliative dimensions of care such as pain control, symptom management, advanced directives), Della is able to promote patient/family well-being and ultimately good end-of-life experiences.

In Box 9.4, Della provides specific ways to collaborate with patients and families by taking a palliative approach.

BOX 9.3

Developing a Palliative Approach to Nursing Care

When asked, most nurses can easily describe the palliative dimensions of care, but when should these dimensions begin to be woven into the nursing care of a person living with life-limiting illness? In acute care, residential care, and home care settings, nurses care for many people living with one or more chronic, life-limiting illnesses such as COPD, congestive heart failure, renal failure, and dementia. These diseases are progressive and known to shorten the lifespan. However, in contrast to people with many forms of cancer for whom there may be a clear trajectory and anticipated time frame until death, people living with chronic progressive diseases often lack a clear prognosis and estimated remaining lifespan. Many people with advanced disease or frailty will have a sudden change in their condition related to a flu or exacerbation of their underlying disease and die in a matter of days. This deprives caregivers of the opportunity to find out what is important to that individual so that care is aligned with their wishes. As importantly, suffering from symptoms such as shortness of breath or pain may not be relieved by medications such as opioids if care focuses only on optimizing disease management therapies.

In contrast, the *palliative approach* is emerging. A palliative approach is an integrated approach that addresses patients' quality of life alongside all the other aspects of care. This approach is gaining recognition as vitally important for people living with chronic illnesses that will limit their lifespans. In countries such as Canada and the United States, where the palliative designation has traditionally been reserved for cases in which patients were determined to have only a few months to live, a palliative approach is gaining increasing acceptance for those with chronic diseases. Supported by the work of the Gold Standards Framework (2011) in the United Kingdom, the Australian Government National Health and Medical Research Council (2006), and iPANEL (2013) in Canada, health care providers who take a palliative approach do not wait until a certain death signal to initiate palliative care. From the time of diagnosis, regardless of whether the person is expected to live 10 days or 10 years, these providers work to ensure that the person and their family collaborate in the care planning and receive the care they need to live as meaningful a life as possible. The palliative approach also ensures that providers, patients, and families have conversations about critical end-of-life issues that would otherwise only have been prompted by news of impending death. (*Della Roberts*).

BOX 9.4

Questions to Ask during Admission into Care

In any setting, consider the following questions:
Is there anything about you or your family member that is important for us to know and be aware of while we care for you?

If you would not be surprised if the person were to die in the next few months:
Can you tell me what you understand about your illness and what you expect over the next months? What hopes and fears do you have about what may come?

When caring for a patient who is frail and whose family is visiting:
What changes have you been noticing in your mother?

Exploring a person's wishes and/or goals:
Can you tell me what is most important to you and makes your days meaningful?

During a conversation when the person has acknowledged that they have a limited time to live:
Can you share with me what is important for you now?

Speaking to someone whose family member can no longer speak for him or herself:
What would your father/mother/partner want if s/he could tell us?

Assessing comfort:
Are you uncomfortable or in pain in any way? Is there anything affecting your ability to be comfortable? Is there anything about which you are anxious or worried?

The following four inquiry checkpoints support this kind of collaborative knowing/not knowing.

RI Checkpoint 3.1: Am I Following the Lead?

Central to the collaborative knowing/not knowing process is following the lead of people and families. Again, they are the experts in their own lives, and it is they who collaborate with us. Thus, as nurses, we must mindfully look and listen to what is of significance to them. Following the lead supports assessment as an inquiry process. As you follow the lead and inquire into a patient or family's living experience and what is of meaning and significance to them, you also focus on picking up on cues (e.g., you notice the person's appearance, facial affect, etc.). Following the lead might also involve sharing your observations in a tentative manner: "I've noticed your skin looks red," or "You seem quiet today" invites people to confirm, expand, or modify those observations. Making inclusive observations, asking open-ended questions, and being interested to know more invites people to lead the way. By approaching assessment in this way, we are able to gain a much fuller understanding of people and families in *their living experiences*. We are also able to identify aspects that we might otherwise miss in our assessment.

To be able to follow the lead, you need to let go of the habit of immediately moving to diagnosing "the problem" and allow people to tell you about their experience. For example, recently I (Colleen) watched a nurse responding to a group of women who had just learned that a woman they knew from the street community had committed suicide by jumping from her apartment window. The women had experienced many personal losses, and there had been many deaths in the community in the previous months. The nurse seemed overwhelmed and said to the women, "Oh, this must be so awful for you! I don't know how you do it. It must be terrible every day!" The women stopped talking and remained very quiet for most of the remaining time. After the group, one woman told me that she felt "othered" by the nurse's response; that is, she felt that it was impossible to express what she really felt (which, in her case, was greater determination to survive her own mental health challenges).

Look back at Box 9.4 to see how Della's questions exemplify following the lead. In many ways, following the lead involves what Flanagan (1996) describes as being a "confident unconfident" (p. 207). As nurses, we are confident in the questions and in our ability to collaborate with people and families and with colleagues to ensure we are as knowledgeable as possible. At the same time, because the way we use our expert knowledge can serve to lessen our sensitivity to people, checking if we are following their lead directs us to be less confident in what we *think* we know.

As an inquiry, assessment proceeds in a focused yet open manner. We begin our assessment by inquiring into what is meaningful and significant to a person, family, group, or community. This enables you to open up the collaborative space for people to include anything relevant and important and at the same time hone in on the most salient aspects of the situation. The inquiry is both interpretive and critical and involves a process of focused exploration into the current health and healing experiences of people and families. For example, in the women's group, another nurse circled back to the situation after a while and asked, "What has it been like for you to hear about the woman's death? I imagine there is quite a range of feelings right now." The women brought up varied responses—certainly grief, but also anger, particularly at the lack of help the woman had received and fear that perhaps it was not a suicide (a couple of months previously a woman had been pushed from a window, but her death initially had been reported as a suicide).

Assessment from this inquiry stance refuses theoretical closure and does not allow theoretical categorizations to dominate. This does not mean that we don't bring our nursing knowledge and have our own nursing concerns. Rather, we are sensitized by the insight our HP and critical lenses offer us as well as the knowledge and research from nursing, biomedicine, and so on. For example, in the next To Illustrate box, Rachelle Lautischer, a nurse who works in maternal/child care, describes a simple adjustment she has made to her practice as she has developed her relational inquiry assessment approach.

TO ILLUSTRATE

Assessing in Maternity

When a patient comes in to have her baby, if she is a smoker, overweight, gestational diabetic, gestational hypertensive, and/or over 35 years old, she is labeled a "higher-risk" patient. Subsequently, her care is determined accordingly and based on disease management, not on what the patient and her family deems significant or meaningful. I concede that I have been guilty of abiding to this practice approach because it is to the point and is also what is expected. However, I now recognize that even though this may meet all of my patient's physical needs, it overlooks what really matters to the patient and family. So now that I understand the powers that live within *me*, I deliberately ask my patients and families what matters to them during their labor and delivery experience—which family member they would like to have present in the room during the birth of their child and other things that might be important to them.

In conducting assessment as an inquiry process, nurses *follow the lead of people and families* and resist "jumping in" with responses. For example, when you learn someone is pregnant, you might be tempted to immediately say something such as, "You must be so excited!" Instead, leave room for the person or family to lead. Try focusing on "what is" in terms of their current living experience, for example, "Wow, that is life-changing news." While many may express joy, excitement, and pleasure, you will create space for ambivalence, fear, uncertainty, and all sorts of other responses.

Some statements and questions you might use to begin inquiring into health and healing experiences include:

- I am interested in how you have been.
- Could you tell me a bit about what has been happening for you?
- What stands out as you think about things in your day-to-day life?
- What stands out to you as really important for me to know about your situation? What has been okay, and what has been challenging?
- What has changed as a result of (your situation or health challenge)?

Following the lead is supported by a *listening attitude*—by *actively listening, respecting,* and *trusting* in people's own knowledge and capacity to discern what is significant to them. It is also supported through genuine concern and empathy for their right to live in ways that are meaningful to them, even if that at times is contrary to the latest research evidence that informs good health practices. As you follow the lead, you can simultaneously use another inquiry checkpoint we refer to as "listening to and for."

RI Checkpoint 3.2: Am I Listening to and for?

> When we are listened to, it creates us, makes us unfold and expand. Ideas actually begin to grow within us and come to life. You know if a person laughs at your jokes you become funnier and funnier, and if he does not, every tiny little joke in you weakens up and dies. Well, that is the principle of it. It makes people happy and free when they are listened to. And, if you are a listener, it is the secret of having a good time in society (because everybody around you becomes lively and interesting), of comforting people, of doing them good. (Ueland, 1992, p. 104)

For many nurses, listening is considered to be a rather passive process, something to be done "pre-action." For example, nurses often listen with one ear while they are busy thinking about what they want to say or do in response. But there is a vast difference between waiting to speak or waiting to act and truly listening. The checkpoint "Am I listening to and for?" draws attention to your listening action—to *how* you are listening.

TRY IT OUT 9.5
Waiting to Listen

The next time you are in conversation—a minute from now, an hour from now, tomorrow—monitor your own listening habits. See if you can catch yourself waiting to speak. See if you can force yourself to stop and *listen* more actively. First, count the number of seconds you allow between when one person finishes speaking and you begin. Then, try to double your pause time and see what happens.

Listening to and for is both a knowledge-generating process and an intervention. It offers an opportunity for people to understand and make sense of their illness experiences, identify specific concerns and what really matters to them, affirm the choices they are making, and/or consider options in light of their beliefs, customs, and their health and healing experiences. This type of listening might indeed be the most effective nursing intervention during a particular situation. As Rogers (1961) contends, when it comes to promoting well-being, listening is a powerful action in and of itself. Ueland (1992) describes listening as a magnetic force that can provide an opportunity for re-creation and discovery.

Although we tend to think of listening as something we do with our ears, to truly listen requires enlistment of all of our senses. We come to know people, families, and colleagues not just from what they say, but from what they communicate energetically, bodily, contextually, and so forth. We also come to know them through what they don't say. When we do a physical assessment, we are listening. For example, palpating someone's abdomen is a form of listening, as is assessing chest sounds, checking reflexes, finding a vein to start an IV, and so forth. Therefore, listening requires attuning all of our senses (not just our ears) and opening the relational space to hear what it is that is being communicated in multiple ways and at multiple levels. The poem in Box 9.5 is a helpful reminder of how important it is to listen.

As we noted in Chapter 7, the way you theorize nursing practice profoundly shapes how you proceed in action—including how you listen. As you connect with a person or family, your own particular theoretical perspective will prompt you to listen to and for particular things. And as your

---

BOX 9.5

Listen

When I ask you to listen to me
and you start giving me advice
you have not done what I asked.
When I ask you to listen to me
and you begin to tell me why I shouldn't feel that way,
you are trampling on my feelings.
When I ask you to listen to me
and you feel you have to do something to solve my problem,
you have failed me, strange as that may seem.
Listen! All I ask, is that you listen,
not talk or do—just hear me.
Advice is cheap—10 cents will get you both Dear Abby
and Billy Graham in the same newspaper.
And I can do that for myself; I'm not helpless.
Maybe discouraged and faltering, but not helpless.
When you do something for me that I can and need to do
for myself, you contribute to my fear and weakness.
But, when you accept as a simple fact that I do feel what I feel,
no matter how irrational,
then I can quit trying to convince you
and can get about the business of understanding what's behind
this irrational feeling.
And when that's clear, the answers are obvious
and I don't need advice.
Irrational feelings make sense when we understand
Perhaps that's why prayer works, sometimes, for some people,
because God is mute and he doesn't give advice or try to fix things.
"They" just listen and let you work it out for yourself.
So, please listen and just hear me.
And, if you want to talk, wait a minute for your turn;
and I'll listen to you.—*Anonymous*

theory shifts or changes, so does what you listen for. This is why it is vital that you are as consciously aware as possible of the theories that are guiding you—so that you can intentionally choose which ones will inform your work with particular people and families. This also emphasizes how important it is to be continually reading, studying, and updating your research and theoretical knowledge. As we have continued to read and conduct research to inform our practice, our theoretical perspectives have evolved substantially. For example, working with Gweneth, I (Colleen) have learned to intentionally listen for capacity. Similarly, in working with Colleen, I (Gweneth) have learned to pay much closer attention to the politics of practice. As we have evolved our theories, what we listen to and for as we go about our work has been extended.

Although listening is certainly integral to any nursing practice, we have found that listening for particular things can enhance our ability to promote health and healing. It is a concrete way of focusing attention both widely and specifically. The lenses described in Chapter 2, the ways of knowing and modes of inquiry in Chapter 6, and the theories described in Chapter 7 highlight particularly important aspects to listen *for*. That is, they offer some road signs for us to look and listen to and for. Below, we offer many suggestions for listening to and for. This list does not constitute a prescription, since in relational inquiry practice, people and families lead the way. Nevertheless, using the different lenses and modes of inquiry can help expand your ability to hear what might be meaningful and significant to people's experiences. The lenses help sensitize us to what *might* be important. This sensitivity can help people, families, and nurses recognize and articulate their health and healing experiences and the challenges they are living as they attempt to exercise their power and choice in order to live a meaningful life. Each lens overlaps with the others, each offering a particular angle on what to listen to and for.

Listening to and for with the HP Lens
An HP lens focuses our attention on living experience. As such, it directs us to listen in the following ways.

Listen for Who This Person or Family Is
Cameron (1992) describes attention as an act of connection. Paying attention to "right now" in this moment.

Listen for Living Experience
What is being communicated energetically? Bodily? Verbally? Contextually?

Listen for What Is Particularly Significant within People's/Families' Experiences
For example, it is helpful to pay attention to what people highlight in their story, what seems to be at the center of what they are talking about, and/or what they keep going back to or repeat as they talk. Our colleague, Karen Mahoney, has pointed out that sometimes what is most significant for people is to not be known; they prefer to remain anonymous or keep many aspects of their lives private. Recently, I (Colleen) interviewed a man for a research study. He wanted to take part in the survey in a study that is aiming to improve primary health care for people marginalized by poverty and other forms of social disadvantage but did not want to tell me his name or

share many aspects of his history. He had been incarcerated in a psychiatric prison and was fearful people would learn about his history. I learned that what was of greatest significance to him was keeping many details of his life private. That is, I could be most responsive by *not* asking probing questions. Our team was able to help him participate while respecting his privacy by giving a code number to a staff member who did know his identity.

Listen for Meaning and What Is of Particular Concern

As you listen, you might pay attention to the "so what." What does all of this mean for them? This involves listening to the details and facts of their stories and descriptions and moving to inquire into what all of those facts and details mean in their lives. What impacts do the things they are describing have on their lives? What specifically and concretely is concerning them in their everyday lives?

Listening for meaning involves listening beyond the surface to pick up cues. For example, sometimes what is of particular concern may not be readily obvious even to the person or family. By inquiring into their experiences and listening carefully, people have the opportunity not only to articulate their experiences but also to gain insight into their situations. For example, years ago, I (Gweneth) was speaking with a man who was recovering from a myocardial infarction. In asking him how he was feeling about things, he commented that he was really going to miss eating French fries ("chips" to some of you!). On the surface, this may seem like a fairly inconsequential thing; however, exploring further, we both came to realize that the French fries symbolized the loss of life as he knew it. As he talked, we both became aware of how he was feeling overwhelmed and powerless in his situation—powerless to the point that he couldn't even choose what food he wanted to eat. That understanding provided the avenue for him to reclaim his power; it opened the door for him to consider what choices he did still have. This example highlights how listening for significance and concern can enhance overall understanding of the health and healing experience. Questions you might consider include:

- What is it like for you?
- What is particularly important, difficult, and/or challenging about what is happening?
- What would you really like to be able to do, change, or address?

Listen for What Is Not Said

Using your nursing knowledge, you can listen for things that people may not be saying yet seem relevant given other things that they have said, what you yourself have noticed, what research has identified as salient, and so forth. Sometimes, people have difficulty naming all of their experiences; they may not have found the "right" words or they may feel it isn't acceptable to feel the way they do. In such cases, it can be helpful to have someone else—a nurse—raise a topic or inquire about a concern. For example, research by Kelli Stajduhar and her colleagues (Stajduhar, 2003; Stajduhar, Funk, Cohen, et al., 2011; Stajduhar, Funk, Roberts, et al., 2011; Stajduhar, Nickel, Martin, & Funk, 2008) on family caregivers (see Chapter 4) informs us that not all families are prepared and/or want to provide care for family members in their homes. If in listening for the families' experience this seems relevant, you could offer that knowledge and inquire into their experience. For example, you could say something like, "Families often get the feeling from health care professionals and others that they should be looking after their ill family members at home, yet for many families that is difficult to do, or they find it is not the best option. What is your experience?"

Listening to and for with the Critical Lens
A critical lens focuses our attention on sociocontextual structures and processes that may be shaping the experiences of people and families. As such, it complements the HP lens, directing us to listen in the following ways.

Listen for How Societal Norms Are Shaping Experience and Choice
Listen for what is being taken for granted; once again, this means listening for what is *not* being said as well as what is being said. Listen for how people are trying to live up to social expectations and dominant norms and how they are resisting these. For example, when you are working with mothers, listen for how discourses about "good mothers" might be exerting an influence. Similarly, as an ER nurse, I (Gweneth) would listen for how societal norms might be shaping the way people presented themselves—how was the "macho" male image affecting how a particular patient describes his level of his pain?

Listen for Dominant Narratives and How People May Be Conforming
People may conform to what they anticipate your expectations are or to what they might think is expected of the role of patient, mother, diabetic, and so on. What stories are people telling, and what are the underlying meanings? How are dominant health care narratives playing out in particular situations? For example, I (Colleen) notice that women who have experienced intimate partner violence speak about having "low self-esteem" as an explanation for why they were vulnerable to this. The idea of low self-esteem may be helpful to women in thinking about their own role in their vulnerability to violence, but this narrative can become dominant to the point that it obscures the role of others (e.g., the perpetrator of the violence), can function as a form of victim-blaming, and/or can disempower or make the person feel hopeless. How are you (and they) embracing taken-for-granted ideas such as the idea of a "good" patient? How do you reinforce these ideas and reward certain behaviors and punish others?

Listen for How Sociocontextual Elements Are Constraining and/or Promoting Choices and Power
Listen for how economics, policies, values, norms, traditions, history, sexism, racism, ageism, and so on are shaping situations and experiences. Discrimination based on these social categories occurs within families as well as within wider social contexts. Listen for how different values and various forms of discrimination are played out within and among people. What are the common forms of stigma in your area of practice, and how are they stratified by social categories?

Listen to Who Is Speaking and for Whom They Are Speaking

Paying attention to who is speaking "for whom" provides insight into the power dynamics within a situation. It also provides direction for nurses on how to proceed. Begin by attending to this along the multiple lines of power inequities such as age (e.g., parents speaking for children, adult children speaking for older persons), gender (e.g., men speaking for women), ability (e.g., others speaking for a person with cognitive impairment or hearing impairment), and so on.

Listening to and for with a Socio-Environmental Orientation

In concert with the above lenses, a socio-environmental health-promoting orientation focuses our attention on listening for capacity in people and their life situations. The *Oxford Dictionary* (1982) defines capacity as "the power of containing, receiving, experiencing, or producing . . . [capacity includes] mental power, faculty, talent, position, character" (p. 136). These descriptors are reflective of what we have come to know about people/families. We have often found ourselves in awe at the strength of the human spirit and the capacity that people have within themselves. We have witnessed people experiencing life challenges such as chronic, life-threatening, or terminal illness; poverty; isolation; prejudice; and trauma. We have seen them draw upon their inner power and faculties to live through those life-challenging experiences. Moreover, we have seen many people and families produce positive personal and social results out of adverse circumstances and experiences.

Although often people's capacity goes unnamed or unrecognized, we have yet to meet anyone who does not have capacity and more potential capacity. Interestingly, it is during times and conditions of adversity that capacity is particularly evident. Yet, it is those times of adversity when capacity is most often overlooked or not recognized. The tendency to focus on the adversity or problem and on servicing or fixing what is lacking overrides both patients' and nurses' ability to see the resourcefulness and capacity patients have to affect their own life situations.

TO ILLUSTRATE
No Crib for a Bed

During a discussion of health-promoting family nursing practice that I (Gweneth) had with a group of public health nurses, one nurse described her experience with a family that included a teenage mother and father and a new baby. Until the time of the birth, the parents had been living on the street. Upon discharge, the public health nurse was notified that this was a "high-risk" family that needed careful following. The public health nurse had made a home visit and described to us what she found when she arrived. The family had just moved into a "very run-down apartment" that had no furniture and few household items. The parents had rigged up a bed for the baby by converting an old solid-looking box into a crib. When I asked

continued on page 363

TO ILLUSTRATE *continued*

No Crib for a Bed

how she had found the parents and the baby, the nurse replied that the baby was in a sleeper that was old and torn but seemed to be well nourished and healthy. The parents seemed "quite attached and interested" in the baby.

What I found interesting was the varying responses of those of us listening to this nurse's story. Some of the nurses listening expressed great concern about the safety of the baby "without a crib to sleep in." Others talked about the teaching the parents would need if they were to be able to meet the needs of the baby. Finally, one of the more senior nurses in the group replied, "I think their resourcefulness is remarkable." Her comment helped turn the conversation to consideration of the capacity of these two young parents. We discussed the obvious commitment they must have to their baby and the resourcefulness they had to be able to go from living on the street to moving into an apartment. We also found ourselves marveling at how in the course of a few weeks, they had not only become parents but had also changed their entire life structure. As we began identifying the capacity we saw, the nurse who had made the home visit commented that on top of that, they had seemed relaxed and happy when she was there— more so than many mothers she visits who are living in comfortable homes and who have economic resources and extended family support.

The story, "No Crib for a Bed" is an important reminder of how easy it is to not look beyond the surface of things. On the surface, these parents may not seem to measure up to parents who have more economic resources. Yet, when you consider what they were willing to do and had actually done with such limited resources, it is clear that they have as much or more capacity than many families who have all of the surface fixtures that are sometimes taken for granted as necessary for a new baby. For example, a crib is often a taken-for-granted necessity for a baby, and in fact, the public health nurses pointed out that ensuring there was a good crib for the baby was a routine part of their well-baby assessment. Without stopping and really thinking about it, a nurse could have easily added "no crib" to the high-risk score. However, according to the nurse, the box was safe and secure and served the purpose well. Thus, from a vantage point of capacity, the box is evidence of the parents' thoughtfulness about the baby's safety and their resourcefulness in providing for the baby. This highlights how easy it is to fall into negative judgments based on preconceived taken-for-granteds and how crucial it is to consciously and intentionally question those taken-for-granteds. In addition, this example highlights that *if we want to find capacity in people and families, we have to look for it and recognize it when we see it.*

Listen with Unconditional Positive Regard

Rogers (1961) maintains that the primary ingredient of any relational connection is unconditional positive regard. Unconditional positive regard involves accepting people as being of unconditional worth and creating an atmosphere in which judgments (e.g., about good, bad, right, or wrong) and expectations do not dominate. Unconditional positive regard requires that we let go of our own preconceived and selective interests and relate to the person before us as a being of worth and dignity.

Listen for Patterns of Capacity

What inner resources do people and families have? Upon what other resources are they drawing? What resources do they have that they might not be seeing? What collaborative resources do you have between you? What external resources might enhance their existing capacities?

Listen for Capacity-Adversity Patterns

What challenges are facing this person or family? How are sociohistorical aspects (such as those that arise with race, economics, and gender) intersecting and intensifying their adverse situation? What has enabled them to live in this adversity; that is, what capacities have they accessed or enlisted as they live with the challenge of this adversity? How are they taking up certain practices within their situation?

TRY IT OUT 9.6

Listening Using Multiple Modes of Inquiry

Each of the modes of inquiry outlined in Chapter 6 (empirical, aesthetic, ethical, and sociopolitical) can be enlisted to enhance your listening. Take one listening area above (e.g., what is not being said, patterns of capacity, ways of conforming, etc.), and jot down how each mode might turn your attention to some specific aspect. Have a particular patient or family in mind.

For example, if you had in mind a pregnant woman who has an abusive partner and chose "Listen for capacity-adversity patterns," what would empirical inquiry suggest? Research has shown that patterns of abuse in pregnancy vary including initiation, escalation, and de-escalation of abuse (Daoud et al., 2012; Devries et al., 2010; Mitra, Manning, & Lu, 2012). Knowing that, you might listen for such patterns in her experience. What would aesthetic inquiry invite you to listen for? How is the woman trying to make her pregnancy experience positive and hopeful within her circumstances? What of ethical inquiry? What values are strengthening the woman? Is her commitment to family helping her to survive? What does sociopolitical inquiry surface? How does this woman's access to material resources shape her possibilities for leaving her partner?

RI Checkpoint 3.3: Am I Looking beyond the Surface?

Throughout the preceding chapters, we have offered examples that illustrate how unexamined assumptions and normative practices can override responsive action. Thus, a key inquiry checkpoint is that of looking beyond the surface to question taken-for-granted knowledge and habits. This is not just a matter of questioning your own habits of thought and practice but also of looking and questioning beyond the surface with people, families, colleagues, and the structures organizing your practice.

Looking beyond the surface begins with the action of *seeing relations*. Looking at people and families and trying to imagine the contexts of their lives *beyond the health care encounter* is a first step. When you next encounter a person or family, try looking over their shoulders to imagine what might have contributed to the situation. Similarly, check your own proximity. Are immediate concerns obscuring longer term concerns? For example, if you are working in pediatrics and are concerned that a child is being abused, does your immediate impulse to rescue the child obscure the fact that the child will always be in relation to the parent? Is the proximal (those factors that are in front of you) obscuring the distal view? Suspecting child maltreatment, do you jump to the conclusion that it is a particular person who is responsible? Are similarities obscuring difference; are differences obscuring similarities? Are you, for example, more likely to be suspicious of child abuse with people who are considerably more impoverished than you?

TO ILLUSTRATE

Looking beyond the Surface to See Red

Red was born in a rural Canadian community in 1954. As an Aboriginal child, she was sent to the Mission, a residential school, at age 6 years, where she remained until she was 12 years old and then off and on until she was 17 years old. She described her life and experience of family as one of continuous rejection, not only because of being removed from her mother's care, but also because of how her mother and grandmother (who had both been in residential school) treated her.

> *My mom would come and get my other brothers and sisters and leave me, and she did it twice. The first time . . . she said she didn't have enough money, and kids came back and said she had lots of money. Another time she said she had no room, and they came back and said she had lots of room. And then when I was 12, she took me, and she said the only reason she took me was to babysit . . . They used to drink a lot and [my mom] was always kicking me out.*

---

continued on page 366

TO ILLUSTRATE *continued*

Looking beyond the Surface to See Red

Red was released from residential school at age 17. Having neither access to further education nor employable skills, and unable to live with her mother, she lived with a series of men. One of her longest relationships was with a man named Edward.

> *I ended up pregnant. I told him and he told me, "Pack your stuff, you're going back to town." He dumped me off and said, "Go have an abortion." And he left me there. And I don't know how I got back, but I went back there, and he said, "As soon as that baby is born, you're giving it up for adoption."*

She had several children, all of whom were either given up for adoption or apprehended by the state and placed in foster care. Although she did not raise her children and doesn't have much contact with them, they remain a primary focus of Red's conversation. Red has always been very poor and as a young woman spent time living on the street.

> *A lot of times we would just go to the dumpsters, you know, and dig around in there for, um, whatever. You know, bread, sometimes they'd throw bread out that was still in bags. Throw out fruit and all kinds of stuff you could just find in there. And other times . . . I went to a few people's places, you know, and they might give me something to eat. But . . . that's pretty much how I lived, you know, and in the end I started living with these two guys. They had a one-bedroom apartment . . . most of the time, we all three of us slept . . . in the living room, because a lot of times if you have a hangover, you're really depressed and so we would just watch TV. That was a spot where everybody came to drink and bring booze or Lysol . . .*

Today she has quit drinking, is struggling to get herself "healthy," and hopes to have more contact with her children someday:

> *I thought, you know, I should write [my son] a letter for his birthday. I thought, no, not until I'm [pause] really to the point, you know, where more rejection isn't going to hurt me. I'm going to get myself healthy. Yeah. And then I might try and find my [pause] daughter.*

As a nurse, you may have cared for Red when she was a pregnant teen, when she was giving birth to one of her children, or when she came to emergency, perhaps with an injury from abuse by her partner. More recently, you might have met Red as a family member when her older sister was admitted to psychiatry following a suicide attempt or when her mother was dying. In those encounters, you might not have inquired in such a way as to learn the above story. Yet, her sociohistorical context is integral to who she is today and how you might best respond to promote her health and healing.

Take a minute and think about Red's story. What stands out for you about that story? What seems to be of concern and significance to Red?

What is the meaning of family to her? What historical, political, economic, and social conditions shaped the experience of Red's family? How are these conditions shaping what is of concern and significance to Red?

To understand Red and her family beyond the surface, they must be understood against the background of colonialism and racism (using a critical lens). However, such understanding must be developed thoughtfully and cautiously, because as we described in Chapter 4, understanding people in their cultural contexts can be a double-edged sword (Razack, 1998). In seeking to understand people's oppression, sometimes people are painted only as victims (and their strengths overlooked), or worse, painted as somehow inferior and responsible for their social circumstances. The history of Aboriginal people in Canada, the background to Red's life, is one of the clearest examples of how people and families are shaped by social, political, and economic contexts. In concert with policies and practices that stripped Aboriginal people of their lands and means of survival, the place where Red grew up was home to one of the most notorious residential schools in Canada, St. Joseph's Mission (Furniss, 1995, 1999). The state's intended project was the assimilation of Aboriginal people into white society. A premise central to this project was that "Aboriginal children would have to be removed for a lengthy period from the 'destructive' influences of their families and communities" (Furniss, 1999, p. 42). For six decades, from 1891 to the 1960s, children of the Secwepemc, Southern Carrier, and Tsilhqot'in people were sent to the Mission, where they were allowed little or no contact with their families and were "subjected to a strict regime of discipline in which public humiliation, beatings and physical punishments were used to maintain their submission" (Furniss, 1999, p. 43). Today, the Aboriginal people of that area often speak of themselves as survivors of generations of residential school as they strive to heal the destruction of family ties, loss of culture and language, loss of parenting skills, and destruction of sense of self that is their legacy.

Red and her family are some of those survivors. Red was not the first generation of Aboriginal children taken by the state. Rather, her mother, her grandmother, and children of earlier generations were taken from their families. These practices wrecked family ties, and entire communities of children grew up in successive generations not knowing their parents, their language, or their customs. Furthermore, the children were subjected to abuse and were taught that they were inferior. These practices were implemented along with other Indian Act policies that forced Aboriginal people into economic dependence and confined them to reservations without means of economic support other than state dependence. Despite the people's amazing strength, resilience, and efforts to heal, the despair and destruction wrought continues to pervade many communities. With this background in mind, Red's mother's "rejection" of her can be seen not as bad mothering but as a direct consequence of state practices over many generations. In turn, Red's loss of her children to the state can be seen as a continuation of state practices in relation to Aboriginal people, and at least in part as a failure of the state to take measures to attempt to remedy generations of abuse. Indeed, it is only recently that lawsuits by Aboriginal people in Canada have drawn attention to these abuses and resulted in some attempts to implement measures such as treatment programs for residential school survivors. Still, despite years of bargaining, few treaty negotiations have been concluded in Canada, with the result that the enforced poverty and dependence of Aboriginal people continues. Had such remedies and treaties been in place, might Red have raised her own children?

For Aboriginal people in Canada, racism is a daily feature of life. In my work on a project in the rural area where Red grew up, I (Colleen) have been overwhelmed by the extent to which the Aboriginal people have been taught that they are inadequate, dysfunctional, and inferior and how deeply these messages have been absorbed. One woman, Rita (a well-educated, accomplished woman) said to me, "When you are told by your family that you are a drunken Indian, that you will never be anything but a drunken Indian . . . then, you are unlikely to be anything but a drunken Indian." Against the backdrop of widespread racism, enforced poverty, and her family's history, Red's life on the street and struggle with alcohol are more comprehensible. And her capacity—her effort to get healthy, to quit drinking, to hope for contact with her children—seems remarkable. As you consider Red's story, you can begin to see the importance of questioning beyond the surface. What questions might have helped you bring the relation of Red's life to larger social structures into view?

In summary, ask below the surface questions. Using the lenses and perspectives that we offered in earlier chapters, ask about gender, race, class, history, and other factors available through sociopolitical inquiry. Although we have emphasized the sociopolitical aspect in our examples, it is also important to look below the surface using ethical and aesthetic and empirical inquiry. Finally, ask what language and assumptions support any given understanding, action, decision, policy, practice, or problem.

RI Checkpoint 3.4: Am I Enlisting Multiple Forms of Knowledge?

Another checkpoint to support your collaborative knowing/not knowing process is to check that you are enlisting the multiple forms of knowledge we described in Chapter 6. Are you intentionally enlisting empirical, ethical, aesthetic, and sociopolitical knowledge? This checkpoint helps you focus on judicious use of generalizable evidence (population, qualitative, quantitative) and to consider what knowledge is needed for informed decision making. For example, think back to Red's story and imagine you are caring for her on a medical unit when she is admitted with liver failure. You will be presented with a wealth of biologic data. What other knowledge will be required, and how can you enlist it?

RI Checkpoint 3.5: Am I Willing to Backtrack?

A final checkpoint for collaborative knowing/not knowing is to ask yourself what you do when you are wrong. That is, when you recognize that you have jumped to conclusions too fast, have not checked your assumptions, have found out that your assumption is wrong, or have missed an important piece of information, what do you do? This is a vital question in nursing practice. We all make mistakes, make incorrect assumptions, and leap to conclusions. However, it is what we do in those moments that distinguishes good nursing, in both the sense of morally good and competent. Being willing to take a stance of not knowing sets you up not to feel you need to claim certainty when you are uncertain or to claim to know prematurely. Following on that stance, being willing to backtrack— to be uncertain, to check your assumptions and conclusions, and to revise your understanding—is central to sound knowledge development.

STRATEGY 4: RECOGNIZING AND RESPONDING TO PATTERNS

Effective action in nursing is focused toward recognizing and responding to patterns. The strategies we have described to this point work in concert to (a) support the discernment of salient patterns playing out in any situation and (b) respond effectively with targeted action. Pattern recognition includes identifying significant patterns of experience, sociopolitical patterns, patterns of response, patterns of capacity, patterns of adversity, patterns of health care practice, and so forth. For example, as described earlier in the story of nurses working in the asthma program, by following the lead and listening for what was meaningful and significant to the families living with asthma, the nurses were able to hear a pattern of inequity of resources. Rather than assuming the families were just not bothering to show up for appointments and becoming frustrated, they learned that socioeconomic limitations hindered access to the asthma program for some families.

Thus, *seeing connections* is an action one can employ to recognize and respond to patterns. Seeing connections involves looking to see how one aspect of the experience might be connected to another and how these relations might be creating and/or sustaining barriers to health.

Noticing discrepancies is a second action that flows from seeing connections. Being alert to discrepancies between what you are hearing or seeing on the surface and what might lie beyond is supported by enlisting the HP and critical lenses. If something does not ring true or seem right, if something feels uncomfortable to you or does not seem to add up, follow that lead and ask questions to figure out if the discrepancy is relevant.

Noticing simplifications is a third action that is integral to the strategy of recognizing and responding to patterns and involves paying attention to signals that something is being glossed over. For example, when someone identifies personality problems or communication problems, we are often alerted to look more carefully—to see what other factors might be at play.

By working collaboratively, patients and nurses can make connections between experiences and discern the implications for action. In recognizing the patterns, it is important to understand how those patterns are meaningfully experienced by the person or family. For example, in the context of family caregiving, one woman may cherish the caregiving role while another might resent it. Either woman might both cherish and resent it, or some family members may feel it is the woman's duty, and she may or may not see it that way herself. Della Roberts offers another end-of-life story to illustrate the pattern recognition process and its importance.

TO ILLUSTRATE
Seeing the Pattern

I was speaking with a friend, Claire, about her mother Jean who had been living with congestive heart failure. A few years earlier, I had given the family the Fraser Health My Voice workbook to have advance care planning conversations. Jean was very open to talking about her end-of-life wishes and this had prompted intimate conversations that gave direction for the care she wished to receive. Now, I heard that Jean had been in and out of hospital three times in the last 6 months, most recently discharged home on oxygen. In conversation with Claire, I gently explored what information Jean and her family had been given about the trajectory of her illness and possibility of death. From my clinical knowledge and experience, hearing her pattern of illness exacerbation over the previous 6 months, I would not have been surprised if Jean died in the next months. I shared this information with Claire and suggested that they speak with Jean's physician. Our conversation prompted Claire to share this information about the possibility of death with her siblings and with Jean. As a result, a son who had been distant in his relationships with his mother and sisters for the past few years urged everyone to gather for a family weekend. During the weekend, the family talked about the possibility of Jean's death and rebuilt connection. Within 2 months, Jean had an exacerbation of her heart failure, was admitted to hospital, and died. Without the information shared about the possibility that time could be short until the mother's death, the family might have missed this time to prepare together.

Important to this pattern recognition process is following the lead of families. For example, had Jean and her family not been open to discussing end-of-life care the knowledge that the change in pattern signaled might have been enlisted differently by Della. This illustrates how recognizing patterns works in concert with following the lead of people and families and how direction for action is determined by enacting the strategies together. For example, in the story of the young couple who didn't have a crib for their baby, it is possible that a nurse could have identified a pattern of adversity and high risk. Yet, from the family's vantage point, that pattern would not necessarily be accurate; from their perspective, they were living a meaningful life with their baby. Because what one person or family may experience as adversity may not be experienced as adversity by another, it is important that the pattern, choice, and action are determined by the particular people in the situation. Moreover, it is important to ensure that our own expert pattern recognition does not get privileged over patient/family perspectives; both forms of knowledge are needed.

RI Checkpoint 4.1: Am I Creating Opportunities for Choice-Making?

Relational inquiry focuses on opening the space for collaborative choice-making. Since it is people/families who are living with any illness conditions, it is they who have to decide how and whether the knowledge and interventions we have to offer are relevant to their health and well-being.

TO ILLUSTRATE

Choosing Medications

My (Gweneth's) cousin whose son is living with a mental health challenge told me about an interaction she recently witnessed between a psychiatrist and a young man. She had found the interaction profoundly meaningful since it stood in such contrast to how her own son had been related to by his health care providers. The young man who had been experiencing symptoms such as auditory hallucinations, flight of ideas, and so forth had refused to take psychotropic medication because of the side effects. As with many people living with mental illness, he had found the medications had caused a lack of coordination, a feeling of depersonalization, drowsiness, drooling, excessive thirst, jitteriness, tremors, and so forth (Hagen, Nixon, & Peters, 2010; National Institutes of Health, 2012). Thus, he had decided that the cost of taking the medications outweighed the benefit. Although the psychiatrist believed that the young man would benefit from pharmacologic treatment, he related to the young man by joining him where he was. He inquired into what was currently happening in his life, asking what was of significance to him and how he might support him in his current situation. The young man replied that at this point, he really wanted a girlfriend, and he was finding it a bit challenging because the voices were interfering with that. However, he was averse to medication because the side effects (e.g., drooling) would also be problematic in terms of getting a girlfriend. Working with what mattered to the young man, the psychiatrist suggested the possibility of starting on a very low dose of medication to see if it might be possible to decrease the voices just enough to make them manageable (from the young man's perspective) without causing noticeable side effects. In telling me this story, my cousin remarked on how simple yet profound the psychiatrist's approach had been. It was simple in that he just "followed the lead" and responded to the pattern the young man described and used the knowledge he had to support the young man in his life aspirations. It was profound in that the approach was in such contrast to what her son had experienced. Seldom had a health practitioner ever *started* by asking what mattered to *him* and how the choices might support him with *his* goals.

RI Checkpoint 4.2: Am I Creating Opportunities for Enhancing Capacities and Addressing Adversities?

Collaborating with people and families to recognize and explicitly name capacity is perhaps one of the most empowering things people can experience. Being situated in a health care system that is focused on problems and the servicing of those problems, combined with the powerlessness that people often experience during times of illness and adversity, sometimes people and families have difficulty seeing the capacity they have. Recognizing, affirming, and/or connecting with the capacity you see living within them can potentiate people's reconnection with the power and choice they have and are living in spite of the adversity they are facing.

Unfortunately, naming strengths and capacities has sometimes been translated as yet another thing to add to the assessment or intervention list—as though acknowledging strengths is one more thing *the nurse* should do. We want to be clear this is not what we are suggesting. Naming and supporting capacities is not one more thing to add on to an assessment or intervention! *Recognizing and affirming capacity is an approach and perspective one takes into one's work; it is a philosophical, theoretical, and practical way of relating and working with people and families that shapes every moment of practice.* This distinction is essential because naming strength and capacity can be done in ways that are noncollaborative and at times even disrespectful. For example, sometimes, nurses identify strengths of patients and families as part of their intervention. Depending upon how that is done, identifying strengths can be comparable to an expert, benevolent nurse giving the person a pat on the back. Patients have told us that they have experienced such action as patronizing and disrespectful. For example, in the earlier story about the women who were discussing the news of how the woman had committed suicide by jumping from window, the statement from the nurse who said "I don't know how you do it" was meant to recognize the women's strength. However, the women perceived it as pitying or pathologizing them.

Recognizing and affirming capacity may not even be something that is necessarily said or done by the nurse. Rather, through their work together, the opportunity is created for both patients and nurses to recognize and come to know the capacities living out in the relational situation. So in the above example of the psychiatrist working with the young man, at the heart of the psychiatrist's approach was an obvious belief in the man's capacity to not only make his own life choices but also to play a central role in titrating the dose of medication to a workable level. In a similar fashion, in considering the previous crib example, the recognition of the family's capacity could arise through a conversation about what babies really need in their first year. The family's resourcefulness and capacity to provide this would have become readily apparent—it could have been the young couple, nurse or all involved naming the capacity. At the same time, the opportunity for them to collaboratively name other things that might enhance that existing capacity likely would have arisen.

The relational inquiry strategies support you to see the capacities that people and families are living in their everyday lives amidst the adverse situation (the lack of choices available to them).

TO ILLUSTRATE
A Heroic Admission

A few years ago, while I (Gweneth) was working on a research project (Hartrick Doane, Storch, & Pauly, 2009; Rodney, Hartrick, Storch, Varcoe, & Starzomski, 2002; Rodney, Storch, Varcoe, & Hartrick Doane, 2002–2005) looking at the quality of care (from an ethical perspective) on a medical oncology unit, the husband of one of the patients told me the following story and gave his permission for me to share it. Although the story has much to say about many things in health care, one of the most striking features for me is capacity. I met the couple when I entered the woman's hospital room to explain the research we were doing and ask their permission to accompany their nurse throughout the day as she cared for them. The woman was lying in her bed looking pale and frail. They told us she had had a restless night that had been further disrupted when she had failed to make it to the bathroom in time. Their first request was that we bring a commode chair in so she would have easier access.

About an hour later, I was standing out in the hallway, and the husband approached me to say he had read the information pamphlet about the study and wanted me to know that he thought the nurses on the unit gave "wonderful care." "It is the health care system and actually being able to get into the hospital to get the care the nurses have to give that is the problem," he informed me. Following his lead, I inquired into their experience of getting into the hospital.

He explained that his wife had been in hospital receiving chemotherapy, but due to the hospital bed situation, she had been discharged even though she was feeling very ill from the chemotherapy and in a lot of pain. After a few days at home and of her being "in such pain and vomiting so badly," he tried calling the emergency department to ask if he could bring her back to be readmitted. The emergency doctor, although sympathetic, told him that the bed situation in the hospital was such that even if he brought her in there would be nothing they could do for her—that she would just end up waiting a long time to be seen and would then be discharged home. Feeling powerless, he hung up the phone and told his wife there was no help and "we will just have to tough it out at home." After helping his wife settle for the night, he went to bed at about 1 a.m.

The next thing he knew, the phone was ringing, and it was the hospital. While he slept, his wife had cut off her hospital identification band and, leaving all identification at home, had left the house in her housecoat and pajamas and started walking to the hospital. For a well person walking at a fast clip, the walk would probably have taken 45 minutes. A taxi driver stopped when he saw her and asked if she needed a ride. She accepted the ride to the hospital where, upon her arrival, the police were called. In spite of their insistence, she refused to give her name, knowing that if she did identify herself they would just take her home. After much persistence on the part of the police and the hospital staff she finally gave a phone

continued on page 372

TO ILLUSTRATE *continued*

A Heroic Admission

number. The husband was awakened by the call asking if he was aware that his wife was at the hospital. A frantic check revealed that in fact his wife wasn't where he had left her. The nurse on the other end of the phone told him that he would have to come and get his wife. "I said okay and hung up, but it was after I hung up that I realized that if I did go down to the hospital I would just defeat her heroic effort. They would just send her home, and all that she had done would have been for nothing. So I just phoned back and told them I refused to come and get her, and that is how she got to be readmitted."

Taking an HP lens to this story, many capacities become evident. First, the supportive relationship between the couple that is serving as the foundation from which they are surviving this incredibly challenging situation comes into focus. The man's care and commitment toward his wife as well as his understanding and support of her "heroism" reveals the depth of understanding and appreciation of what it is like for her to live with her cancer and through the treatment process. Taking a critical lens to the situation, it is possible to see the capacity the woman has drawn upon to challenge the system that is seemingly refusing to provide the care she feels she needs. Even with her existing physical limitations, she drew upon her capacity and strategically thought about how she might march in protest to receive the resources she felt she needed to get through this experience. What is important to highlight is how this story could be read from many different vantage points. For example, through a critical lens, it is possible to challenge the discourse of the good patient who does what she is told or the discourse that says there is a scarcity of health care resources and depicts the health care crisis as due to the inevitable need to limit expenditures rather than due to corporate decisions about how to spend the resources available (Bourgeault, 2006; Rodney & Varcoe, in press). Similarly, it is possible to challenge the dominant societal narrative of family as a safe haven that should look after their own and to question the values that are dominating our society and health care system, resulting in this incredibly ill woman having to leave her home in the middle of the night in a desperate attempt to receive hospital care.

Relational Inquiry Takes and Is an Ongoing Practice

While for the purpose of description we have outlined the actions of relational inquiry (the strategies and inquiry checkpoints) separately and in a somewhat linear way, it is important to emphasize that in practice they are *not* separate and linear. The different strategies and checkpoints work in concert with and shape each other. They are enacted in an interwoven way and work in concert with the inquiry lenses and the theoretical ideas and approaches we have described throughout the book.

At this point, we want to emphasize that to integrate relational inquiry into your nursing practice, you need to practice. That is, to develop your nursing practice (as a noun) you need to practice (as a verb). Nursing practice as a *noun* refers to nursing as a form of professional action that includes a particular professional role and capacity that is enacted in accordance with disciplinary values, knowledge, and goals. In speaking of nursing practice as a *verb*, we are highlighting the importance of doing that particular form of action repeatedly to both polish and habituate the capacity for good action—that is, to hone and cultivate your skill as a nurse.

As a nurse, one has a professional practice mandate and role (noun), but to undertake that nursing practice role in a skillful manner, one has to practice (verb). We emphasize both forms of practice because often once nurses are out practicing their profession (noun), they are not necessarily supported or directed to practice (as a verb). They are considered and expected to be competent actors as if competence is a constant state of being—as if once you are competent you are always competent. However, as our discussion in the previous chapters has highlighted, good nursing practice (as a professional role enactment) requires continual practice (honing and embodying of knowledge and skill), because regardless of the years of experience or amount of knowledge you have, without conscious practice, you can automatically fall into the habit of using normative practices that are not aligned with nursing values and commitments.

By describing the relational inquiry strategies and checkpoints, we are giving you support to cultivate a practice of (a) focusing your attention to consciously look for and be mindful of the values, ideologies, power dynamics, knowledge, truths, normative practices, structures, and so forth that are at play; (b) critically examining the relational interplay occurring within a situation (including the five Cs and five Ws of your own relating); and (c) consciously choosing how you yourself will relate and act.

THIS WEEK IN PRACTICE
Practicing Relational Strategies

Explore some of the relational strategies we have presented in your clinical work with people and families this week. Regardless of where you are working and who the people are that you are nursing, choose one inquiry checkpoint with which to practice. Notice if it changes your approach in any way. If you are not actually in a practice setting this week, identify someone with whom you have a relationship (your grandmother, friends, a neighboring family, etc.) and consciously try the checkpoint out when you are with them.

YOUR RELATIONAL INQUIRY TOOLBOX

Add the following tools to your relational inquiry toolbox.

- Use checkpoints to assess whether you are using the strategies of relational inquiry.
- Enlist knowing and not knowing collaboratively.
- Listen specifically for what is of meaning and significance.
- Listen specifically for how social norms and expectations, social structures, and power are operating.
- Look for and respond to patterns of adversity and capacity.

REFERENCES

Australian Government National Health and Medical Research Council. (2006). *National palliative care program. Guidelines for a palliative approach in residential aged care.* Canberra, Australia: Author.

Benner, P. (2000). The roles of embodiment, emotion and lifeworld for rationality and agency in nursing practice. *Nursing Philosophy, 1*, 1–4.

Bourgeault, I. (2006). The provision of care: Professions, politics and profit. In D. Raphael, T. Bryant, & M. Rioux (Eds.), *Staying alive: Critical perspectives on health, illness and health care* (pp. 263–282). Toronto, Ontario, Canada: Canadian Scholar's Press.

Cameron, J. (1992). *The artist's way.* New York: G. P. Putnam's Sons.

Centers for Disease Control and Prevention. (2012). *Chronic diseases and health promotion.* Retrieved August 13, 2013, from http://www.cdc.gov/chronicdisease/overview/index.htm

Daoud, N., Urquia, M. L., O'Campo, P., Heaman, M., Janssen, P. A., Smylie, J., et al. (2012). Prevalence of abuse and violence before, during, and after pregnancy in a national sample of Canadian women. *American Journal of Public Health, 102*(10), 1893–1901.

Devries, K. M., Kishor, S., Johnson, H., Stöckl, H., Bacchus, L. J., Garcia-Moreno, C., et al. (2010). Intimate partner violence during pregnancy: Analysis of prevalence data from 19 countries. *Reproductive Health Matters, 18*(36), 158–170.

Flanagan, O. (1996). *Self expressions: Mind, morals, and the meaning of life.* New York: Oxford University Press.

Furniss, E. M. (1995). *Victims of benevolence: The dark legacy of the Williams Lake residential school.* Vancouver, British Columbia, Canada: Arsenal Pulp Press.

Furniss, E. M. (1999). *The burden of history: Colonialism and the frontier myth in a rural Canadian community.* Vancouver, British Columbia, Canada: UBC Press.

Gendlin, E. T. (1992a). The primacy of the body, not the primacy of perception. *Man and World, 25*(3–4), 341–353.

Gendlin, E. T. (1992b). Thinking beyond patterns: Body, language, and situations. In B. den Ouden & M. Moen (Eds.), *The presence of feeling in thought* (pp. 21–151). New York: Peter Lang.

Gold Standard Framework. (2011). *Gold Standard Framework in care homes.* Retrieved August 7, 2012, from http://www.goldstandardsframework.org.uk/GSFCareHomes

Hagen, B. F., Nixon, G., & Peters, T. (2010). The greater of two evils? How people with transformative psychotic experiences view psychotropic medications. *Ethical Human Psychology and Psychiatry, 12*(1), 44–59.

Hartrick, G. A. (2002). Beyond behavioral skills to human-involved processes: Relational nursing practice and interpretive pedagogy. *Journal of Nursing Education, 41*(9), 400–404.

Hartrick Doane, G. A. (2004). Being an ethical practitioner: The embodiment of mind, emotion and action. In J. Storch, P. Rodney, & R. Starzomski (Eds.), *Toward a moral horizon*. Toronto, Ontario, Canada: Pearson.

Hartrick Doane, G. A. (in press). Cultivating relational consciousness in social justice practice. In P. Kagan, M. Smith, & P. Chinn (Eds.), *Philosophies and practices of emancipatory nursing: Social justice as praxis*. New York: Routledge.

Hartrick Doane, G. A., Stajduhar, K., Bidgood, D., Causton, E., & Cox, A. (2012). End-of-life care and interprofessional communication: Not simply a matter of more. *Health and Interprofessional Practice, 1*(3), eP1028.

Hartrick Doane, G. A., Storch, J., & Pauly, B. (2009). Ethical nursing practice: Inquiry-in-action. *Nursing Inquiry, 16*(3), 232–240.

iPANEL. (2013). *Initiative for a palliative approach nursing education and leadership*. Victoria, British Columbia, Canada: Michael Smith Foundation for Health Research.

Lakoff, G. Z., & Johnson, M. (1999). *Philosophy in the flesh: The embodied mind and its challenge to Western thought*. New York: Basic Books.

Merleau-Ponty, M. (1962). *Phenomenology of perception*. (C. Smith, Trans.). New York: Humanities Press.

Mitra, M., Manning, S., & Lu, E. (2012). Physical abuse around the time of pregnancy among women with disabilities. *Maternal and Child Health Journal, 16*(4), 802–806.

National Institutes of Health. (2012). *Mental health medications*. Retrieved August 13, 2013, from http://www .nimh.nih.gov/health/publications /mental-health-medications /nimh-mental-health-medications.pdf

Nepo, M. (2005). *The book of awakening*. San Francisco: Canari Press.

Newman, M. A. (1994). *Health as expanding consciousness* (2nd ed.). New York: National League for Nursing.

Oxford Dictionary of Current English (6th ed.). (1982). Oxford, United Kingdom: The Clarendon Press.

Razack, S. (1998). *Looking white people in the eye: Gender, race and culture in courtrooms and classrooms*. Toronto, Ontario, Canada: University of Toronto Press.

Rodney, P., Hartrick, G. A., Storch, J., Varcoe, C., & Starzomski, R. (2002). Ethics in action: *Strengthening nurses' enactment of their moral agency within the cultural context of health care delivery*. British Columbia, Canada: Social Sciences and Humanities Research Council, University of Victoria.

Rodney, P., Storch, J. L., Varcoe, C., & Hartrick Doane, G. A. (2002–2005). *Ethics in action: Strengthening nurses' enactment of their moral agency within the cultural context of health care delivery*. British Columbia, Canada: Social Sciences and Humanities Research Council, University of Victoria.

Rodney, P., & Varcoe, C. (in press). Constrained agency: The social structure of nurses' work. In F. Baylis, J. Downie, B. Hoffmaster, & S. Sherwin (Eds.), *Health care ethics in Canada* (3rd ed.). Toronto, Ontario, Canada: Nelson.

Rogers, C. (1961). *On becoming a person*. Boston: Houghton Mifflin.

Stajduhar, K. (2003). Examining the perspectives of family members involved in the delivery of palliative care at home. *Journal of Palliative Care, 19*(1), 27–35.

Stajduhar, K., Funk, L., Cohen, S. R., Williams, A., Bidgood, D., Allan, D., et al. (2011). Bereaved family members' assessments of the quality of end-of-life care: What is important? *Journal of Palliative Care, 27*(4), 261–269.

Stajduhar, K., Funk, L., Roberts, D., McLeod, B., Cloutier-Fisher, D., Wilkinson, C., et al. (2011). Home care nurses' decisions about the need for and amount of service at the end of life. *Journal of Advanced Nursing, 67*(2), 276–286.

Stajduhar, K., Nickel, D. D., Martin, W. L., & Funk, L. (2008). Situated/being situated: Client and co-worker roles of family caregivers in hospice palliative care. *Social Science & Medicine (1982), 67*(11), 1789–1797.

Thille, P. H., & Russell, G. M. (2010). Giving patients responsibility or fostering mutual response-ability: Family physicians' constructions of effective chronic illness management. *Qualitative Health Research, 20*(10), 1343–1352.

Ueland, B. (1992). Tell me more: On the fine art of listening. *Utne Reader, November/December*, 104–110.

Varcoe, C., Doane, G., Pauly, B., Rodney, P., Storch, J. L., Mahoney, K., et al. (2004). Ethical practice in nursing: Working the in-betweens. *Journal of Advanced Nursing, 45*(3), 316–325.

10 Nursing Is Collaborative

LEARNING OBJECTIVES

By engaging with the material in this chapter, you will be able to:

1. Explain how taking a nursing standpoint can help you translate your nursing commitments into action in multidisciplinary health care settings.

2. Develop clarity and confidence in the unique role of nursing and a nursing standpoint.

3. Negotiate differences within interprofessional teams with increasing confidence and competence as you experience hard spots in health care situations.

In this chapter, we focus specifically on the complex process of collaborative nursing practice within contemporary health care contexts. We consider the distinct role that nursing plays within health care teams, how to effectively nurse within the realities of diverse teams, particularly interprofessional teams, and how relational consciousness and the relational inquiry toolbox might be enlisted to support confident, competent action in day-to-day practice.

BEGINNING FROM A NURSING STANDPOINT

In previous chapters, we have discussed how nurses might work collaboratively with patients and families. In this chapter, we turn our attention to how nurses might collaborate effectively with colleagues. When collaborating with other health care professionals, you need a clear understanding of your own expertise, responsibilities, and role. You also need to be able to communicate the value of that role and contribution to others. Subsequently, a central strategy to add to your relational inquiry toolbox is that of consciously inquiring into and articulating the distinct role and function of nursing in particular health care situations. We call this strategy "practicing from a nursing standpoint."

How Do You See Your Role as a Nurse?

As we suggested in Chapter 1, each nurse comes to nursing with a unique set of influences and motivations. Perhaps one of the most important influences to consider as you develop your collaborative practice and nursing

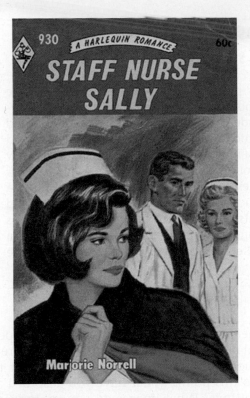

Stereotypical images of nursing.

standpoint is how you think of yourself as a nurse and how you think of nursing within the health care process (Benner, Sutphen, Leonard, & Day, 2010). While there are multiple influences specific to each person that shape one's thinking about nursing, there are also a number of contextual elements that shape our thinking. For example, shaped by larger social contexts, nurses, and nurses' workplaces are often influenced by stereotypical images, gender, race and ethnic privilege, Eurocentrism, liberalist ideology, and so forth. Together, these forces serve to shape the experiences and thinking of all nurses, regardless of their genders, appearances, or identities.

TO ILLUSTRATE

Images and Symbols Shape Our Views of Nursing

Having an older sister who had gone through a traditional hospital nursing program, I (Gweneth) entered nursing school with images of a white dress uniform, nursing cap, and black cape similar to that worn by the nurse in the picture above. It was quite a shock and disappointment when I arrived in my college program and found that these symbols had been eradicated. Wanting to move beyond the traditional view of nurses as

continued on page 380

TO ILLUSTRATE *continued*

Images and Symbols Shape Our Views of Nursing

handmaidens to physicians, our program had been developed with the explicit intent to reject any symbols that would associate us with that former image. So, for example, students were required to wear a bright red tunic and identify ourselves as "student health workers." We were informed that we were a new generation of nurses, and our work was to forge a new image of nursing. However, although we were in an educational program that disavowed traditional images, we were simultaneously working in a health care context that was structured according to traditional roles and images. Subsequently, as students we struggled to meet the expectations of two contradictory contexts and value systems. How I was deemed a worthy and competent nurse differed depending on the context and the people within those contexts.

Stop for a minute, and consider the various influences that have shaped *your* understanding of nursing and of yourself as a nurse. What aspects drew you to nursing? Are they congruent with how you have been taught to think about yourself as a nurse to this point? What have you absorbed as you have been in your clinical settings? What images do you try to work toward and/or enact as a nurse? What images do you find yourself countering in practice settings or in social settings?

Perhaps one of the most powerful influences on our nursing images is that of gender stereotypes. Although the gender composition of nursing is changing in many countries, nursing has long been feminized, seen as quintessentially feminine work in many societies. This feminization is revealed in common stereotypes of nurses as "angels of mercy," sexually promiscuous, and controlling and domineering. For example, in a review of 280 feature films portraying nurses, Stanley (2008) found that early films portrayed nurses as self-sacrificial heroines, sex objects, and romantics, whereas more recent films increasingly portrayed nurses as strong and self-confident professionals. However, Beal (2012) recently analyzed depictions of nursing on YouTube and concluded that marketing pieces, TV show clips, and cartoons objectified or sexualized nurses, trivialized their work, and reinforced negative stereotypes. Also, analyzing YouTube postings, Kelly, Fealy, and Watson (2012) examined the 10 most-viewed videos depicting nurses and nursing and concluded that these postings constructed three distinct nursing identity types: the nurse as a skilled knower and doer; as a sexual plaything; and as a witless, incompetent individual.

The feminization of nursing shapes both male and female nursing stereotypes. Male stereotypes range from exaggeratedly effeminate to hypermasculine. Reviewing 13 feature films (12 of which were made in the United States), Stanley (2012) found that most films "portrayed male nurses negatively and in ways opposed to hegemonic masculinity" (p. 2526). Negative portrayals included depicting male nurses as homicidal, corrupt, or incompetent. Few film images showed male nurses as clinically competent or self-confident. Moreover, male nurses were predominantly portrayed as gay and rarely shown in traditional masculine roles. Very little has been published or portrayed about gay, lesbian, two-spirited, or transgendered persons in nursing. Heterosexism and stereotypical forms of femininity and masculinity influence everyone, including nurses and the public we serve.

Gendered dynamics affect different nurses differently and vary with context. For example, Prebble and Bryder (2008) argued that in New Zealand, different gender and class dynamics dominated psychiatric nursing with unionized men resisting the influence of female-dominated general nursing. However, across contexts, these various dynamics shape how nurses think about themselves (Fletcher, 2007) and influence public perceptions (Morris-Thompson, Shepherd, Plata, & Marks-Maran, 2011), including the perceptions of those who become "patients" and those who govern nursing, such as policy makers and administrators.

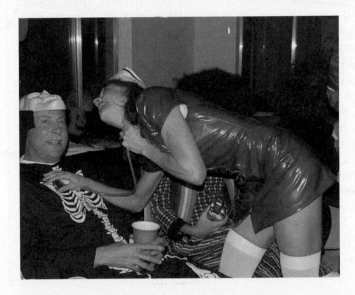

Gender dynamics. (Photograph by Colleen Varcoe.)

Gender dynamics profoundly impact the experience of people of all genders and identities in nursing. Partly because women were the norm in nursing until recently when economics and social attitudes began to shift the gender composition of nursing, the gendered experiences of men have received considerable attention. Research in diverse contexts shows that gendered stereotypes have significant effects on male nursing students' educational experiences (Bartfay, Bartfay, Clow, & Wu, 2010; Dyck, Oliffe, Phinney, & Garrett, 2009; Ierardi, Fitzgerald, & Holland, 2010; McLaughlin, Muldoon, & Moutray, 2010; Meadus & Twomey, 2011; Morris-Thompson et al., 2011), on their experiences in practice (Evans, 2002; Fisher, 2009), and their choice of practice areas (Snyder & Green, 2008). Evans and Frank (2002, 2003) showed that sexuality is routinely in question for male nurses and, regardless of their personal sexual preferences, they can be cast simultaneously as gay and as heterosexual predators. Such depictions have served as barriers to men entering nursing and positioned male nurses as having to defend their career choices, contributions to nursing, and their sexuality (Evans, 2004; Evans & Frank, 2003; Hanvey, 2003).

TRY IT OUT 10.1

What Nursing Images Are Shaping You?

To consider the images and ways of thinking about nursing that are operating within you and shaping how you identify, think about, and act as a nurse, it is also crucial to attend to how others—including other nurses and non-nursing colleagues, are relating to these images and ways of thinking and how these dynamics shape your experience.

First, take a piece of paper and write down the first words that come to mind when you think of an ideal nurse. Also jot down any images that pop up. Are these images gendered, raced, classed, abled? Next, think about yourself as the ideal nurse. Imagine yourself in action, and write down what you see. How are you acting? How are you feeling? What are you thinking? What are you doing? What are you prioritizing? What qualities do you see yourself having? What knowledge and skills do you possess? What is it that makes you feel good about yourself and your work? Who else is in the picture, or do you see yourself as alone and going about your work?

Second, find a non-nursing colleague to talk to. Ask if you can get the person's opinions about nursing, and then ask them the questions you considered in the exercise above. Ask: What comes to mind when you think of an ideal nurse? What images? What do you know about what a nurse "does?" What knowledge and skills do nurses bring to health care? What is the nurse's role in relation to your role?

Finally, compare your understanding with that of the person with whom you spoke. What are the differences and similarities, and what do you think accounts for those? What is the influence of the person's own positioning?

I (Colleen) did this activity inadvertently when I was developing some policies for a burn unit. As part of the process, I met with radiology technicians to get their opinions on the proposed policies. One was clearly speaking for the group when he said, "Do you know how unusual it is for a nurse to ask our opinion? Most nurses act like they barely see us and just want us to get out of the way as quickly as possible."

I (Gweneth) also had this experience when I worked as a psychologist in an acute care setting. On the first day, the psychologist who was orienting me said, "If you want to get anything done for your patients, you have to get the nurses on board—they are the ones who determine what gets done and doesn't get done." Yet, in interprofessional team meetings, I observed how the nurses rarely spoke unless they were asked direct questions by another team member. I happened to know some of the nurses, having taught some of them, so I took the opportunity to ask them how they saw their role on the interprofessional team. They saw themselves at the bottom of the hierarchy and with little decision-making power.

What images of nursing have you embodied in your own practice? How do you think others have been influenced by the images and stereotypes? Did the person you spoke to in Try It Out 10.1 reflect on any such images or stereotypes? Popular images and dominant stereotypes provide part of the backdrop against which nurses, other health care providers, and the public develop understanding of the nursing role.

Developing Role Clarity

While you bring your own images of nursing to your work, the role of nursing is continuously changing in response to myriad social, political, technologic, and economic changes. At the same time, rather than being puppets on the strings of change, nurses can be active agents influencing the direction of change for themselves as practitioners and for the profession. Taking an active role in guiding your own practice requires continuing to pay attention to what is influencing you as a nurse.

For example, Duchscher and Myrick (2008) describe how the dramatic changes and restructuring of health care and nursing that have taken place in North America during the last few decades has resulted in role ambiguity for new nurses. With corporatization, contemporary health care has evolved to a highly complex system of medicalized treatment that is economically based, hierarchically driven, and often in contrast with the humanistic, social-justice values of the nursing profession. This corporatization has required nurses to take up new and expanded roles. At the same time, some of the direct care work that traditionally constituted the domain of nursing has shifted to others. As a result, articulating the distinct role and contribution of nursing has become increasingly important. Risjord (2010) describes that one strategy undertaken to distinguish the nursing role has been to articulate the distinct area of intellectual knowledge and substantive expertise within nursing. The theories and metaparadigm concepts (health, people, nursing, environment) discussed in Chapter 7 are examples of such intellectual work.

This work of clearly articulating the art and science of nursing has several goals, including identifying appropriate nursing roles and resisting inappropriate ones (Risjord, 2010). It has also been undertaken with the intent to distinguish nursing from other disciplines. However, while there is some agreement about the values and conceptual domains inherent to nursing, the ephemeral nature of nursing has made the task of distinguishing it from other professional disciplines somewhat challenging. Thorne (2011) offers insight into this difficulty by explaining that "the central paradox of nursing is that it is a professional-practice discipline at once so mundane that some of its technical aspects can be performed by almost anyone, yet so cognitively sophisticated and mysterious that its excellent application requires advanced education, extensive reflective clinical practice, and an ongoing commitment to inquiry" (p. 86). Sometimes, the mundane tasks are foregrounded, obscuring the complexity of nursing practice. For example, consider how something as mundane as giving a bedpan includes the complex integration of limiting embarrassment for patients, fostering physical comfort and cleanliness, incorporating physiologic observation into health data, and so forth.

Given the complex, multifaceted nature of nursing, the wide range of places nurses work, and the vast array of people and situations to which nurses respond, it seems unlikely that we could fully define nursing and/or the role nurses play in any comprehensive way. Thus, how do we confidently communicate and enact our role within the health care world? How do we identify ourselves and understand our unique role? How do we determine our place and distinct contribution as we work within health care teams? How does nursing stand apart from other disciplines in terms of the particular knowledge and expertise we have to offer?

Risjord (2010) suggests that, by shifting our attention toward outlining the unique *function* of nursing at point-of-care, it is possible to distinguish the nursing role from other professions. This requires moving beyond static definitions of nursing to conceptualize and articulate the nursing role in a relational, functional way. By focusing attention on the *function* nursing plays at point-of-care, the goal of defining and delineating nursing becomes a very practical endeavor. It requires that we inquire into the distinct role of nursing in each health care situation. The more consciously you ask that question in each encounter throughout each day, the more your substantive nursing knowledge and expertise enables you to articulate the specific role and function nursing might serve in any situation. It also enables you to develop and further the knowledge and expertise you might need to carry out that function competently and/or enlist the knowledge and expertise of other disciplines. Through such a process, you also gain clarity about the unique role you have as a nurse and the confidence to articulate your role and obligations as you work collaboratively with others.

In Try It Out 10.1, we asked you to examine your own thinking about the nursing role and to explore how others see nursing. We have suggested that the most effective way to gain clarity about your role as a nurse and articulate the distinct contribution you have to make when you collaborate interprofessionally is to focus on the *function* nursing has at point-of-care. A helpful strategy to assist you in that pragmatic discernment—to articulate the unique role and function of nursing in a particular health care situation—is to consciously practice from a nursing standpoint.

What Is a Nursing Standpoint?

Risjord (2010) describes how the idea of standpoint can be traced to social/political theorists who contend that human activities (what people do) are shaped by power relations that are determined by those with the most power. These theorists assume that power is never equal; rather, it is manifested in the practical ways in which people relate to each other (Risjord, 2010). Risjord gives the example of a factory owner who has power over the workers and creates and shapes what people do, the way they relate to each other, and how the system is organized and functions.

Specifically, Risjord (2010) uses standpoint theory to identify four characteristics of roles and functions within work relationships:

- One role is more dominant and has more power relative to another.
- The relationship between the roles is structured according to the needs and interests of the dominant role.

- The practices of the subordinate role make the activities of the dominant group possible, and this is assumed to be normal (and is largely invisible) to the dominant group.
- In order to fulfill their role, those who occupy the subordinate role need to understand the domain of both the dominant group and of their own.

Stop for a moment to consider these four conditions in terms of the collaborative power relations that make up most health care settings. For example, can you identify similarities between what Risjord describes and how nurses work in health care organizations? Risjord (2010) contends (and we agree) that these four standpoint conditions are evident in the biomedically dominated health care system and have a significant impact on how nurses enact their role. For example, in line with the four conditions, the role of the nurse is most often subordinate to the role of the physician and increasingly to managerial staff, and nurses work in systems that are largely determined by the biomedical needs and interests of physicians and the corporate entities within which health care is delivered. The nursing role is necessary for biomedical activities (treatment protocols to be administered, surgeries to occur, etc.), yet the importance of the nurses' role, expertise, and work is often unseen and/or unacknowledged. In addition, while nurses need to understand patient care from the physician's perspective, mobilize biomedical knowledge, and anticipate physician concerns, the nurse's understanding cannot be limited to that biomedical knowledge because the health needs to which he or she responds as a nurse are far more comprehensive.

Also consider these four conditions in terms of the power relations between nursing and staff other than physicians. How are nurses typically positioned in relation to technicians, pharmacists, security staff, housekeeping or janitorial staff, administrative clerks, aides, dieticians, and so on? Practicing from a nursing standpoint means developing role clarity for nursing that will be effective with all members of the health care team.

Consistent with how we have outlined relational inquiry, Risjord (2010) suggests that there is no one specific nursing standpoint. Rather, a nursing standpoint arises from nurses' lives—from the questions and concerns that come up in their practice. In a relational inquiry approach, to speak of a nursing standpoint does not presuppose an essential, timeless nature of nursing. Rather, a nursing standpoint requires that you make a political commitment to:

- Ground your nursing practice in the commitments, values, and obligations of nursing
- Recognize the value of all forms of knowledge
- Understand difference as an essential feature of nursing situations
- Develop the knowledge and skills necessary to navigate the social/relational interplay of health care situations

When you practice from a nursing standpoint, you are better able to traverse that in-between place where nursing is most often positioned (between biomedical knowledge and other forms of knowledge, between patients/families and biomedical interventions, etc.). This process involves continual attention to what is happening, what needs to happen for the patient, and what your role as a nurse is in that moment of care. It also requires you to consider how a nursing standpoint might inform the care process and the deleterious implications to patients of subordinating your nursing standpoint.

We have found that this understanding of standpoint—in particular examining how power relations shape the social/relational process of health care and nursing—can be very helpful when considering how nurses might effectively articulate and enact the nursing role within health care. As we have described earlier, as a nurse you are shaped by the contexts and power relations within which you work. Thus, to collaborate effectively, you need to strategically consider those power relations. Yet, nurses are often so used to working in a relational dynamic where their knowledge and expertise is subordinated to managers and physicians that they just participate in it without really questioning how this contextual level "habit" is affecting them and patient care. For example, in Chapter 9, I (Colleen) gave the example of a turning point in my career while I was looking after Mr. Gray and his family. That turning point was characterized by my decision to not subordinate nursing knowledge in my practice any longer.

At the same time, nurses can become used to enacting their power in ways that subordinate the knowledge of others—including non-nursing professionals, other health care providers, volunteers, and patients and family members. Enacting power through reinforcing professional boundaries, defending professional turf, and subordinating others can become habits that drain energy and prevent collaboration. Those nurses who are aware of these dynamics often struggle with how to work in such a way as to address their nursing concerns effectively. We believe that committing to a nursing standpoint and enlisting the relational inquiry toolbox can offer a way forward.

Committing to a Nursing Standpoint

Nursing standpoint begins with commitment to the idea that nursing and nursing knowledge makes a difference to health care (Risjord, 2010). For that commitment to occur, nurses must value their knowledge and expertise and believe in the importance of their nursing contribution. We emphasize this because often, this is not the case. For example, Coombs's research (as cited in Risjord, 2010) found that both nurses and physicians treated nursing knowledge as a second-class form of knowledge. "The physicians' knowledge was treated as the more important form, and the areas of nursing expertise were marginalized . . . the nurses' expertise was treated as a 'superficial' addition" (Risjord, 2010, p. 71). Even when the nurses and physicians recognized their distinct expertise and it was evident that all areas of knowledge (biomedical and nursing) were important to informed clinical decision making about patient treatment, physicians, and to some extent nurses, disvalued nursing knowledge and expertise (Risjord, 2010). Nursing knowledge and expertise were considered "clinically superficial," and as such, it was routinely dismissed (as cited in Risjord, 2010, p. 71).

Stop for a moment and think about your own experience of nursing knowledge in health care. Have you witnessed a knowledge hierarchy in which biomedical knowledge trumps other forms of clinical knowledge? How does that knowledge hierarchy shape your own commitments and how you enact those commitments? Do you tend to privilege biomedical knowledge over other forms of knowledge? Do you subordinate your nursing knowledge to medical knowledge? And how does that shape your commitments and your actions? For example, I (Gweneth) have often witnessed how nursing students can unconsciously begin to work more in concert with biomedical imperatives than their own nursing commitments. Practicing in a health care context that privileges biomedical knowledge and imperatives, nurses get confused and unsure about how biomedical knowledge and nursing knowledge work in concert—and how drawing upon both can support them to better meet their nursing commitments. Many begin to see biomedical knowledge as crucial while other forms of knowledge are seen as "nice to know," not necessarily "need to know." This shapes how they evaluate their own knowledge base (according to how much biomedical/empirical knowledge they have) and how they subordinate their nursing knowledge and commitments.

Last term, the third-year BSN students I (Gweneth) taught were experiencing this confusion. Having just completed clinical rotations in acute care settings, they expressed great frustration at having to take a nursing inquiry course and learn about nursing theory. How could abstract nursing theories written by academics have any relevance to what they had been doing in acute care? As we discussed their frustration and what was important to them, it quickly became evident that they were equating "health care" with biomedical imperatives. From that biomedical standpoint, it made sense that they could not see the relevance of nursing theories to their day-to-day actions. However, as we looked at actual health care situations and began to identify the *nursing care* that was needed in those situations and what they as nurses needed to know, be, and do to provide that care, the nursing theories took on a whole new meaning. What made the difference was exploring health care from a *nursing* perspective.

One day, one of the students exclaimed, "This is a whole new way of looking at my practice—it is like how to *nurse* patients is the focus, not just biomedical treatments—and that totally changes how I look at things and understand my role." That statement was a sign that the students were beginning to develop a *nursing* standpoint. Gaining clarity of their nursing role and looking at health care situations from a nursing standpoint served to guide their actions and give them confidence in the value and contribution they as nurses had to make—and how it was both distinct from and worked in concert with the other disciplines with whom they collaborated. Importantly, they began to realize that the health needs to which a *nurse* responds are more comprehensive than just disease treatment.

As we discussed in Chapter 6, there is no doubt that biomedical knowledge is vital to health care, and to be competent, you need to be informed by biomedical knowledge and respond to biomedical imperatives. However, valuing biomedical knowledge and imperatives *over* other forms of knowledge and health care is highly problematic both in terms of meeting your nursing commitments and effectively enacting your full scope of practice as a nurse. Moreover, not grounding your practice in a nursing standpoint can severely limit your views, your choices, your confidence, your actions, and your contributions.

TRY IT OUT 10.2

From the Mundane to the Profound through a Nursing Standpoint

Pick a nursing task, skill, or action, such as suctioning, turning a patient, diapering a neonate, giving out meds, helping a patient use a urinal, staunching the flow of blood from a wound, or changing a dressing. Brainstorm the relevant physiologic and biomedical knowledge. Then brainstorm "what else" is required from a nursing standpoint. For example, we have said that relational inquiry nursing practice is oriented toward the living experience of the person. If you orient your attention in that way, what other nursing concerns arise? What empirical, ethical, sociopolitical, and aesthetic knowledge would you as a nurse need to enlist? What questions do you need to ask to translate your nursing values and commitment into action?

Developing Confidence in Your Nursing Standpoint

Within nursing, confidence has been identified as a central component for competent, effective clinical performance (Mavis, 2001). In doing a concept analysis of confidence, Holland, Middleton, and Uys (2011) define confidence as "a dynamic, maturing personal belief held by a professional or student. This includes an understanding of and a belief in the role, scope of practice, and significance of the profession and is based on their capacity to competently fulfill these expectations, fostered through a process of affirming experiences" (p. 222). Let's consider this definition in light of developing confidence in your nursing standpoint. It appears that confidence rests in the valuing of nursing—in a strong belief that the nursing profession has a significant role to play in health care. Also central to confidence is the ability to competently fulfill that role in your professional capacity.

There is a vital connection between confidence and competence. "Professional confidence underpins competence and is inextricably linked to professional identity" (Holland et al., 2011, p. 214). For example, research has shown a link between students' confidence development and their increasing ability to make clinical decisions (White, 2003). As Bandura (2001) contends, "Unless people believe they can produce desired results and forestall detrimental ones by their actions, they have little incentive to act or to persevere in the face of difficulties" (p.10).

Box 10.1 includes two statements from national level nursing organizations, the National League for Nursing (NLN) in the United States and the Canadian Nurses Association (CNA), that highlight the importance of believing in the value and impact nursing can have. Notice how both statements emphasize the promotion of health and well-being beyond biomedical interventions. In each statement, it is possible to see how competence and confidence are intricately intertwined. By consciously aligning your nursing actions with these nursing competencies, you can have more confidence in the contribution you have to make as a nurse. As you read the statements, what elements stand out? How might they inform your own nursing standpoint? How might you enlist them to have confidence in the significant role that you as a nurse have to play in health care?

Although confidence in the nursing role is crucial to competent practice, Orchard (2010) contends that nurse educators often give little attention to helping nursing students understand and/or articulate their

---

BOX 10.1

Competencies for Nurses

The National League for Nursing (NLN) identifies the following competencies for BSN graduates:

Human Flourishing
Incorporate the knowledge and skills learned in didactic and clinical courses to help patients, families, and communities continually progress toward fulfillment of human capacities.

Nursing Judgment
Make judgments in practice, substantiated with evidence, that synthesize nursing science and knowledge from other disciplines in the provision of safe, quality care and that promote the health of patients, families, and communities.

Professional Identity
Express one's identity as a nurse through actions that reflect integrity, a commitment to evidence-based practice, caring, advocacy, and safe, quality care for diverse patients, families, and communities as well as a willingness to provide leadership in improving care.

Spirit of Inquiry
Act as an evolving scholar who contributes to the development of the science of nursing practice by identifying questions in need of study, critiquing published research, and using available evidence as a foundation to propose creative, innovative, or evidence-based solutions to clinical practice problems.

The CNA describes the competencies of registered nurses as follows:

Registered nurses are self-regulated health care professionals who work autonomously and in collaboration with others. RNs enable individuals, families, groups, communities, and populations to achieve their optimal level of health. RNs coordinate health care, deliver direct services, and support clients in their self-care decisions and actions in situations of health, illness, injury, and disability in all stages of life. RNs contribute to the health care system through their work in direct practice, education, administration, research, and policy in a wide array of settings. (Canadian Nurses Association, 2007, p. 6)

unique contribution and the various roles nurses perform. Subsequently, Schwartz, Wright, and Lavoie-Tremblay (2011) found that at the outset, many new nurses expressed a lack of confidence in even interacting with interprofessional colleagues to disseminate patient information and/or voice their opinions. Similarly, Chesser-Smyth and Long (2013) found that nursing students did not have the confidence or know-how to effectively respond to the dominant culture when challenges arose.

TRY IT OUT 10.3
What Is Shaping Your Confidence?

Developing confidence begins with yourself and your nursing commitments. White (2009) describes how a primary characteristic of confidence is the explicit personal belief that one can achieve an affirmative outcome in a certain situation. Thinking of this idea, can you identify beliefs you have that serve to support or undermine your confidence as a nurse or the confidence you have in your nursing contribution? Self-awareness is also an antecedent to confidence. As we described in earlier chapters, undertaking intrapersonal inquiry to become aware of your own beliefs and clear in your vision and goals and in the obligations and commitments that are central to your nursing work (clarifying the five Cs) offers you an internal locus of control from which to practice.

Thus, we invite you to try to identify some of the beliefs and assumptions that might be shaping your confidence as a nurse. For example, what assumptions do you hold about your place in the power hierarchy? Do you believe that nurses are second class citizens (next to physicians or other professions)? How do you respond when someone asks you why you didn't go into medicine instead of nursing (given that you are so smart)? While at times medical intervention might need to be more urgently prioritized, do you believe it is more important than nursing interventions? To help you to identify your beliefs, recall a time when you have felt lacking in confidence. Try to remember what you were thinking and feeling inside. Can you identify any beliefs or assumptions that were giving rise to those thoughts and feelings? Next, identify a time when you felt and acted with confidence as a nurse. What was the difference?

To continue to develop and nurture your confidence as a nurse, it can be helpful to practice engaging in intrapersonal, interpersonal, and contextual inquiry and to enlist the other strategies in the relational inquiry toolbox. They can be used to help you identify the contribution nursing has to make in a particular situation and how you as a nurse might confidently collaborate. As Davidhizar (1993) contends, "Nurses who are really confident in their skills and values do not have to *act* powerful, they *are* powerful" (p. 218). Thus, the more confident you are in your nursing standpoint, the more confidently and competently you can act!

Focusing Your Attention through a Nursing Standpoint

Practicing from a nursing standpoint requires that you focus your attention in intentional and conscious ways. Consciousness is a powerful force to bring to your nursing work (Hartrick Doane, in press). For example, have you ever had the experience of becoming so engrossed in a good movie that you completely lose consciousness of yourself and your surroundings? This offers a good example of the power of consciousness. We actually have the ability to focus our attention outwardly in such a way that we can literally forget ourselves. Or we can focus so directly on ourselves and our own experience that we are not aware of what is going on around us.

Singer (2007) explains that at the most basic level, consciousness is determined by what you focus your attention on. As we have described earlier, how and why you focus your attention shapes the way you act. Let's think about this in the context of your nursing practice. When you begin working on a new nursing unit, you probably focus your attention on specific things to create a sense of orientation (e.g., you might pay attention to the physical surroundings and look for familiar things to help you orient yourself). In all likelihood, you are more conscious of your actions and relate to your surroundings differently as a new person on the unit than if you have been working on the unit for a long time and know your way around. Similarly, as a nurse, you might use external objects or specific aspects (e.g., risk indicators) to orient and know a patient. Or you might use internal structures such as values, goals, or interpretations to narrow your focus. Depending on the situation, you might focus your attention on contextual aspects to orient and know. Simply put, "Consciousness is a dynamic field of awareness that has the ability to either narrowly focus or broadly expand" (Singer, 2007, p. 128). This dynamic nature of consciousness is an important feature since it enables you to adapt your focus of attention to look at something narrowly and/or broadly.

To consider how you focus your attention, stop reading for a moment and look up from where you are sitting. Scan the room slowly until something grabs your attention. Now consider why your attention rested on that particular thing. What was it that drew you toward it? Once you focused your attention on that one object, what happened? Did your relationship to the object and/or to the other things in the room change? Once that particular thing became the focus of your attention, how did you relate to the other things in the room? If you try this exercise, you will see how conscious attention and how you relate and act are connected. *Namely, our consciousness determines the five Ws (how we act and relate), and our relational action determines our consciousness* (Hartrick Doane, in press). As we focus on one element, we may be relationally oblivious to other intrapersonal, interpersonal, and contextual elements. For example, when we focus our attention narrowly (as we do when watching a movie or reading a book), we lose the broader sense of ourselves and what is going on around us (Singer, 2007).

TRY IT OUT 10.4

Focusing Attention from a Nursing Standpoint

This dynamic of focusing attention on particular things and not on others is happening continually as we go about our nursing work. Moreover, as you go about your studies and/or work in clinical settings you are developing specific habits for structuring and orienting your conscious attention. For example, as you study pathophysiology, aseptic technique, and practice skills such as dispensing medications, starting IVs, and doing catheterizations, you are being schooled to structure your attention in specific ways. Similarly, as you enlist assessment tools or best-practice protocols to guide your nursing actions, your consciousness and the way you structure your attention is being shaped and patterned.

The relational inquiry lenses, strategies, and checkpoints are intended to help you cultivate a nursing standpoint and the habit of focusing your attention from that nursing standpoint. They offer specific ways you can develop and practice acting from a nursing standpoint.

Revisit the tools identified in each of the chapters (e.g., lenses, five Cs, forms of inquiry, five Ws, nursing theories, etc.). Consider how they can serve to orient you in a *nursing* standpoint. What *nursing* questions do they draw to your attention? How might they help you discern what is significant in terms of *nursing* care? How might they also support you with making clinical decisions from a *nursing* standpoint?

Making Conscious Choices from a Nursing Standpoint

Throughout this book, we have emphasized that every moment of nursing and every action you take as a nurse is a relational one. We also explained that relational inquiry helps you see how you are focusing your attention and making your nursing choices. At this point, we want you to consider how a nursing standpoint might support you to focus your attention in ways that help you make good nursing choices.

Stop for a minute, and think about how you make choices as a nurse. What kinds of things do you focus on as you consider how to respond in a situation? What questions do you ask yourself? When you make choices do you tend to privilege thinking? Feelings? Other people's opinions? Do you find yourself spending quite a bit of time carefully weighing your choices as you deliberate your actions? Do you feel pressured to make choices and act quickly?

Drawing upon decades of behavioral science research in psychology about how people make choices, Thaler and Sunstein (2009) state, "The picture that emerges is one of busy people trying to cope in a complex world in which they cannot afford to think deeply about every choice they have to make. People [therefore] adopt sensible rules of thumb that sometimes lead them astray" (p. 37). These rules of thumb are ways of thinking and orienting that serve to structure (and determine) the choice architecture that frames how you see the choices available to you (Thaler & Sunstein, 2009).

Earlier, we discussed how, based on their own social locations and backgrounds, people develop particular reference points that shape how they interpret and decide the value or meaning of something. The automatized rules they use to make choices arise out of those reference points and serve as "shortcuts" in thinking that can be both helpful and limiting. They are informal and often unconscious rules or structures from which we work. For example, the definition of health that you work from is a reference point that creates a particular way of orienting and focusing your attention. In essence, it provides the framework that determines the automatic rules from which you work and the choices you consider as you go about promoting health.

Thaler and Sunstein (2009) describe that because people are so busy and have limited attention to give to the choice-making process, they tend to work from their own reference points and rules, accepting the *choice questions as they are posed*. In addition, people are often conscripted into a particular choice architecture. For example, nurses will often make clinical decisions using the choice architecture that dominates the health care setting. As such, nursing care may or may not include responding to specific concerns of patients and families. It is important to be aware of the reference points and rules from which you are working because they can limit your choice options. To illustrate this, I (Gweneth) describe an experience I had a few years ago when I was hospitalized following a motor vehicle accident.

TO ILLUSTRATE
Conscripted into Power Relations

I sit up and reach for the nasal prongs, turn the oxygen on, and take some slow, deep breaths. Funny, my breathing has been so stable over the past couple of days—why am I suddenly feeling so short of breath? Sitting upright, I take my pulse and go over the possibilities in my mind. The cardiograms have been normal; my pulse is strong and steady. Maybe it's just tightness from the fractured ribs. But why now? It could be an embolus—or maybe it's just the contused lungs from the steering wheel trauma. I reach for the call bell and wait for the nurse. My nurse walks in smiling. "What can I do for you?" she asks cheerfully.

"I am feeling quite short of breath. It's different than it has been. I'm due to go home this afternoon so I am wondering if maybe I could get it checked before I leave just in case something has developed."

The nurse frowns. "It's probably nothing—just your fractured ribs." She takes my vital signs, shrugs, and says, "Don't worry about it. It's nothing."

continued on page 394

TO ILLUSTRATE *continued*

Conscripted into Power Relations

"Well yes," I reply, "it may be just my ribs, but I wonder if I could get it checked out before I leave just to be on the safe side."

Suddenly, the friendly demeanor is gone. In an authoritative tone, she states, "I'll think about it." With that she turns and walks out of the room. I wait.

An hour later she has not returned, my breathing has eased somewhat, and lying in my bed I contemplate my next step—do I let it go or do I persist? An x-ray porter calls out my name as she wheels a stretcher into the room. I raise my head to identify myself. "I'm having an x-ray?" I ask.

The porter looks surprised. "That's what the requisition says."

"Great," I reply as I attempt to move to the stretcher before she can question further; I want that x-ray!

Half an hour later as I settle in my bed after returning from x-ray, the nurse walks in. "Oh, there you are. I just wanted to check that you were back and everything is okay." She smiles at me. "You know I didn't make the connection earlier."

"The connection?" I ask, confused.

"Yes, I read your articles when I was a nursing student—about relational practice. I so believe everything you write about." With great conviction in her eyes she declares, "And I practice exactly as you describe."[1]

---

[1] This story has been previously published in Doane, G. H., & Varcoe, C. (2008). Knowledge translation in everyday nursing: From evidence-based to inquiry-based practice. *Advances in Nursing Science, 31*(4), 283–295 and is reprinted with permission from Lippincott Williams & Wilkins.

How is it that this passionate nurse, who was so committed to the values and commitments of relational inquiry and a relational nursing standpoint, acted so out of alignment with those values and commitments? Her actions were grounded in evidence and theory; she carried out an assessment and made a clinical decision to request an order for an x-ray. Yet, the evidence she drew upon was quite limited. For example, her actions did not reflect the nursing theories or ways of relating she had studied and with which she had obviously deeply resonated. She "knew" the relational inquiry nursing approach well enough to actually identify it with a specific author, yet in that particular situation, those values, commitments, and the knowledge she espoused were not evidenced or translated into nursing action. Yet, she believed she *was* acting in a way that was congruent.

Our reason for telling you this story is to highlight how nurses can practice with the best of intentions and be deeply committed to nursing in responsive and equitable ways yet inadvertently move away from their nursing standpoints as they work in collaborative contexts. For example, the nurse's enactment of power, evident in her statement "I'll think about it," does not merely reflect *her* actions. It also reflects her social conditioning into understandings and normative practices that dominate health care settings—understandings regarding what knowledge is relevant, who is knowledgeable, how knowledge should be used, and so forth. The nurse's actions reflect how this particular nurse was *acting from* the reference point of the expert professional who knows and has control over what knowledge should be used and how. That identity and way of acting was not only justified by her position within the health care hierarchy—it was modeled.

Paul Ricoeur (1991) describes this social conditioning process as automatization. Automatization is the conscription of individuals into the actions of the social group. A consequence of this automatization process is the inability of the actor to see how his or her action has been conscripted or to see the impact of those actions on others. Just as the nurse in the story could not see the inconsistency of her actions, we all act in ways that are inconsistent with our intentions and values. Simply put, we have all been conscripted in some way—whether in line with colonial privilege, expert power-over stances, efficiency processes of organizations, or a multitude of other possibilities. Given that we are relational beings who are both situated in and constituted by our surroundings, it is impossible to not be.

Thus, consciously examining how you make choices is vital. It can ensure the choices you make are consistent with your nursing goals and commitments. It can also enable you to *be more confident in the choices you make and open up the range of choices available to you*. For example, time is a precious commodity in busy health care settings. As a result, nurses continually have to ration their time and set priorities. If you speak with nurses, one of the common refrains you will hear is, "I don't have time to give the care I want to." They often feel so pressured to get tasks done that their choices are made as they move from one task to another.

Can you think of any particular rules you have seen nurses use in the name of time and efficiency? For example, situated in a health care system that prioritizes biomedical imperatives, often, the working rule is "symptoms and treatment first." In other words, nurses prioritize and use the time they have to address the biomedical disease efficiently. Of course, this way of working is completely understandable. When a patient arrives with an acute asthmatic attack in a busy ER, biomedical intervention takes priority. However, having a working rule that prioritizes biomedical assessments and treatments *instead of* other concerns can be limiting.

Thus, their actions can be shaped by contextual conditions and collaborative relations to the point that they can be conscripted into normative practices that are contrary to their nursing values and commitments.

What is important about working from normative reference points and automatized rules is that in doing so, nurses do not stop to consider other possibilities for action. That is, they answer the "time" question just as it is posed: "What symptoms and treatment will I address in the little time I have?" They may not think beyond the routines to see the particular situation in its entirety—or to the broader and/or specific *nursing* aspects. Thus, they do not consider alternative formulations—other ways of posing the "time" question that offer different and expanded possibilities. For example, alternative formulations of the question that include a more holistic nursing view could be: "How can I respond effectively to this particular person or family *and* get the required treatments done in the time I have?"

Just by posing the question differently, you are "nudged" toward alternative ways of thinking and/or acting (Thaler & Sunstein, 2009). For example, think of how you reframed problems in Chapter 9. Kelley Doucette, the ER nurse we told you about in Chapter 8, describes how a relational inquiry approach (and looking at her work from a *nursing* standpoint) has enabled her to consciously extend her choice architecture in the ER.

> In the ER, we deal with people in acute situations whether it be physically, medically, emotionally, or mentally, and we have minimal time to develop meaningful relationships with our patients. Yet, now I realize that due to the vulnerability of these people in their acute state, it is more important than ever to establish an open, working relationship in order to provide safe, ethical, and relevant care each and every time to every patient that presents to the department. In order to be able to do this, I have identified significant developments and changes in my practice—the ability to be present with each patient and give them my undivided attention for the brief time I have with them; being able to connect with them without bias or judgment, and relating to the person and who they are in this time and place in their life.

As we described earlier, one specific change Kelley has made by extending her choice architecture is to be fully present with people when they come to the triage desk. In the 1 or 2 minutes she has with each person, she has decided to consciously engage in a way that communicates that they and their health concern matters and that someone (she) is going to do what is possible to attend to their health concerns. Just by shutting the pocket door between the triage area and the waiting room to make the moments she has with the patients meaningful, her practice has changed dramatically. This is a clear example of extending one's choice architecture. Looking beyond the automatized rules that govern the ER, Kelley could see other possibilities for action. While the busy ER context limits the time she has with people, she has extended her options for how she spends the time she has. Moreover, she is acting in ways that are more aligned with her nursing values and commitments.

Simply put, by consciously taking a nursing standpoint and considering the reference points and automatized rules that are shaping your actions, the options for nursing action are extended. Moreover, being aware of the rules from which you are working and considering the choice architecture that is shaping your choices can enable you to more confidently act in a way that aligns with your nursing commitments and obligations.

As Risjord (2010) describes, "In nursing, the commitment is to the values at the core of nursing practice . . . [and playing a central role in] embedding the view of human health as disease and dysfunction into a larger picture that includes the psychological, social, and personal elements of health. This attempt to synthesize physiology, pharmacology, patients' experiences, is the science of nursing . . . [and through this synthesizing work,] the nursing standpoint can provide a less distorted view of human health" (p. 72). *Nursing standpoint requires that we make the practical and political commitment to consciously "stand" in nursing at the point-of-care and inquire how the values and commitments that are at the core of nursing practice (e.g., the well-being of patients, nurses, the health care system) can be articulated and acted toward.*

TRANSLATING NURSING COMMITMENTS INTO ACTION: A COLLABORATIVE PROCESS

Safe, competent health care is something that is accomplished within contextual conditions that include physical layouts, staff mixes, resource allocation, organizational policies, knowledge hierarchies, and so forth. In the midst of these contextual conditions, nurses work in ongoing collaboration with others. While collaboration is an essential feature of nursing work and is seen as a central nursing competency (Miller et al., 2008), nurses often find that collaborative practice can be challenging within contemporary health care settings. For example, in their examination of nurses' participation in interprofessional collaboration (IPC) on medical units, Miller and colleagues (2008) found nurses often tried to avoid or ignore the collaborative aspect. Lack of reciprocity and equity of status and knowledge sharing between nurses and interprofessional colleagues "elicited in nurses individual anxiety, avoidance behaviors, and defensive professional efforts. Nurses 'voted with their feet' and whenever possible abstained from structured IPC. Professional consequences included nurses' poorer comprehension and participation in care planning, as well as ongoing disengagement with unstructured IPC" (p. 340). Overall, these researchers found that, for a variety of reasons, nurses did not collaborate effectively in their day-to-day practice.

Yet, while nurses may not know how to collaborate effectively, their action is strongly influenced by collaborative relations. For example, Hamilton and Campbell (2011) describe nurses' "constant conversation" with physicians and other practitioners through which nurses "keep an image of the patients' doctors and their expectations in mind as they conduct their therapeutic interventions, tend monitors, make observations, and compare what they see happening to what they know should be happening. They conduct this virtual dialogue as work in preparation, not just for reporting to doctors and to subsequent shifts of nurses, but to determine how to act correctly at each moment" (p. 284). Within this collaborative process, nurses also turn to colleagues to enlist their expertise and enhance their own knowledge to better respond to health care challenges (Hamilton & Campbell, 2011).

A Relational Understanding of Collaborative Practice

So how does one practice from a nursing standpoint *and* work effectively within collaborative spaces of care? What might help nurses work between differing and competing interests and within hierarchical power relations and be as effective as possible in addressing their nursing concerns? Because your nursing actions in any particular moment are strongly influenced by the relational interplay that is occurring, bringing a relational understanding to your collaborative practice is crucial.

A relational understanding highlights the way in which difference is an essential feature of nursing and of collaborative practice. Differences arise between colleagues (nursing and/or interprofessional) due to any number of reasons—differences in professional values, roles and status, lack of common purpose and goals, differing social and professional behaviors, lack of trust, differing and competing professional agendas, differing levels of power or control and/or differing organizational policies, and so forth (Beales, Walji, Papoushek, & Austin, 2011; Miller et al., 2008). Within health care teams, it is also not uncommon to have differing understandings about what each team member has to offer. Similarly, there is often uncertainty or disagreement about who is competent and has the authority to do different things. The following story, told to us by a fourth-year nursing student during an ethics research project (Rodney, Hartrick, Storch, Varcoe, & Starzomski, 2002) illustrates these differences.

TO ILLUSTRATE
Bouncing back and forth

I listened to a child's . . . chest, who was in for pneumonia, and he was due to be discharged that day or the next day. And I had listened to his chest in my assessment, and he was clear in my opinion . . . And he had been ordered Ventolin, and I didn't think he needed it . . . so I discussed it with the medical student who had ordered it . . . "Oh, give it to him anyway" was the response. And so I went to the RN, and I said, "This is the issue and I don't think he should get it." And she said, "Well, go and talk to the medical student again."

So I went again to the medical student, and I said, "I don't feel comfortable giving this Ventolin. I don't feel he needs it." Because I think that kind of medication, unless it's needed, does some major flip flops with the heart rate and all sorts of things. It's pretty traumatic to have this mask thrust in your face.

And again, the medical student said, "I think he needs it. Give it to him." So I went back to the RN and I said, "You have to give it to him. I'm not giving it to him." And I felt very confident that my opinion was correct. And so I felt frustrated in the end, because as it turned out, I was in the room with him and the parents when the RN gave him the Ventolin, and she just walked out. She put the mask on with him screaming and fighting and carrying on, and I was the one who was distracting him in the end while he had to sit there for 15 minutes.

From a collaborative practice perspective (and from a nursing standpoint) the question that needs to be asked in situations such as these is: *What would be the best, most responsive, patient care?* It is evident that the student is drawing on empirical and biomedical knowledge ("*His chest . . . was clear*"; Ventolin "*does some major flip flops with the heart rate*") and combining ethical knowledge about autonomy with experiential knowledge about children ("*It's pretty traumatic to have this mask thrust in your face*"). Bringing her nursing standpoint and the emphasis on human flourishing and well-being, she has (as outlined in the NLN competencies) synthesized nursing knowledge and knowledge from other disciplines to make a clinical judgment about what might be the most responsive approach to care. But clearly in this situation, knowledge and sound clinical decision making is not enough. Importantly, the primary difference at issue in this example is not "which" knowledge should be privileged. Nor is it a simple example of difference in which bio medical knowledge is privileged. Rather, by focusing on the "relational inter-play," it is possible to see that the difference at issue is a difference in power relations. And these power relations result in less effective intervention for the patient. Ironically, while the physician wields the power and determines what transpires, the normative routines are even subordinating good use of biomedical knowledge. At the same time, the power dynamics are such that the student is unable to practice in a way that she believes to be best for the child's well-being. Because the knowledge and clinical judgment of the nurse who is monitoring the patient is subordinated, evidence-based clinical deci-sion making is thwarted, and patient care is negatively impacted.

Richardson, West, and Cuthbertson (2010) found that this pattern of subordinating nursing knowledge in clinical decision making is com-mon. These researchers describe how despite a move toward interdiscipli-nary collaboration, clinical decision making continues to be perceived as a top-down and authoritative process in which nurses and nursing knowl-edge are subordinated. But it is not just biomedicine that subordinates the nursing standpoint. Hamilton and Campbell (2011) describe how within contemporary health care settings, the experientially based professional knowledge of direct care nurses is also being downgraded and bypassed as a result of the managerial turn toward objective, institutionally organized health information. For example, while nurses may voice concerns based on what is happening at the bedside, managers tend to favor data gath-ered from quality control measurement tools and so forth. The researchers state that "the standpoint of the nurse at the bedside is critically important to consider when re-forming health care to achieve greater safety, quality, and effectiveness, [however] our findings suggest that far from having their knowledge valued, direct-care nurses are being persuaded to see things dif-ferently, to get on board with institutional priorities and actions designed in the boardroom. This happens not because individuals on boards or in administrative positions do not value safety, quality, or effectiveness but because they see these qualities from a different standpoint" (p. 295).

As Hamilton and Campbell (2011) emphasize, the standpoint of direct-care nurses is crucial. Nurses have a unique vantage point and form of knowledge. They bring multiple forms of research and theoretical knowl-edge to their practice. Given their around-the-clock view and through the daily activities of nursing practice, they also bring temporal knowledge that can inform recognition of patterns, trends over time, immediate concerns, and so forth. Because of their position in relation to patients and families in everyday clinical care, nurses cultivate knowledge that no one else in the organization has.

Practicing from a nursing standpoint and a relational view of collabo-ration focuses your attention on difference and how difference is not only an essential feature of collaborative practice, it is a resource. As the HP and critical lenses illustrate, depending on how people are positioned and the contextual/sociohistorical background they bring to each situation, they will bring differing understandings, and their attention will focus on dif-ferent priorities and concerns. It is this breadth and depth of knowledge and skill that can offer the most holistic and informed approach to collaborative care. However, to effectively enlist and integrate these differing forms of knowledge requires valuing them. Relationally orienting enables you to consciously (a) pay attention to the differences that are part of the collaborative interplay, (b) bring and maintain a nursing standpoint, and (c) extend the choices you see available to you (your choice architecture). In so doing, it can serve to enhance the confidence and clarity you have in terms of the particular contribution you have to make as a nurse and provide effective strategies for collaborative action.

Simply put, being confident in your nursing standpoint enables you to work across difference more effectively. It also enables you to more effectively navigate the relational interplay of authority, commitment, and privilege. Beales and colleagues (2011) point out that, although health care professionals might adopt and support the premise of IPC, often, their frames of reference have not been developed to the point where they actually know how to work collaboratively. For example, when differences arise in challenging or uncertain situations, health care professionals are much more likely to fall back on their own professional culture and their mono-professional lens—to get into an "us and them" stance where they see difference as a problem ("we powerless nurses" versus "those arrogant doctors" or "those overbearing administrators").

Relational inquiry offers a way of working across differences—a way of practicing collaboratively even when others are not being particularly collaborative. Conceptualizing difference relationally, we are able to look at differences and problems from multiple vantage points simultaneously. Difference implies more than one perspective and thus draws attention to the place *in between* different perspectives. Using a relational inquiry approach, "hard spots" (areas of disagreement, conflict, uncertainty) become cues to look relationally at the in-between spaces—to inquire and discern the significant elements that are at play. Viewing and approaching difference relationally promotes responsibility rather than blame, understanding rather than defensiveness, connection rather than guilt or anger, and responsiveness rather than a sense of powerlessness and frustration.

TO ILLUSTRATE
Racializing Death

I (Colleen) have been trying to train myself to respond in a constructive way to racializing processes. Yesterday, the head of housekeeping at an organization with which I am affiliated asked me for some advice. She said that she was having trouble with a couple of "Filipino" nurses. When a patient dies, the nurses are supposed to provide care until the person's body is taken to the morgue and then strip the beds. There are often deaths on this unit, but recently, these nurses have been leaving such work to the day shift staff, causing a backlog of work for the housekeeping staff. She said, "Filipinos don't like to have anything to do with death."

continued on page 401

> ### TO ILLUSTRATE *continued*
> #### Racializing Death
>
> My immediate feelings are anger and frustration. I find such simplistic ra-
> cialized explanations overwhelmingly frustrating. Yet, she was asking my ad-
> vice because I supposedly know something about culture, and she sincerely
> wanted help. Expressing frustration and anger would not help. To give my-
> self a chance to "let it be," I asked what I thought were innocuous questions
> intending to stall for time before I responded: Is this a new pattern? Have
> there been other big changes on the unit? As she answered, I think she real-
> ized before I did that the number of deaths, the level of staff on sick leave,
> and other staffing issues might have been contributing to the situation.

Understanding Collaboration as an Adaptive Challenge

A relational view highlights the way in which collaboration is an adaptive challenge. Heifetz (1998) distinguishes technical challenges (in
which it is possible to clearly identify a problem, a clear solution, and
the knowledge or skill set needed to address the challenge) from adaptive challenges (ones that lie within people and situations and require
something beyond the incorporation of knowledge, technical skills, or
solutions). "Technical problems reside in the head; solving them requires
an appeal to the mind, to logic, and to the intellect. Adaptive challenges
lie in the stomach and the heart. To solve them, we must change people's values, beliefs, habits, ways of working, or way of life" (Heifetz &
Linsky, 2002, p. 35).

While most situations pose a combination of technical and adaptive
challenges, Heifetz (1998) asserts that the biggest error made in efforts to
effect change in action (e.g., improve collaboration) is to identify the technical aspect and apply technical means without attending to the adaptive
elements. In looking at the research and literature related to collaborative
practice in health care, the emphasis on technical solutions is evident. For
example, two technical solutions that have been identified include teamwork and communication.

While it makes sense that teamwork is necessary to collaboration,
understanding the adaptive challenges of teamwork in health care is crucial. For example, while technically a "health care team" approach makes
sense, making this a reality is not a straightforward process. Richardson,
Wright, and Cuthbertson (2010) emphasize the distinction between a
team whose members work in concert and engage in interdependent tasks
toward the accomplishment of shared and meaningful goals via coordinated processes and an ad hoc grouping of health care providers who each
provide some form of health care to a particular patient population. These
researchers highlight how collaboration rests upon a particular definition
of team as (a) two or more individuals who (b) socially interact (face-to-face
or increasingly virtually); (c) possess one or more common goals; (d) are
brought together to perform organizationally relevant tasks; (e) exhibit
interdependencies with respect to work flow, goals, and outcomes; (f) have

different roles and responsibilities; and (g) are together embedded in an encompassing organizational system with boundaries and linkages to the broader system context and task environment (p. 79).

Similarly, good communication has been identified as essential to collaborative practice. Research suggests that effective interprofessional communication can positively influence patient satisfaction, symptom control such as pain management, and patient outcomes (Curtis, Tzannes, & Rudge, 2011; Sargeant, MacLeod, & Murray, 2011). Yet, research also suggests that poor communication and team collaboration between health care providers is a persistent challenge (Bokhour, 2006; Bronstein, 2003; DeLoach, 2003; Hartrick Doane, Stajduhar, Bidgood, Causton, & Cox, 2012; Reese & Sontag, 2001; Wittenberg-Lyles, Parker Oliver, Demiris, & Regehr, 2009). While it is possible to teach the technical aspect (e.g., communication skills training), the adaptive challenge of communication needs to be considered. For example, SBAR (situation, background, assessment, recommendation) is a communication tool that is widely used to help nurses organize their thoughts prior to calling physicians. It is a structured way of communicating that provides a brief, organized, predictable flow of information so nurses can be clear and concise when speaking with physicians. In other words, it offers a technical solution. In recommending the use of SBAR, Thomas, Bertram and Johnson (2009) contend that nurses and physicians are educated differently and thus communicate differently. They suggest that this difference arises because nurses are taught to be descriptive in their thought and spoken language, whereas physicians are concise in thought and speak in shorter sentences. Thus, they propose that nurses should use SBAR to better align their communication with physicians to improve communication and team functioning. This assumption that the best solution is for nurses to align their communication style with that of physicians is interesting from a power relations perspective. What is also interesting is how the technical solution (SBAR) is being employed to address the adaptive challenge (differing education and language practices).

Without doubt, teamwork and communication are important ingredients of effective collaborative practice, and many of the technical solutions being employed are helpful. However, a relational perspective draws your attention beyond the technical strategies that are typically suggested to examine how both teamwork and communication are adaptive challenges that are contextually influenced and arise from historical, economic, sociopolitical, and linguistic contexts and power dynamics.

From a relational perspective, merely addressing the technical aspects of communication or teamwork is not sufficient. Simply "adding" communications skills training or tools or integrating team building exercises will not result in effective collaborative practice if other adaptive issues are not considered. For example, while tools like SBAR might be helpful, as Curtis and colleagues (2011) describe, historical factors have shaped each profession's roles, responsibilities, and the power relations between them. And these traditional structures and relations can lead to fundamental differences that arise in areas of conflict and disagreement. For example, while there may be an overlap in the focus and content of medical and nursing education, just as with communication styles, each profession brings differing perspectives, values, and approaches to their work (Woodhall, Vertacnik, &

McLaughlin, 2008). Thus, even if they are both working toward the "health care" of a particular person or population, the focus and priorities perceived by each may be quite different (Curtis et al., 2011). Even what is considered to constitute effective teamwork might differ. For example, Finn (2008) found that nurses in the OR equated teamwork with a "relational repertoire" of respect, appreciation, and courtesy while physicians equated the more technical-instrumental aspects, including efficiency and coordination, as markers of effective teamwork. Similarly, Nathanson et al. (2011) describe how, in researching teamwork and collaboration in ICUs, nurses consistently gave more negative responses on every survey question than did physicians. While nurses experienced the amount of collaboration as inadequate, physicians were satisfied. The views between the two groups were most divergent on questions about overall satisfaction with team decisions, which points to differences in power and how decisions were made. These researchers concluded that a different collaborative effort between physicians and nurses is needed to improve nurses' satisfaction on a critical care team.

Once again, this is where the relational perspective—and relational inquiry specifically— can be helpful. Relational inquiry draws attention to adaptive challenges and the many levels of difference that shape interprofessional communication and teamwork. The value of a relational inquiry view was illustrated during recent research that I (Gweneth) was involved in with a team of colleagues (Hartrick Doane et al., 2012). During our research, which focused on improving end-of-life care in acute medical and long-term care (LTC) facilities, participants (including nurses, physicians, and allied health practitioners) told us that they needed "to work as a team" and "to communicate more." Yet, we had observed and our data confirmed that there was not a *lack* of communication or coordinated teamwork. Rather, the problem seemed to be *the nature and patterns* of communication and teamwork that were constraining collaborative palliative care. As we researched the factors shaping and informing existing patterns of communication and the consequences of those existing patterns, we discovered that the complex interworking of people, roles, differing knowledge bases, and power relations were creating relational disjunctures that were constraining collaboration.

TO ILLUSTRATE

Working Together When We Have to

In listening to the health care providers, we came to recognize that they understood teamwork as an either/or—either people worked as a team (and communicated) or they did not work as a team (and did not communicate). However, in observing their communication/teamwork in action, it was possible to see a far more complex relational process at play.

continued on page 404

TO ILLUSTRATE *continued*

Working Together When We Have to

While all of the health providers espoused the importance of team, a central feature of their work was the autonomous way that each practitioner worked within his or her professional purview and attended to his or her individual patient assignment. This juxtaposition of teamwork and autonomy was highly significant. Specifically, while the team members worked autonomously, they simultaneously worked in concert with the team's normative pattern of staying out of each other's way.

For example, to enable their interprofessional colleagues to do their respective jobs, the nurses quite literally left the room to "get out of the way" when other team members entered patient rooms. Paradoxically, they related to each other (worked as a team) by staying out of each other's way. And it was evident that this way of working within and through interpersonal spaces of care served to reinforce the gap between them. Although they wanted more collaborative teamwork, working collaboratively was only really sanctioned when it was not possible to proceed autonomously. Thus, there was a disjuncture between what they were wanting and how they were actually enacting teamwork.

This way of working as a team also shaped communication practices. For example, team members only communicated when it was required for their particular aspect of patient care. Moreover, it didn't really matter how skilled a practitioner was at communicating since on both units there was a knowledge hierarchy that profoundly affected the communication processes and determined how a particular member's questions and/or information was received and how it was valued and/or used. This knowledge hierarchy also shaped whether a team member was informed, whether and how much time was allotted to them to communicate, the nature and amount of communication that occurred, and to which resources they had access. Everyday examples included distinctions about who gave report to whom and in what form, who charted where, who was invited to attend clinical care meetings, who waited to speak to whom, and so forth.

Interestingly, this knowledge hierarchy was experienced and perpetuated all the way down the hierarchy. While in some cases RNs expressed distress that their knowledge was not being valued by physicians or administrators (they were not communicated to), the care aides often described the way in which RNs wielded the same kind of knowledge authority over them. For example, while care aides were expected to have the knowledge to manage and respond to residents, because they were seen as "only aides," they often were not given important information about residents, nor were communication avenues available for them to share their knowledge (e.g., they were not allowed to chart what they knew about the resident in the formal health record).

The analogy of playing hockey without a game plan was used to describe their "team" experience. *"If you think of, oh, let's say a hockey team right now where you only tell certain people on the team certain things about the*

continued on page 405

TO ILLUSTRATE *continued*

Working Together When We Have to

game and the rest you say, 'That's OK, you just go out there and skate the best you can. You hit the puck whenever you can and that's all. But you don't need to know the strategy and all that.' I mean you wouldn't be able to play the game. And so when you leave people out of that and kind of say, 'No, no, you don't need to know, you just get information and feed it back to us,' it doesn't allow you to be part of the team" (Hartrick Doane et al., 2012, p. 7).

This knowledge/communication dynamic also played out between RNs and physicians. For example, physicians often did not inform RNs about advance care plans for patients so that the nurses were at times left in the dark as to the specific direction care was taking. Yet at the same time, the physicians experienced frustration when the nurses did not meet their expectations in terms of being knowledgeable practitioners when they phoned for information about a patient. This dynamic was further exacerbated by time restraints. As members were positioned according to role distinctions, they were subsequently allotted varying levels of "legitimacy" to take time to communicate. For example, a physician could request information and take the time from anyone on the hierarchy, while those in other positions within the hierarchy did not have the same privilege.

In the above description, notice how knowledge, power, and authority are relationally connected in collaborative practice—and how this relational dynamic can enhance and/or constrain teamwork and communication. For example, in the study, pain control was one of the primary nursing concerns. The nurses on the medical units described numerous situations where they had watched a patient have a "bad death" because of inadequate analgesia. These situations were frequently filled with tension and poor collegial collaboration between the physicians and the nurses, and the nurses felt powerless in getting what they considered to be adequate symptom control for their patients. It was evident that enhancing effective collaborative practice required careful consideration of how knowledge, power, and authority were shaping response-ability to the patient concerns nurses were trying to address—and how collaboration was an adaptive challenge.

The Challenges of Collaboration

Heifetz's (1998) emphasis on adaptive challenges is in line with what we think nurses need to collaborate effectively in health care. While technical solutions such as SBAR might be helpful, nurses also need to intentionally relate to the adaptive challenges that are part and parcel of collaborative practice. And a relational view can help them do so. For example, because of the relative lack of interprofessional education in undergraduate curricula, new nurses and other professionals often start their careers with little understanding about each other's professional vocabulary, culture, values, strengths, roles, and approaches (Schwartz et al., 2011). How then do practitioners learn to adapt their practice to work across those professional differences?

To address the adaptive challenges, many nursing programs and health care organizations are now offering interprofessional educational opportunities for health care providers. A key premise behind these programs is that developing the ability to understand the differences and interact with other practitioners early on might serve to facilitate collaboration. Maureen Ryan, a nursing instructor involved in developing interprofessional educative opportunities describes her own work in this area.

TO ILLUSTRATE
Learning Interprofessionally

One of the teaching strategies that I have recently incorporated into the fourth year consolidated practice experience is a high-fidelity simulation learning activity. The learning activity is designed to gather both subjective and objective data from the registered nursing student and first-year medical resident about their confidence, knowledge, and skill in assessing and managing (through effective decision making and actions) complex patient care situations. What we have learned to date about the possibilities of promoting interprofessional practices was summed up well recently by my physician colleague who stated, "We need the nurses in our simulation scenarios. It just doesn't work for one of the residents to play a nurse; we really do not know the role of the nurse."

I agree and note that incorporating residents into nursing simulations offers us the same opportunity. It is in the working through of the assessment and planning of interventions for patients' presenting symptoms that our students share how each "sees" the patients, the priorities in their assessment and planning, and the forms of knowledge that support those priorities.

For example, in one case simulation, a nursing student cares for a man who presented to the emergency department with acute abdominal pain and distension, nausea, periumbilical pain, diarrhea, and anorexia. The student's task is to assess the patient and act according to his/her assessment. As part of the process, the nurse discovers that a routine order exists for Tylenol plain, and she, the patient, and his wife do not think that is enough. The student must call the medical resident who then assesses the patient. They both engage in discussion about how to best manage the patient's pain while in the hospital. In a controlled and safe environment, the students have an opportunity to work through the hot spots, for example, when the nurse and physician role do not seem to be on the same page. As facilitators, we have an opportunity to help the students recognize the importance of clearly communicating to each other expectations about patient care.

Maureen describes one of the most important requirements for effective collaborative practice—that of understanding the differences between team members by gaining more understanding and role clarity to work across those differences. Understanding different professional roles is referred to as "role sharing" in the interprofessional literature (Barrett, Greenwood, & Ross, 2003; Pearson & Pandya, 2006). The intent in role sharing is to enable practitioners to gain the role clarity needed for effective collaboration.

Similar to Maureen's description, Orchard (2010) contends that providing opportunities for nurses to talk about their roles and consider the complementary nature of their knowledge and skills with other interprofessional colleagues is crucial. At the same time, Orchard (2010) describes how "this seemingly simple task, which by the way if you try it, you will learn how difficult a task this is to provide, is a means to correct myths and help all team members learn how others with similar skills sets can assist in providing care" (p. 251).

How Can Relational Inquiry Support Collaboration?

Relational inquiry brings "what" has been identified as the important constituents of effective collaborative practice together with "how to" proceed toward more effective collaboration. Taking a relational inquiry approach to collaborative practice enables you as a practitioner to practice more confidently from your nursing standpoint and simultaneously act in respectful and collaborative ways with colleagues. Earlier in the book, we used the analogy of a nurse being like a boat that has all the workable parts yet is missing a navigational system—which relational inquiry provides. Within that navigational system, our nursing commitments and standpoint serve as the anchor and power source. As nurses busily rush around trying to meet the multiple demands and obligations that are pressing in upon them, it is their commitments to the well-being of people/families, to their own well-being and that of their colleagues with whom they work, and to the well-being of the health care system that both ignites and orients them to the "right" action. *Being a committed, competent effective nurse* requires a continual checking in with what it is that you are working toward. It requires paying attention to the choices you are making and noticing when you may be acting out of alignment with a nursing standpoint and your own values and goals.

As nurses, you will practice in all sorts of contexts, and in each context there will be dominant ideologies, normative practices, competing interests, and relational challenges. Relational inquiry directs you to (a) consciously look for and be mindful of the values, ideologies, reference points, power dynamics, knowledge, truths, normative practices, and automatized rules that are at play, (b) critically examine the relational interplay occurring within a situation (including the five Ws of your own relating), and (c) consciously choose how you will relate and act from your nursing standpoint. To help you do so, we outline some specific strategies targeted toward collaborative practice in the hard spots.

STRATEGIES FOR COLLABORATIVE PRACTICE IN THE HARD SPOTS

Beales and colleagues (2011) contend that to practice effectively, health care providers need to build collaborative competencies (e.g., role clarity, effective communication). Similarly, Sargeant, Loney, and Murphy (2008) suggest that shared understandings of the differing professions and respect for the unique contributions of each, a commitment to work at teamwork, and having the practical "know-how" for sharing patient care are necessary ingredients for effective collaborative practice.

In Table 10.1 we outline four working strategies that can guide your action when collaborating in hard spots when differing values and interests are at play. These strategies are not really different from what we have already presented in Chapter 9, but they are ones that are specifically oriented to navigating hard spots. Basically, they are like a condensed version that you can keep in your back pocket and pull out when you find yourself in the midst of challenging situations. These strategies and the collaboration checkpoints we identify under each one provide a way of orienting and responding in your day-to-day work and in the hard spots that arise as you work across differences. They support the cultivation of a compassionate, inquisitive approach through which you do not just have to rely on your own view and/or settle for how things are. The strategies and collaboration checkpoints offer a way of engaging in an open-minded inquiry into situations and possibilities.

As you work within challenging situations, the strategies and checkpoints we have outlined in previous chapters can also serve you well, and we encourage you to draw on them. The HP and critical lenses, five Cs and five Ws, ideals, values (including nursing theories and ethics), and processes offer direction for questions to help you cultivate your nursing standpoint and the habit and practice of responsive collaboration. It is important to keep in mind that practice is both a noun and a verb—that disciplined, effective nursing action takes ongoing practice. It requires a willingness to be challenged, uncertain, to experience emotions without projecting and labeling, and to not turn away from difficulty as differences arise. It also requires that you are compassionate with yourself and others when you or they act in less-than-perfect ways.

As with the strategies we have previously outlined, each of the strategies and collaboration checkpoints below can serve as questions or cues to guide action.

Table 10.1: Collaborative Practice in the Hard Spots

Strategy 1: Relate to What Is

Collaborative Checkpoint 1.1: Relate to the emotion, not the trigger.
Collaborative Checkpoint 1.2: Remember the five Cs.
Collaborative Checkpoint 1.3: Don't throw the second dart or set up the target.
Collaborative Checkpoint 1.4: Stay in the present moment.

Strategy 2: Relate Appropriately in Inappropriate Situations

Collaborative Checkpoint 2.1: Enlist the five Ws.
Collaborative Checkpoint 2.2: Don't eat the poison.
Collaborative Checkpoint 2.3: Don't "thing" it.
Collaborative Checkpoint 2.4: Be discerning and deliberate.

Strategy 3: Act to Promote Well-Being

Collaborative Checkpoint 3.1: Look for capacity.
Collaborative Checkpoint 3.2: Take in the good.
Collaborative Checkpoint 3.3: Look for the "join."

Strategy 4: Be a Transforming Presence

Collaborative Checkpoint 4.1: Be the change you wish to see.
Collaborative Checkpoint 4.2: Play the cards to the best of your ability.

Strategy 1: Relate to What Is

We have already emphasized "relating to what is" as part of the relational inquiry approach. As we described in Chapter 9, relating to what is can be particularly challenging when in hard spots of conflict or when we experience other forms of difference. Thus, we include it as the first strategy of collaborative practice both as a reminder and as a way of orienting yourself. Orienting to "what is" can be supported by the following four checkpoints.

Collaboration Checkpoint 1.1: Relate to the Emotion, Not the Trigger

When we experience differences between ourselves and others and find ourselves in hard spots, most often, emotions are triggered—both our own and those of others. Importantly, we often respond to these emotions by avoiding relating to them. For example, we might try to free ourselves from the intensity of having to feel the emotion by projecting it onto someone else, swallowing it, distracting ourselves by "doing" something, and so forth, or we might focus our attention on what triggered the emotion (we focus our attention on what or at whom we are mad).

Relational inquiry directs you to consciously and intentionally relate to the emotion as itself—to actually stop long enough to feel what you are feeling and let it dissipate. If we let the emotion run rampant (just react) or if we focus attention on the trigger (on the event that sparked it), we are far less likely to relate to the actual situation appropriately. Moreover, the emotion and our subsequent actions will probably have a harmful impact on well-being.

Thus, an important checkpoint when you find yourself in the midst of a hard spot is to consciously choose to relate to emotions. As we described in Chapter 3, emotions can serve as value antennae; they can draw attention to what really matters to us or to things we are holding within us that need healing. Thus, the more effectively you relate to the emotion, the more effectively you can deal with the event and orient to the well-being of all involved. The same goes with other people's emotions. If a physician lashes out in anger, often, we try to avoid that anger or do something with it. By simply letting the anger be and relating to it just as it is—as an emotion that a particular person is feeling at that moment in time—you can more thoughtfully consider your options. Rather than lashing back in anger, retaliating, or getting defensive, you can take a moment to think before you respond. Importantly, if you "let the emotion be" by not adding anything else onto it (e.g., making interpretations of yourself or others—I am right, you are wrong) or becoming embroiled in it, it will have a chance to dissipate.

Collaboration Checkpoint 1.2: Remember the Five Cs

The five Cs can aid you as you attempt to relate to emotions and hard spots more consciously. The five Cs remind you to:

- Be compassionate with yourself and others—to relate human being to human being.
- Be curious, interested, inquisitive, and open to what is and to the uncertainty of the situation.

- Actively and consciously choose the values and concerns that will orient your response and continually monitor how your actions are aligning with those commitments.
- Competently use your knowledge, judgment, skills, energy, and capacities to respond effectively to promote the well-being of all involved and adequately address the demands of your professional responsibility.
- Correspond to the situation by relating to and with people in a way that takes the differing meanings and concerns into consideration—that enables you to connect across difference.

One example of how we might check in with ourselves in this way was given by a nurse who participated in an ethics research project our team conducted (Rodney et al., 2002). The nurse described that she monitored her practice by asking herself each day, "If I were a patient on this ward, would I want me for my nurse today?" Asking herself this question and realizing that sometimes the answer was "no" helped her more consciously decide how she wanted to be in practice and constantly reminded her to respond to the people she was caring for and those with whom she was collaborating.

Collaboration Checkpoint 1.3: Don't Throw the Second Dart or Set up the Target

Hard spots can be unpleasant and even hurtful. We have had experiences and witnessed colleagues saying derogatory or cruel things, acting in disrespectful and demeaning ways, and generally being uncollaborative. We are sorry to say that we have also been that way ourselves at times. When others throw the first dart (act in hurtful or disrespectful ways), we can often be triggered to respond by throwing a second dart (Chodron, 2002). In doing so, we inadvertently set ourselves up as a target. As Pema Chodron (2002) explains, each time we retaliate with aggressive words and actions, we actually strengthen negative behaviors, and as long as we do so, plenty of arrows will come our way. As we become increasingly irritated by others, we also become more like a walking target.

This does not mean that you should not respond to problematic behavior—rather it is a question of *how* to respond effectively. Focused on ultimately enhancing well-being, you respond by not throwing a second dart and/or setting yourself up as a target for further harm.

Collaboration Checkpoint 1.4: Stay in the Present Moment

One way to not set yourself up as a target is to stay in the present moment. From a relational inquiry perspective, there is a temporal aspect to experience; our present time experiences are shaped by what has occurred in the past and what we anticipate in the future as much as what is occurring in the moment. If you pay attention to yourself in any current moment, you will find that it takes a great deal of disciplined attention to stay in the present moment. Often, you are oriented toward your next step; you focus attention on what it means, on responding, and so forth. The distinction we made in Chapter 9 between listening and waiting to speak is a great example of how our attention can be future-oriented. In essence, Strategy 1 reminds you to bring mindful attention to the present moment—to really tune in to the here and now and "let be" so you can be as informed and responsive as possible.

TRY IT OUT 10.5
Washing Your Hands to Focus

Lesley Moss, a nurse colleague who is currently the executive director of occupational health and safety in the health region where I (Gweneth) live, offered a wise suggestion to the students I am teaching this term. In discussing the challenges of working in hectic health care settings, Leslie suggested that one effective way to build in a timeout (and reset your bearings when you are feeling frazzled) is to wash your hands. "No one is ever going to criticize you for washing your hands—they might criticize you for stopping for a timeout, but they will never question hand washing." Leslie's suggestion is a great example of one way you might stop for a minute and check in with yourself to consciously focus your attention. Pausing even for 60 seconds and purposefully stepping out of the frazzle to slowly and gently wash your hands can give you the relational space to do a quick attention check. You can pause to notice what is happening intrapersonally, interpersonally, and contextually, consciously consider your choices, and more consciously decide how to focus your attention and action within the situation as it is.

Strategy 2: Relate Appropriately in Inappropriate Situations

A helpful working strategy to keep in mind when you find yourself in hard spots is to try to relate appropriately even in inappropriate situations. To illustrate this strategy, we describe a situation that I (Gweneth) experienced a few years ago when I did an observation shift on a medical unit as part of our research into nursing ethics (Hartrick Doane, Storch, & Pauly, 2009).

TO ILLUSTRATE
Relating to a Chipped Cup

The observation shift involved buddying with one of the staff nurses so I could get to know the nurses and develop more of an inside view into the everyday work on the unit. The shift began with the team convening in the meeting room to listen to a recorded report from the previous shift. Five minutes into report, one of the nurses who had been on the night shift burst through the door carrying a yellow coffee cup. Slamming the cup onto the table, the nurse who was visibly upset demanded to know, "Who chipped my cup?" There was a stunned silence as everyone looked

continued on page 412

TO ILLUSTRATE *continued*

Relating to a Chipped Cup

up in surprise. Getting no response, the nurse exclaimed, "I want whoever did this to own up to it." Looking at the faces of her colleagues, I could see their shock at the inappropriateness of her behavior.

After report, I enlisted my relational inquiry strategies to inquire further into the situation. My understanding expanded as I learned that the nurse had worked a 12-hour shift caring for a number of very ill patients with only a junior nurse with little experience to assist her. As a result, there were things left undone for the day staff in spite of the fact that the nurse had had no breaks during the entire night. Her chipped coffee cup was an apt metaphor for how she herself was feeling—the combination of exhaustion, feeling like she had let the other staff down, and the response of the day staff to the uncompleted tasks left her feeling like a chipped cup.

As our team continued to do observation shifts on the unit, we came to view the chipped cup as a symbol for what was happening on the unit overall. We observed everyone working hard to keep things going and ensure good care for patients. We also observed a growing pattern of inappropriate situations leading to inappropriate actions—there was a gradual chipping away of resources, of energy, of pride, of well-being, and of relationships, and as a result, the nurses' behavior began to change.

Collaboration Checkpoint 2.1: Enlist the Five Ws

The five Ws can serve as a helpful orienting checkpoint when you are in hard spots and want to relate appropriately. They enable you to both monitor your experience and actions and to consciously focus your attention on the "who, what, why, when, and where" of the situation so you can more effectively respond. They also can help you identify colleagues who may be in need of support and/or problematic patterns that are developing and impeding the well-being of patients, of staff, and contexts.

Collaboration Checkpoint 2.2: Don't Eat the Poison

Another helpful checkpoint is to pay attention to our own responses—to what we are saying to ourselves, how we are responding to our own emotions, and the impacts of our inner processes on our actions. For example, often, we "hold" the remnants of an upsetting experience because we don't quite know what to do with them. Someone does something we experience as hurtful or disrespectful, and the leftover emotion serves as a trigger or fodder for future experiences—for how we see and relate to that person in the future (e.g., we are fearful of that physician who yelled at us, hold a grudge against that colleague who judged us, etc.). While most of us tend to hold tight to our reactions, ironically, it is most often ourselves who suffer when we do so. Chodron (2002) exemplifies this in her example of holding a grudge—as if holding a grudge were going to make us happy and ease our pain. She contends that holding a grudge is comparable to eating rat poison and thinking the rat will die. When we hold a grudge, the one most hurt is ourselves.

Therefore, a helpful checkpoint is to remember not to eat the poison (Chodron, 2002). Not eating the poison does not mean we stifle our own responses. It means that we respond with compassion to ourselves and to others—that we feel and respond to whatever arises and stay open enough to heal and let it go. While sometimes, as in the case of the chipped cup, there are rational explanations for people's behavior, at other times we may not understand why people act as they do. Regardless of what your inquiry illuminates (whether you can empathize or someone is just being ornery), in all cases, well-being requires that we heal and let go of negativity. As Nepo (2005) contends, sometimes nothing can be done except to give the wound air, "which in the case of the heart means saying deeply, without aversion or self-pity, 'Ouch'" (p. 44). In those times, it is a matter of focusing our attention on how to relate in ways that leave our own integrity intact and that do no further harm.

Collaboration Checkpoint 2.3: Don't "Thing" It

One helpful checkpoint to help us avoid eating the poison is to listen to our thing-thinking—to how we name or identify people and situations. Comparable to the distinction between still shots and moving pictures, we often relate to people and situations by freezing or "thinging" them (Hartrick Doane, in press; Holecek, 2009). We look through our own interpretive frames and turn complex relational living experience into still shots as we define, judge, label, and assign meaning to people and circumstances (people are good, bad, arrogant, disrespectful, incompetent, etc.). Regardless of the accuracy of our interpretations (e.g., some behavior *is* harmful), what is relationally significant is the way in which this process of "thinging" solidifies our understandings and hinders our relational responsiveness (Hartrick Doane, in press).

An example of how thing-thinking can limit us is offered by Vietnamese Zen master Thich Nhat Hanh in his book *Being Peace*. He tells the story of a man who was rowing his boat upstream on a misty morning when he saw another boat coming downstream. The boat was coming directly at him so he shouted, "Be careful! Watch out!" But the boat ran right into him. The man became very angry and began to shout at the other person, giving him a piece of his mind. But when he stopped yelling and looked closely, he saw that there was no one in the other boat. His reaction to the same situation completely changed when he realized that the boat had just gotten loose and drifted downstream. When the "thing" was a runaway boat rather than a careless boatsman, the man's experience completely changed. He went from anger to laughter in a single moment (laughing at himself for shouting at an empty boat). The actual happenings did not change—his boat had still gotten hit—what made the difference to his reaction was the "thing" he created in his mind. By paying attention to how we are interpreting and labeling (how we are thing-thinking) people and situations through our own selective and limited frameworks, we can extend our relational effectiveness substantially.

Collaboration Checkpoint 2.4: Be Discerning and Deliberate

The fourth checkpoint to help us relate more appropriately is that of being discerning and deliberate. Paying attention to the normative ways of relating (our own and others) and the competing interests and concerns that may be at play in any situation enables you to be more discerning and deliberate—to identify the salient aspects, discern your most appropriate response, and act accordingly. When you are in hard spots, consider the following questions:

- What is the primary concern in the situation?
- What are the primary nursing commitments?
- What are the important factors to consider in identifying those concerns and commitments?
- What am I obligated to address?
- What is challenging for me in this situation?
- How might I best promote well-being?

Strategy 3: Act to Promote Well-Being

From a nursing standpoint, the overriding goal of any action is to promote well-being. As we have discussed throughout this book, relational inquiry is focused on promoting the well-being of patients/families, health care providers, and the health care system. Thus, an important working strategy to bring to your collaborative practice is that of acting to promote well-being.

Collaboration Checkpoint 3.1: Look for Capacity

Throughout the earlier chapters, we have discussed the idea of bringing a capacity orientation to your nursing work. That same half-full view can serve you well as you collaborate in the hard spots. Often in hard spots, our attention focuses on what is not going well, on the difficulties we are experiencing, and/or what we are not able to do. While of course you need to clearly discern the challenges you are facing, looking for the capacities in the situation can help you address those challenges. For example, reread the opening story in Chapter 1 looking for capacity. While obviously there were challenging collaborative relations affecting the care of the man and his wife, what capacities can you identify in the nurse? When I (Gweneth) first heard that nurse's story during our research, I was struck by her capacity to maintain her nursing standpoint and provide such responsive nursing care in the midst of such difficult circumstances. From a capacity perspective, I was also struck by the deeper stirrings that were rumbling within her—the questions she was asking herself were sites from which to consider how the capacity within herself, her nursing unit, and the organization to care for patients and families at end-of-life might be extended.

You can enlist your focus on capacity to promote well-being. For example, in my earlier example of talking to the head of housekeeping, I (Colleen) noted that she had begun to solve the problem ("It sounds as though you think something else is going on") and mentioned her generally good rapport with the nursing staff as a way of supporting her intention to discuss the problem directly with the nurses.

Collaboration Checkpoint 3.2: Take in the Good

Looking for capacity enables you to take in the good that is present in your nursing work. Hanson (2009) describes how the brain preferentially scans for and registers unpleasant or negative aspects: "It's like Velcro for negative experiences and Teflon for positive ones" (p. 68). Certainly, as a nurse working in health care settings that are ripe with competing interests and values—where corporate decisions can trump decisions about well-being—you will find yourself experiencing many challenges. That makes it all the more important to consciously take in the good—to take in those moments when you see a patient responding to treatment and growing in strength, when you share a joke or a moment of heartfelt connection. When I (Gweneth) was working as a nurse at the bedside, one of the "goods" that I would intentionally take in was looking for a moment at the seriously ill patients after I had given morning care, visually seeing them relax into the freshness of clean linens and the feeling of having bathed and been cared for—savoring that feeling of having helped ease their illness experience if only briefly.

Collaboration Checkpoint 3.3: Look for the Join

Using a relational inquiry approach to connect across difference directs you to look for the "join"—that meeting space in between differences where ambiguity and ambivalence reside (Bhabha, 1994). Differences, whether they are differences in values, beliefs, privileges, practices, concerns, or experiences, both challenge and offer us the greatest opportunities to learn about ourselves, learn about others, and learn about contexts. Like the point where one metal part is soldered to another, a join can be a place of weakness or a place of strength greater than that of the original materials. Focusing on the join creates the opportunity for significant differences to be attended to and acknowledged. It can also shift us from an adversarial relationship (a contest of wills or working "against") to a place of commonality from which to collaborate. It enables you to look for what you might hold in common. For example, in the research focused on improving end-of-life care that I (Gweneth) mentioned earlier (Hartrick Doane et al., 2012), it became evident that one place where all of the health care providers were joined was in their desire to ensure good end-of-life care. They were also in agreement that the way they were working as a team was not serving that purpose. These joins offered sites from which to consider how they might enhance their collaborative practice.

Strategy 4: Be a Transforming Presence

Presence is accepted as a core aspect of relational engagement in nursing and has been defined as a nursing intervention that takes the form of being with and being there (Covington, 2003; McMahon & Christopher, 2011). Covington (2003) describes that presence can provide a context "to put thoughts and feeling into words . . . [and to] see new perspectives and make decisions. Implicit here is the understanding that presence is an existential way of being-with another consistent with the professional value of commitment and authenticity within the nurse-patient relationship" (p. 306).

While nursing presence tends to be equated with nurse–patient relationships, relational inquiry extends the understanding and enactment of presence. Presence is a form of consciousness one brings to situations—mindful attention enacted through positive regard, genuineness, and involvement. As we explained using complexity theory in Chapter 8, as a nurse, you always have a relational impact of some sort. Relational inquiry instructs you to make a conscious choice about the potential of that impact. Specifically, the intent underlying relational inquiry is that you will be a transforming presence—transforming in the energetic sense of resonating and creating a relational space in which well-being can flourish.

In Chapter 4, we invited you to do an "influence experiment" to try intentionally to influence a social situation with your presence, energy, and action. Now we invite you to take that capacity to influence purposefully into every moment of care.

Collaboration Checkpoint 4.1: Be the Change You Wish to See

To borrow the words of Mahatma Gandhi, one of the most powerful ways to be a transforming presence is "to be the change you wish to see in the world." That question: "Am I *being* the change I wish to see?" offers a simple and direct way to check in with yourself—to take a deep breath when in the midst of a hard spot, and center in your nursing standpoint in the commitment and obligation to promote well-being as you discern and make a deliberate decision about how to proceed.

Collaboration Checkpoint 4.2: Play the Cards to the Best of Your Ability

The final checkpoint that can be helpful when working in hard spots is (to use the metaphor of a card game) to play the existing cards to the best of your ability. As we have described, currently, nursing is positioned in a power and knowledge hierarchy that tends toward subordinating nursing knowledge and concerns. Although we might prefer a different hand of cards (and there are certainly settings in which the power relations are more equitable and collaborative), coming from a nursing standpoint of relational inquiry enables you to see the cards as they are in any moment. In doing so, you are well-positioned to use your knowledge, skills, and compassion to act in ways that are responsive and just.

TRY IT-OUT 10.5
Dog Bite and a Hard Spot

The following story was told to me (Gweneth) by an emergency room nurse, Karin Kim-Yang, who recently took a relational inquiry course. As you read the story, put yourself in Karin's place, and consider how you might enlist the working strategies and checkpoints to act in this "hard spot" situation.

I was triaging a woman who had been bit by a pit bull in her right hand. She had visible puncture wounds in her hand, along with swelling and redness. She told me that her fingers were completely numb and that her hand was in pain. I decided that because of the hand numbness,

continued on page 417

TRY IT OUT 10.5 *continued*
Dog Bite and a Hard Spot

possible tendon damage, the amount of pain she was in, and the wounds on her hand, this patient should be made a level 3 and stay in the emergency room instead of the urgent care area. I called over the radio for a level 3 dog bite and was assigned a room. The nurse that was going to receive this woman as her patient [we will call her Mandy], marched into my triage room, picked up this woman's hand, and said to me, "Why can't she go to urgent care?" I politely excused myself and walked to the nurse's station with Mandy and told her why she was staying in the emergency room. Mandy looked at me and said, "You know she is just a drug seeker, she comes here all the time." There was nothing more I could say to Mandy; she was convinced that this woman was faking her pain. I was left with a sobbing patient because her nurse caused more pain by picking up her hand and a coworker who was angry that she was being "given" a so-called drug seeker.

Choose one checkpoint from each of the four strategies, and explain in writing how it might apply to this situation.

THIS WEEK IN PRACTICE
Practicing Collaborative Practice

This week in practice, intentionally take the ideas from this chapter with you to try out. First, look for differences and points of contention. Pay attention to who is involved, what seems to be the source of contention, and how power is playing out. Consider how those involved are differently positioned within the knowledge hierarchy. See what emotions you can observe. To what extent are anxiety, anger, defensiveness, frustration, and avoidance evident? What role are nurses playing? Can you identify one strategy that might move the situation more effectively toward collaborative practice?

YOUR RELATIONAL INQUIRY TOOLBOX

Add these tools to your relational inquiry toolbox.
- Consciously center your practice in a nursing standpoint.
- Commit to your nursing values and goals.
- Value your nursing knowledge.
- Pay attention and relate to the adaptive challenges.
- Enlist the collaborate inquiry strategies and checkpoints.

REFERENCES

Bandura, A. (2001). Social cognitive theory: An agentic perspective. *Annual Review of Psychology, 52*, 1–26.

Barrett, G., Greenwood, R., & Ross, K. (2003). Integrating interprofessional education into 10 health and social care programmes. *Journal of Interprofessional Care, 17*(3), 293–301.

Bartfay, W. J., Bartfay, E., Clow, K. A., & Wu, T. (2010). Attitudes and perceptions towards men in nursing education. *Internet Journal of Allied Health Sciences & Practice, 8*(2), 1–7.

Beal, E. (2012). Nursing's image on YouTube. *American Journal of Nursing, 112*(10), 17.

Beales, J., Walji, R., Papoushek, C., & Austin, Z. (2011). Exploring professional culture in the context of family health team interprofessional collaboration. *Health and Interprofessional Practice, 1*(1), eP1004.

Benner, P., Sutphen, M., Leonard, V., & Day, L. (2010). *Educating nurses: A call for radical transformation*. San Francisco, CA: Jossey-Bass.

Bhabha, H. (1994). *The location of culture*. London, United Kingdom: Routledge.

Bokhour, B. G. (2006). Communication in interdisciplinary team meetings: What are we talking about? *Journal of Interprofessional Care, 20*(4), 349–363.

Bronstein, L. R. (2003). A model for interdisciplinary collaboration. *Social Work, 48*(3), 297–306.

Canadian Nurses Association. (2007). Framework for the practice of registered nurses in Canada. Ottawa, Ontario, Canada: Author.

Chesser-Smyth, P. A., & Long, T. (2013). Understanding the influences on self confidence among first-year undergraduate nursing students in Ireland. *Journal of Advanced Nursing, 69*(1), 145–157.

Chodron, P. (2002). *The places that scare you. A guide to fearlessness in difficult times*. Boston: Shambhala Press.

Covington, H. (2003). Caring presence: Delineation of a concept for holistic nursing. *Journal of Holistic Nursing, 21*(3), 301–317.

Curtis, K., Tzannes, A., & Rudge, T. (2011). How to talk to doctors—A guide for effective communication. *International Nursing Review, 58*, 13–20.

Davidhizar, R. (1993). Self-confidence: A requirement for collaborative practice. *Dimensions of Critical Care Nursing, 12*(4), 218–222.

DeLoach, R. (2003). Job satisfaction among hospice interdisciplinary team members. *American Journal of Hospice & Palliative Care, 20*(6), 434–440.

Doane, G. H., & Varcoe, C. (2008). Knowledge translation in everyday nursing: From evidence-based to inquiry-based practice. *Advances in Nursing Science, 31*(4), 283–295.

Duchscher, J., & Myrick, F. (2008). The prevailing winds of oppression: Understanding the new graduate experience in acute care. *Nursing Forum, 43*(4), 191–206.

Dyck, J. M., Oliffe, J., Phinney, A., & Garrett, B. (2009). Nursing instructors' and male nursing students' perceptions of undergraduate, classroom nursing education. *Nurse Education Today, 29*(6), 649–653.

Evans, J. (2002). Cautious caregivers: Gender stereotypes and the sexualization of men nurses' touch. *Journal of Advanced Nursing, 40*(4), 441–448.

Evans, J. (2004). Men nurses: A historical and feminist perspective. *Journal of Advanced Nursing, 47*(3), 321–328.

Evans, J., & Frank, B. (2003). Contradictions and tensions: Exploring relations of masculinities in the numerically female-dominated nursing profession. *Journal of Men's Studies, 11*(3), 277–292.

Finn, R. (2008). The language of teamwork: Reproducing professional divisions in the operating theatre. *Human Relations, 61*(1), 103–130.

Fisher, M. J. (2009). "Being a chameleon": Labour processes of male nurses performing bodywork. *Journal of Advanced Nursing, 65*(12), 2668–2677.

Fletcher, K. (2007). Image: Changing how women nurses think about themselves. Literature review. *Journal of Advanced Nursing, 58*(3), 207–215.

Hamilton, P., & Campbell, M. (2011). Knowledge for re-forming nurses' future: Standpoint makes a difference. *Advances in Nursing Science, 34*(4), 280–296.

Hanson, R. (2009). *Buddha's brain: The practical neuroscience of happiness, love, and wisdom*. Oakland, CA: New Harbinger.

Hanvey, L. (2003). *Men in nursing*. Ottawa, Ontario, Canada: Canadian Nurses Association.

Hartrick Doane, G. A. (in press). Cultivating relational consciousness in social justice practice. In P. Kagan, M. Smith, & P. Chinn (Eds.), *Philosophies and practices of emancipatory nursing: Social justice as praxis*. NewYork: Routledge.

Hartrick Doane, G. A., Stajduhar, K., Bidgood, D., Causton, E., & Cox, A. (2012). End-of-life care and interprofessional practice: Not simply a matter of more. *Health and Interprofessional Practice, 11*(3), EP1028.

Hartrick Doane, G. A., Storch, J., & Pauly, B. (2009). Ethical nursing practice: Inquiry-in-action. *Nursing Inquiry, 16*(3), 232–240.

Heifetz, R. A. (1998). *Leadership without easy answers*. Cambridge, MA: Harvard University Press.

Heifetz, R. A., & Linsky, M. (2002). *Leadership on the line. Staying alive through the dangers of leading*. Boston: Harvard Business Review.

Holecek, A. (2009). *The power and the pain*. Ithaca, NY: Snow Lion.

Holland, K., Middleton, L., & Uys, L. (2011). Professional confidence: A concept analysis. *Scandinavian Journal of Occupational Therapy, 19*(2), 214–224.

Ierardi, J. A., Fitzgerald, D. A., & Holland, D. T. (2010). Exploring male students' educational experiences in an associate degree nursing program. *The Journal of Nursing Education, 49*(4), 215–218.

Kelly, J., Fealy, G. M., & Watson, R. (2012). The image of you: Constructing nursing identities in YouTube. *Journal of Advanced Nursing, 68*(8), 1804–1813.

Mavis, B. (2001). Self-efficacy and OSCE performance among second-year medical students. *Advanced Health Science Education, 6*, 93–102.

McLaughlin, K., Muldoon, O. T., & Moutray, M. (2010). Gender, gender roles and completion of nursing education: A longitudinal study. *Nurse Education Today, 30*(4), 303–307.

McMahon, M. A., & Christopher, K. A. (2011). Toward a mid-range theory of presence. *Nursing Forum, 46*(2), 71–82.

Meadus, R. J., & Twomey, J. C. (2011). Men student nurses: The nursing education experience. *Nursing Forum, 46*(4), 269–279.

Miller, K. L., Reeves, S., Zwarenstein, M., Beales, J. D., Kenaszchuk, C., & Gotlib

Conn, L. (2008). Nurses' emotion work and interprofessional collaboration in general internal medicine wards: A qualitative study. *Journal of Advanced Nursing, 64*(4), 332–343.

Morris-Thompson, T., Shepherd, J., Plata, R., & Marks-Maran, D. I. (2011). Diversity, fulfilment and privilege: The image of nursing. *Journal of Nursing Management, 19*(5), 683–692.

Nathanson, B. H., Hennerman, E. A., Blonaisz, E. R., Doubleday, N. D., Lursadi, P., & Jodka, P. G. (2011). How much teamwork exists between nurses and junior doctors in the intensive care unit? *Journal of Advanced Nursing, 67*(8), 1817–1823.

National League for Nursing. Competencies for graduates of baccalaureate programs. Retrieved March 16, 2013, from http://www.nln .org/facultyprograms/competencies /comp_bacc.htm

Nepo, M. (2005). *The book of awakening*. San Francisco: Canari Press.

Orchard, C. A. (2010). Persistent isolationist or collaborator? The nurses role in interprofessional collaborative practice. *Journal of Nursing Management, 18*(3), 248–257.

Pearson, D., & Pandya, H. (2006). Shared learning in primary care: Participants' views of the benefits of this approach. *Journal of Interprofessional Care, 20*(3), 302–313.

Prebble, K., & Bryder, L. (2008). Gender and class tensions between psychiatric nurses and the general nursing profession in mid-twentieth century New Zealand. *Contemporary Nurse, 30*(2), 181–195.

Reese, L. E., & Sontag, M. A. (2001). Successful interpersonal collaboration on the hospice team. *Health and Social Work, 26*(3), 167–175.

Richardson, J., West, M. A., & Cuthbertson, B. H. (2010). Team working in intensive care: Current evidence and future endeavors. *Current Opinion in Critical Care, 16*, 643–648.

Ricoeur, P. (1991). *From text to action: Essays in hermeneutics, II*. Evanston, IL: Northwestern University Press.

Risjord, M. (2010). *Nursing knowledge: Science, practice and philosophy*. Oxford, United Kingdom: Wiley Blackwell.

Rodney, P., Hartrick, G. A., Storch, J., Varcoe, C., & Starzomski, R. (2002). *Ethics in action: Strengthening nurses' enactment of their moral agency within the cultural context of health care delivery.* British Columbia, Canada: Social Sciences and Humanities Research Council, University of Victoria.

Sargeant, J., Loney, E., & Murphy, G. (2008). Effective interprofessional team: Contact is not enough to build a team. *Journal of Continuing Education in the Health Professions, 28*(4), 228–234.

Sargeant, J., MacLeod, T., & Murray, A. (2011). An interprofessional approach to teaching communication skills. *Journal of Continuing Education in the Health Professions, 31*(4), 265–267.

Schwartz, L., Wright, D., & Lavoie-Tremblay, M. (2011). New nurses' experience of their role within interprofessional health care teams in mental health. *Archives of Psychiatric Nursing, 25*(3), 153–163.

Singer, M. A. (2007). *The untethered soul.* Oakland, CA: New Harbinger.

Snyder, K. A., & Green, A. I. (2008). Revisiting the glass escalator: The case of gender segregation in a female-dominated occupation. *Social Problems, 55*(2), 271–299.

Stanley, D. J. (2008). Celluloid angels: A research study of nurses in feature films 1900–2007. *Journal of Advanced Nursing, 64*(1), 84–95.

Stanley, D. J. (2012). Celluloid devils: A research study of male nurses in feature films. *Journal of Advanced Nursing, 68*(11), 2526–2537.

Thaler, R. H., & Sunstein, C. R. (2009). *Nudge.* New York: Penguin books.

Thomas, C. M., Bertram, E., & Johnson, D. (2009). The SBAR communication technique: Teaching nursing students professional communication skills. *Nurse Educator, 34*(4), 176–180.

Thorne, S. (2011). Theoretical Issues in nursing. In J. C. Ross-Kerr & M. J. Woods (Eds.), *Canadian nursing: Issues and perspectives* (5th ed., pp. 85–104). Toronto, Ontario, Canada: Elsevier.

White, A. H. (2003). Clinical decision making among fourth-year nursing students: An interpretive study. *Journal of Nursing Education, 42*(3), 113–120.

White, K. A. (2009). Self-confidence: A concept analysis. *Nursing Forum, 44*(2), 103–114.

Wittenberg-Lyles, E. M., Parker Oliver, D., Demiris, G., & Regehr, K. (2009). Exploring interpersonal communication in hospital interdisciplinary team meetings. *Journal of Gerontological Nursing, 35*(7), 38–45.

Woodhall, L. J., Vertacnik, L., & McLaughlin, M. (2008). Implementation of the SBAR Communication Technique in a tertiary center. *Journal of Emergency Nursing, 34*(4), 314–317.

11 Leadership in Every Moment of Practice

LEARNING OBJECTIVES

By engaging with the material in this chapter, you will be able to:

1. Distinguish leadership from management.

2. Compare and contrast transactional and transformational leadership styles with other styles.

3. Describe a relational view of leadership.

4. Relate core leadership practices to quality work environments and good nursing care.

5. Discuss the workplace environmental conditions that can lead to workplace bullying, moral distress, and burnout and the role of leadership in reducing these problems.

6. Create a leadership development plan for your career trajectory.

In this chapter, we address leadership as integral to every moment of nursing practice. We consider how nursing leadership is essential for achieving optimal health care outcomes and healthy workplaces. The chapter begins by distinguishing between leadership and management and presenting some of the ways that styles of leadership typically have been thought about in nursing. We then offer a relational view of leadership in nursing. Our goal is to demonstrate that leadership skills are required not only for those in formal leadership and managerial roles, but for all nurses throughout all career trajectories.

THE IMPORTANCE OF UNDERSTANDING LEADERSHIP IN NURSING

All nurses are leaders. Some nurses may not see themselves as leaders or feel comfortable thinking about other nurses in this way, but each day, nurses lead patients and families, unit committees, interdisciplinary rounds, and more. (Pate, 2013, p. 186)

Nursing leadership is required to achieve optimal outcomes for individuals, families, and groups in health care (Hutchinson & Jackson, 2013; Institute of Medicine, 2011; Pate, 2013). As we showed in Chapter 10, nurses bring a standpoint to the interprofessional team that is unique, reflecting the commitments, values, and obligations of nursing; multiple forms of knowledge; and an understanding of the complex relational interplay of health care situations. Pate (2013) argues that nurses "serve as vital interpreters at the critical interface of the reality of patient care and the health system" (p. 187). She says nurses are needed in discussions that challenge the status quo as it relates to patient and family care. She explains that because nurses understand the experiences of patients and families, bring "bedside savvy," and the ability to translate and interpret to those in administration, they have the potential to transform health care. However, she says that "this transformation can happen only if nurses are skilled as leaders and empowered to take on these new challenges as they take charge of their careers as a whole, not just their current jobs" (p. 187).

The 2011 Institute of Medicine report, "The Future of Nursing," claims that although nurses are essential to advancing health, multiple barriers impede nurses from being able to respond effectively to rapidly changing health care settings and an evolving health care system. Nurses need to understand those barriers, address the barriers that they can influence, and develop leadership skills for every moment of practice across their career trajectories. One barrier to nurses enacting effective nursing leadership is how leadership is usually conceptualized.

Distinguishing Leadership from Management

In nursing, leadership has often been understood as being fused with or part of management (Hutchinson & Hurley, 2013). However, the two are not the same. Pate (2013) points out that although both are needed in health care, management brings "stability to complex workplaces by actions such as planning, staffing, controlling, organizing, and problem solving" whereas leadership focuses "on creating a vision for the future, aligning people, and motivating and inspiring. Nurses with formal management titles may not have fully developed leadership skills, whereas a formal title is not necessary for those choosing to lead" (p. 186).

The skills required for effective management and those required for leadership are also different. Management requires the skills to manage budgets, allocate human resources, delegate, and so on. As opposed to these technical skills, leadership abilities are broad capacities; for example, to articulate a guiding vision and inspire others to commit to that vision. That said, the precise abilities required for leadership vary according to how leadership is conceptualized. The two most commonly recognized leadership styles are transactional and transformational.

Leadership as Transactional or Transformational

The theory of transformational leadership was introduced in research into political leadership in the 1970s and then extended into organizational leadership (Hutchinson & Jackson, 2013). The essence of this theory is that there are three types of leaders: nonleaders who practice a laissez-faire style; transactional leaders who achieve performance through contingent rewards and negative feedback; and transformational leaders who motivate others through vision and inspiration. In nursing, leadership has been understood almost exclusively through this theory (Hutchinson & Jackson, 2013) and historically has been characterized as transactional (Hutchinson & Hurley, 2013). In a critical review of nursing literature on transformational leadership theory, Hutchinson and Jackson (2013) identified a number of interrelated limitations of transformational leadership theory that are problematic for nursing:

- *Conceptualizing leadership as dichromatic*. Leaders are often seen as either transactional or transformative. Although some theorists claim a more "relational" view of transformational leadership that would account for a greater diversity of approaches and factors, the focus continues to be on either task- and goal-oriented leadership or visionary change. This binary (either/or) view seems inadequate to support nursing's potential contribution to health care that requires a broad range of approaches to change.

- *Privileging commitment to organizational goals*. Both transactional and transformative leaders are considered to be role models who reflect existing organizational values and ideally promote productivity and efficiency. These values may work well in the corporate world but have a less easy fit with the promotion of health. Stewart, Holmes, and Usher (2012) show how nursing leaders across the globe are working within tensions "between the caring aspect of nursing practice and the bureaucratically imposed requirement for efficiency-focused health care administration in the context of unprecedented sociological and technological change affecting nursing work" (p. 224). They argue that communication becomes exclusively strategic, oriented to achieving greater economic efficiency, and bringing followers into line with corporate goals.

- *Conceptualizing power as top-down*. Transactional and transformative leaders are seen as holding power and as bringing followers into line. This approach quells dissent and is contrary to the call for nurses to challenge the status quo that reinforces barriers to health and health care access. It also overlooks the power and possibilities inherent in all members of the health care team.

- *Privileging stereotypical male charisma and ethnocentrism*. Transformational leadership was initially based on the characteristics of male politicians in the United States, then male executives (Hutchinson & Jackson, 2013). The model was then tested on male officers in the U.S. military. There is an uneasy relationship between this orientation and nursing, which is feminized (in the sense of being associated with stereotypical ideas about feminine characteristics), dominated by women, and increasingly diverse in terms of ethnicity in most countries. Although women represent the majority of the health care workforce (Fontenot, 2012; Pate, 2013), "they are significantly underrepresented in leadership positions, particularly at the executive and board levels" (Fontenot, 2012, p. 11). It may be that the dominant understanding of leadership as aligned with characteristics stereotypically associated with masculinity contributes to this underrepresentation. Stereotypical masculine leadership styles include an emphasis on problem-solving and delegating; stereotypical female leadership includes being supportive and consultative, mentoring, and team building. Pate (2013) cites the characteristic of warmth being perceived as a female trait and associated with incompetence as an example of how the dynamics of stereotyping may undermine nursing leadership and exclude nurses from organizational level leadership roles. However, Mary Robinson, the former president of Ireland and the former United Nations High Commissioner for Human Rights, says that women should be proud of the nurturing characteristics often associated with female leadership and should use those characteristics particularly to foster leadership in others (Ghomeshi, 2013).

■ *Romanticizing charisma and relying on self-report.* The transformational leadership model emphasizes charisma as a key characteristic, and much of the research on transformational leadership has relied on leaders' self-reports of their charisma (Hutchinson & Jackson, 2013). The research has also shown that the ratings of followers often are much less positive than the leaders' own ratings of their charisma. As Isadore Sharp, the owner and leader of Four Seasons Hotels and Resorts, has famously said of leaders, "*We are only what we do, not what we say we are.*" Moreover, some authors argue that when leaders are coercive, charismatic leadership can undermine the sense of self of followers (Bass & Riggio, 2006; Stewart et al., 2012).

■ *Emphasizing formal leadership roles.* Leadership is viewed as a quality and role of those formally designated by the organization as leaders. In health care, this reinforces the tendency to privilege organizational goals, even when they are counter to good patient care and outcomes, and it overlooks the tremendous leadership resource in nurses who are closest to those receiving care. Hutchinson and Jackson (2013) point out that there has been no attention to "followers as constructors of leaders, followers as moderators of leader impact, and followers as co-constructors of leader success or failure" (p. 18).

■ *Overlooking integrity and effectiveness.* Transformational leaders may be charismatic yet self-serving and ineffective in achieving meaningful outcomes. Hence, contemporary leadership theorists have begun to emphasize integrity as a key element of leadership.

■ *Overlooking commitment to employee welfare.* Hutchinson and colleagues (Hutchinson & Hurley, 2013; Hutchinson, Vickers, Jackson, & Wilkes, 2009) argue that a transactional style of leadership can undermine genuine commitment to the welfare of employees and result in "subcultures that tolerate or even reward bullying. In this environment, actors are more likely to be rewarded when they obtain desired outcomes and performance outputs, and those in positions of power are likely to be more concerned with furthering their own interests through obtaining desired goals than addressing the welfare of employees" (Hutchinson et al., 2009, p. 228).

Other Styles of Leadership

Given the limitations of transformational and transactional styles of leadership, a number of alternative styles have been suggested. These styles rely less on individual charisma and emphasize values, ethics, leader integrity, and the leader's capacities to generate and communicate hope, compassion, and motivation (Hutchinson & Jackson, 2013). Hutchinson and Hurley (2013) explain that leadership styles with the capacity to inspire and empower others value emotional intelligence. By this they mean a set of abilities including:

- The ability to perceive emotions in oneself and others accurately,
- The ability to use emotions to facilitate thinking,
- The ability to understand emotions, emotional language, and the signals conveyed by emotions, and
- The ability to manage emotions so as to attain specific goals (p. 554).

Hutchinson and Hurley (2013) then discuss several forms of leadership that emphasize emotional intelligence.

Authentic Leadership

The idea of *authentic leadership* has been proposed as a central aspect of all positive leadership styles (Laschinger & Smith, 2013; Laschinger, Wong, & Grau, 2012). Authentic leadership refers to "authentic transformational" leadership in contrast to charismatic transformational leadership, which can be exploitive, manipulative, and self-aggrandizing (Hutchinson & Jackson, 2013). Avolio, Walumbwa, and Weber (2009) define authentic leadership as "a pattern of transparent and ethical leader behavior that encourages openness in sharing information needed to make decisions while accepting followers' inputs" (p. 423). Authentic leadership emphasizes building on people's strengths and explicitly pays attention to values, particularly leader integrity.

Resonant Leadership

A style of leadership that focuses on minimizing the emotional impact of organizational change upon staff is *resonant leadership*. Hutchinson and Hurley (2013) describe resonant leaders as empathetic and supportive of the needs of their teams. They are also able to effectively manage their own emotions and develop effective relationships with others.

Congruent Leadership

Congruent leadership is a style of nursing leadership that emphasizes emotional intelligence, especially those abilities related to interpersonal relations, integrity, and communication (Hutchinson & Hurley, 2013). It also values a correspondence between the clinical leaders' actions and their values and beliefs about care and nursing (Stanley, 2008). Hutchinson and Hurley (2013) argue that nursing requires a leadership style that is congruent with nurses working within clinical environments, and they propose that congruent leadership can offer a firm theoretical foundation for clinical nurses. Distinguishing clinical leadership from other forms of nursing leadership suggests that clinical nurses should be seen as leaders in their own right (Stanley & Sherratt, 2010).

Each of these alternative styles is consistent with Parks's (2005) assertion that leadership requires learning how to pay attention with compassion. It involves "the formation of a seeing heart, an informed mind, and a little courage" (p. 244).

TRY IT OUT 11.1

Think about the Most Ideal Leader You Have Known

Think about the various leaders you have known. If you have been in nursing for a while, think about nursing leaders; if not, think about other leaders with whom you have worked in workplaces, in college, on sports teams, or in political, faith-based, or other social organizations. Identify the person you consider to have been the best leader.

Jot down the words that come to mind about this person. What qualities, values, achievements, or ways of being did you list? What stood out? Think of your list in relation to the ideas above regarding leadership style. What characterized the person's leadership style, and to what extent does that style align with the styles described above?

A RELATIONAL VIEW OF LEADERSHIP

From a relational view, leadership is understood to be a relational process that occurs and is enacted among people and within contexts. At its core, relational leadership involves shaping and shifting how individuals and groups attend to and subsequently respond to situations—that is, how they relate to and within situations (Scharmer, 2008). Relational leadership focuses explicit attention on the interplay of intrapersonal, interpersonal, and contextual elements; critically considers how those elements are converging; and responds and works within that convergence to promote positive outcomes. In particular, a relational view takes the sociopolitical, historical, economic, linguistic, and physical contexts, including the organizational power dynamics, into account.

From a relational perspective, it is understood that the influence of both formal and informal leaders is shaped by the specific contexts within which they are working, the people with whom they work, and the relationships among them. It acknowledges that although formal leaders may be positioned to have more influence, each person can have influence—and be a leader—regardless of that person's position within the organizational hierarchy. From a relational view, nursing leadership is enacted by engaging with others in such a way that the well-being of patients, families, health care providers, and the health care system is supported and enhanced.

A Relational View Helps You to Better Understand Formal Leadership

While all nurses have a leadership role, formal leaders are required. Indeed, Storch, Schick Makaroff, Pauly, and Newton (2013) have pointed out that the rhetoric of "Every nurse is a leader" has been used to delete formal leadership roles, leaving nurses without effective communication to other levels and departments, support for clinical leadership, and representation at organizational levels. Thus, formal leaders are also essential to nursing and health care.

Enlisting relational inquiry strategies can help you analyze the styles and practices of formal leaders throughout your organization. As you know, formal leaders and staff nurses are positioned differently within an organization. That different positioning shapes the nature of their leadership as well as their specific concerns. Those in formal leadership roles have role expectations and designated responsibilities that extend beyond the immediate practice unit. Often, they are simultaneously subject to the expectations of staff and to the expectations of those to whom they report. This sandwich position can create tensions. For example, a common concern among staff nurses is the limited visibility of formal leaders in the practice setting. Leaders often share the same concerns but must balance practice concerns with the demands of the organization. Interviewing nurses in leadership positions, Hartung and Miller (2013) identified multiple work processes that often hindered a leader's abilities to set a positive tone and stay connected to the staff, ensuring effective communication while meeting multiple unit and institutional challenges. Often, meeting all expectations is difficult, especially when workloads are high and roles poorly defined. A relational view helps you understand the complexities a formal leader may face within the organizational context and to consider multiple ways to work effectively with them.

The ability to analyze others' leadership is crucial for many other reasons as well. First, because leadership is a key determinant of workplace quality, when you are seeking a new job, it is important to consider what forms of leadership will be provided in the new setting—both formal and informal. Second, analyzing the leadership of others in your work setting provides you with a map of the resources and barriers to creating better workplaces. This can enhance your ability to work more effectively with formal leaders and cultivate your own leadership so that you can provide better care and enhance your own job satisfaction. As you come to appreciate the different positioning of individuals within your organization, you'll be able to work more effectively with the different forms of leadership. Third, one way of furthering your own leadership skills is to learn from others, including your colleagues and those who are in formal leadership and management roles. By enlisting the relational inquiry strategies, you can more effectively learn from others and further your own skillfulness.

TO ILLUSTRATE
Matching Styles

When I (Colleen) began working as an educator within the cardiac care unit, the nurse manager was quite different from previous managers with whom I had worked. She had a very personal style of getting to know each staff member individually, did not exert much control over others, and supported the staff to make decisions. Initially, I found her indecisive and thought her friendly, personal style was somewhat unprofessional in contrast to others who were more directive and distant from staff. However,

continued on page 428

TO ILLUSTRATE *continued*

Matching Styles

once I realized that she encouraged me to work directly with staff and that there would be no negative repercussions for doing so (my previous manager did not like any initiatives without her prior approval), I realized that her style was effectively engaging the staff. Once I adjusted my style to complement hers, I became more effective as well.

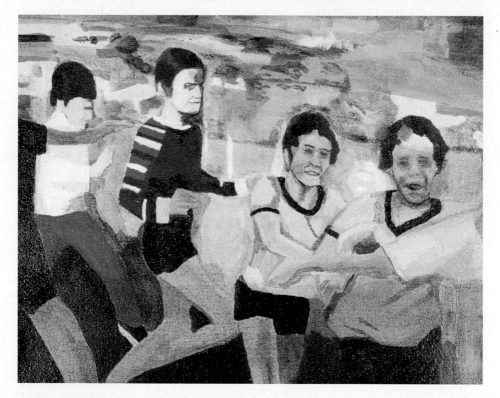

Follow the leader. (Acrylic painting by Alex Grewal.)

TRY IT OUT 11.2

Analyze Formal Leaders

First, from your thinking and reading about leadership in nursing to this point and drawing on the list you started in Try It Out 11.1, generate a list of characteristics you think are important in leaders. The above discussion of leadership styles suggests that being fair, being supportive, having emotional intelligence, and having integrity might be important.

continued on page 429

TRY IT OUT *continued*

Analyze Formal Leaders

Next, generate questions you might ask of formal leaders and of their followers to assess the extent to which any given person leads in the way you think is important. Box 11.1 suggests some possible questions.

Pick a setting in which you have a vested interest. Perhaps select your current workplace or a workplace in which you are interested in working. Find out "who" is seen as a leader in the setting, and then get a sense of the style and quality of that leadership. Try your questions out with at least one formal leader (e.g., the manager, clinical nurse leader, or an administrator) and one person who is not in a formal leadership role. Ask each person about themselves and about others in both formal and informal leadership roles. Next, consider how you enact leadership within that setting through your relational actions. You might revisit the discussion of the five Ws in Chapter 8 to prime your thinking.

BOX 11.1

Suggested Questions for Analyzing Leadership

Who?
- Who is providing leadership in this setting?
- Who is positioned as following whom?
- Who is in a formal (designated by the organization) leadership role?

Where?
- Where is a given leader positioned within the organization?
- Where is that leader positioned relative to the formal authority designated by the organization?

Intrapersonal
- What appear to be the leader's values and goals?
- What are the leader's key characteristics? To what extent does the person seem to exhibit the characteristics commonly identified with positive leadership (e.g., vision, integrity, emotional intelligence)?

Contextual
- What goals are mandated for the leader by the organization?
- How do the goals align with the goals of nursing?
- How do the goals align with the resources available?
- How do the leaders' goals align with those of the organization and the goals of nursing?

continued on page 430

> **BOX 11.1** *continued*
>
> ## Suggested Questions for Analyzing Leadership
>
> Interpersonal
> - How does a given leader relate to their followers, leaders, and peers?
> - How does the leader facilitate leadership in followers?
> - How does the leader enact power? How does the leader reconcile differences?
> - How does the leader motivate others to achieve goals?

A Relational View Helps You Recognize Your Own Leadership

From a relational inquiry perspective, every moment of nursing action involves leadership. Whether you are a student nurse or an experienced registered nurse, you exercise leadership by virtue of the choices you make in every situation. Particularly important are your choices about how you relate—on what you focus your attention, what you privilege, to what you respond, and what you ignore. As we described in Chapter 8, your actions always have an impact of some kind. Thus, the overall leadership question you need to ask yourself is: What will you support and foster through your nursing actions?

Relational inquiry provides you with the tools to (a) see yourself as a leader, (b) critically consider how you are exercising leadership in any particular moment, and (c) consciously cultivate your leadership practice. As you know, relational inquiry involves reflexively considering your own values, attitudes, beliefs, and actions and their impacts; how those are shaped by yourself, others, and the contexts of practice; and evaluation of your practice in relation to the commitments and obligations of nursing. Successful leadership depends on the quality of attention and intention that the leader brings to any situation (Scharmer, 2008). Seeing yourself as a leader in each moment of practice is simply an extension of the relational view of knowing that you are always having an impact on others and being even more purposeful and deliberate in exerting that influence. It requires routinely enlisting the distal view (introduced in Chapter 3) to consider the well-being of individuals, families, nurses, and the organization beyond your immediate view and the immediate moment. Of course, knowing yourself and being clear about your goals is a prerequisite to doing so.

Knowing Yourself Is Important to Leadership

In many ways, relational leadership is a continuation of the process we have been outlining throughout the book. Effective leadership requires you to continually work across the three levels of inquiry (intrapersonal, interpersonal, and contextual) as you simultaneously keep your eye on the ball—on promoting the well-being of patients, health care providers, and the health care system. As we have been emphasizing, intrapersonal inquiry is central to that relational process. In exercising leadership, it is critical to pay attention to how your own values and beliefs shape your actions and how you in turn influence others. For example, Heifetz and Linsky (2002) contend that "The most difficult work of leadership involves learning to experience distress without numbing yourself" (p. 227). These authors identify how we are hardwired with default settings through which we interpret and respond to situations. Thus, active intrapersonal inquiry is vital to help you stay attuned to those default settings and perhaps even reset them. For example, what particular loyalties trigger strong reactions in you? What is your level of tolerance for chaos, conflict, confusion—all of which are inherent aspects of adaptive leadership practice (Heifetz, Grashow, & Linsky, 2009)? What is your emotional makeup and your hardwired way of dealing with emotions, criticism, and uncertainty? When you consider these insights (and what Heifetz and colleagues [2009] describe as your "personal system") in light of the contextual system and the forces acting upon and through you, you are better positioned to identify resources and constraints on your ability to make things happen. You can also assess how well suited you are to take action toward a particular challenge (Heifetz et al., 2009). In leading, you consciously consider the intrapersonal dynamics as you simultaneously expand your attention to others and purposefully use your influence to help others work more effectively toward the well-being of patients, families, health care providers, and the health care system. This means you extend your sense of responsibility beyond yourself and are increasingly aware of others' responses, including their stress.

Knowing Your Nursing Goals Is Important to Leadership

Developing a relational consciousness regarding the goals of nursing and how they are being achieved within any given context sets the direction for leadership. A relational perspective of nursing practice is based on the assumption that nursing is guided by obligations to promote well-being. From the same perspective, leadership should be oriented toward the well-being of individuals and families, the well-being of nurses and other health care providers, and the well-being of health care environments. Keeping these goals in mind provides the grounding for effective leadership practice. Rather than leading others to adhere to practices and policies regardless of their impact, a good leader evaluates the consequences of any action or policy in terms of those goals.

In Chapter 3, we drew upon John Caputo's words to describe how, from a relational perspective, obligations are matters of flesh and blood. Often, our obligations as nurses and as leaders arise in moments when we find ourselves in the midst of a situation and feel compelled to respond. Yet, while we might know "what" needs addressing, often we do not necessarily know "how" to actually address it. The first step in those situations is to admit you don't know and work from that not knowing—to stop, look, and proceed thoughtfully. Proceeding thoughtfully involves asking the orienting questions about nursing goals—how can the well-being of individuals, families, nurses, and the health care system be served?

When the well-being of all people is the goal, equity and social justice become key concerns. That is, all people are seen as deserving of health and health care to promote their well-being. Because the ethic of market justice and the discourses of personal responsibility and choice are dominant in health care, leadership in nursing requires that you consciously focus on promoting well-being despite the constant influence of such discourses. As the saying goes, keep your eye on that ball at all times. Key checkpoints to support you in this process include:

- Look for the five Ws (who is relating to what, how are people's actions in or out of sync with espoused goals, etc.).
- Pay attention to values and make them visible (what is being privileged and what is being ignored).
- Make the intrapersonal, interpersonal, and contextual influences visible (identify the values, habits, historical, economic, sociopolitical, linguistic, and physical environmental factors shaping the situation, make them visible to others, and name the implications for well-being).
- Respond constructively to language that is being used to stereotype, label, or make assumptions in harmful ways or to acquiesce (e.g., when you hear people say, "That's just the way things are, and we are powerless to change it").

TRY IT OUT 11.3
Review Your Recent Leadership

First, recall your most recent day of practice. With whom were you working? Which team members, leaders, patients, clients, and/or residents were involved in your day? What was going on in the setting? How did you feel about your day, and why? Did you feel that you provided good care?

Now, can you recall a time during that day when you tried to influence someone to provide better care? How did you do that? Did you make a suggestion? Offer information? Offer a new viewpoint on something? Role model? How were you thinking about "better care?" Whose well-being was in the foreground of your intentions? Was the goal of well-being being challenged in some way?

Analyze how well your influence "worked." That is, did your influence contribute to better care? And why did your influence work or not? Did you follow any of the checkpoints listed above? How did you use power? Language? You can likely think of multiple times in any day when you try to exert influence toward better care. Now, can you see how you are doing that and how you might be even more purposeful and deliberate in engaging others?

A Relational View Helps You Lead from Any Position

Throughout your career, you will be in relation to others in formal leadership. Regardless of whether you take a formal role yourself, you will usually have a formal leader. You can lead by relating to your formal leaders in ways that shape their leadership, moderate their impact, and shape their success or failure (Hutchinson & Jackson, 2013). How you view your own leaders and how you choose to relate to those leaders can have a significant impact.

Point-of-care nurses can have a powerful influence on leaders. Optimizing that influence requires deepening your understanding of formal leadership. The greater your understanding of the context for formal leaders and the challenges and opportunities they have, the better you will be able to exert influence toward nursing goals. Even when you are not in a formal leadership role, you can lead by virtue of how you focus your attention and how you relate. For example, when I (Gweneth) was in a formal leadership position, I found a great variation in how people related to me. Some would approach me in an adversarial manner, others like salespeople, trying to sell me on an idea, and still others would relate by ignoring the formal structures and roles. I came to realize that what determined their approach often had more to do with them than with me. That is, they related to me based on the assumptions they carried about administrative power relations, formal role distinctions, organizational protocols, and so forth.

Thus, since you can relate to your nurse manager in more or less effective ways, it is important to consider what you yourself bring to the relational interaction. For example, knowing the background of your formal leaders and understanding their philosophies and styles will enable you to better participate in decision making and take up your leadership role as a nurse. Such an understanding will also help you understand the transition from informal to formal leadership that nurses undergo, enable you to better support leadership in others, and subsequently to make such a transition yourself. Furthermore, better understanding formal leadership roles will help you better evaluate whether, how, and when you would like to take on such a role. It will help you to evaluate your existing skills and interests in light of the skills required for leadership.

Nurses who move to formal leadership roles often experience considerable difficulty making the transition from their role as a nurse to their role as a leader. Stewart and colleagues (2012) explain this difficulty as arising from two interlocking aspects of the health care system—the "life world" which is the everyday world in which health care providers relate to one another and provide care, and the "system" comprised of the economic and administrative components of health care. They explain that the "system" aspects can invade and overpower the "life world" aspects in which all processes are understood as technical processes to be controlled. For nurses, this means that values related to good care, humanizing care, and fairness can be overridden. The researchers say that consequently, "Increasingly, nurse leaders, at the cost of denying their humanity, faithfully follow system directives while privately experiencing a distressing dissonance between personal values and public behavior" (p. 226).

TO ILLUSTRATE
Feeling Like an Outsider

When I (Colleen) first moved into a formal leadership role, I went from being a staff nurse in the open heart ICU to being an assistant head nurse. I was shocked to find that I went from being "one of the gang" with

---

continued on page 434

TO ILLUSTRATE *continued*

Feeling Like an Outsider

many friends among the staff to feeling like an outsider. For years, I could not explain the shift. I didn't feel that I had changed as a person. I didn't really think other staff nurses were envious of my role; many had strongly encouraged me to take the role. It was not until later when I formally studied leadership from a critical perspective that I was able to see that my allegiances had changed. Although my colleagues had encouraged me to take the role because I was a strong patient and nursing advocate, as soon as I stepped into a formal leadership role, I aligned with "the system," focusing on rules and efficiencies that did not necessarily privilege patient well-being and rarely considered the impact on nursing practice. In the words of Stewart and colleagues (2012), I had been invited to move from an exclusive nursing identity to a managerial identity that was almost impossible to resist because it was integrated with ideas about good leadership, and my ability to keep the job and thus advance my career depended on my conforming to expectations that I serve the "system" rather than patients or nurses.

As this story illustrates, being a good nursing leader requires keeping nursing goals in view and knowing yourself well enough to align with those goals, regardless of whether you are in an informal or formal leadership role or are transitioning between formal and informal roles. Good leadership can then be enhanced by developing effective core leadership practices.

CORE LEADERSHIP PRACTICES

Good leadership is relational and improvisational (Heifetz & Linsky, 2002). You may have a clear vision, orienting values, and be anchored in your nursing commitments, but what you actually do from moment to moment cannot be scripted (Heifetz & Linsky, 2002). But just as actors in an improvisational troupe cultivate fundamental skills and techniques for successful performances, you can cultivate a set of relational practices that support effective leadership. We offer these here.

Eight Practices of Relational Leadership

Here, we discuss eight practices that effective leaders often enlist and cultivate to support their leadership practice. They are summarized in Box 11.2. We have created this list by drawing on *The Practice of Adaptive Leadership* as described by Heifetz and colleagues (2009), Zander and Zander's (2000) *The Art of Possibility*, and other leadership literature.

In Chapter 1, we described the idea of *getting on the balcony* to extend your relational view. Heifetz and colleagues (2009) use the metaphor of "getting on the balcony" above the "dance floor" to depict what it means

BOX 11.2
Eight Practices of Relational Leadership

1. Get on the balcony.
2. Find out where people are.
3. Listen to the song beneath the words.
4. Distinguish technical from adaptive challenges.
5. Anchor yourself.
6. Diagnose the situation.
7. Create a sanctuary.
8. Enlist your relational inquiry toolbox to help you choose your actions.

to gain the distanced perspective you need to see what is happening at all levels. As you get on the balcony, you can see how the contextual surroundings contribute to what is occurring interpersonally and so forth.

Another core practice that supports relational leadership is *to find out where people are at*—to undertake a targeted inquiry to extend your understanding of what is of meaning and concern to different people in the situation or context. As you inquire and develop understanding of people and their perspectives, it is important to *listen to the song beneath the words* (Heifetz et al., 2009). This includes listening to what is *not* being said, noticing behaviors that seem at odds with people's statements, and/ or considering seemingly disproportionate reactions to situations (Heifetz et al., 2009).

It is also important to *distinguish technical from adaptive challenges*. Technical problems "have known solutions that can be implemented by current know-how . . . Adaptive challenges can only be addressed through changes in people's priorities, beliefs, habits, and loyalties . . . [they require] shedding certain entrenched ways, tolerating losses, and generating the new capacity to thrive anew" (Heifetz et al., 2009, p. 19). As we described in Chapter 10, a common mistake leaders can make is to address adaptive challenges with technical solutions.

Anchoring yourself by connecting to your nursing purpose and commitments enables you to thoughtfully consider how you might *be* a contribution. It can also help you resist leaping to action without fully *diagnosing the situation* and considering the best option given the complexities and tensions that may be shaping current circumstances. When dealing with complex situations, it is important to hold the space open long enough so you can "know what is" and see how best to let things be before jumping to an intervention.

To nurture and sustain yourself in your leadership practice, it is important to *create a sanctuary* (Heifetz et al., 2009). This means looking for allies so you are not alone (remember leadership is a relational process). One important caveat is that of distinguishing allies from confidants—not making the mistake of treating an ally like a confidant (Heifetz, et al., 2009). Allies are people in your work setting who share some of your values and concerns and who you can work with to create a positive workplace or address a particular issue. Someone may be an ally in one situation and not in another. Thus, allies are not necessarily confidants. Confidants "provide you with a place where you can say everything that's in your heart, everything that's on your mind, without being predigested or well packaged" (p. 199). Often, confidants are people outside of the situation, such as a trusted colleague or friend who works in a different setting and is not directly involved.

Finally, *enlisting your relational inquiry toolbox* can provide processes and strategies to thoughtfully choose your actions. As Heifetz and colleagues (2009) emphasize, effective leadership requires engagement with people "above and below the neck" (p. 37). These authors contend that leadership involves the convergence of multiple intelligences (intellectual, emotion, spiritual, and physical) through which you intentionally connect with the values, beliefs, and anxieties of the people with whom you are working. Your relational inquiry toolbox enables you to do just that.

TO ILLUSTRATE

The Concern of Co-Ed Rooms

In a research study our ethics research team undertook a few years ago, a central finding was the way in which "good" care was affected by the physical layout of the hospital unit, bed utilization practices at the organizational level, and the integral connection between those two (Hartrick Doane, Storch, & Pauly, 2009). The physical layout of the unit did not enable easy maneuvering or privacy (e.g., there were no doors on some of the bathrooms), and the organization had a policy of co-ed rooms. The nurses were concerned about the ethics of the co-ed policy, which meant putting men and women in the same room to increase the efficiency of bed utilization. Yet, in checking with their professional nursing association, the nurses were informed that the policy did not violate the code of ethics. In fact, the organization justified the policy by saying it enabled more patients to be admitted more quickly. However, the nurses themselves had concerns. For example, there were a number of elderly people on the unit and many of the elderly women found it quite distressing to be put in a four-bed room with men (especially when there was no door on the bathroom). The nurses decided that while the professional association and the hospital did not see an ethical issue with this practice, from their perspective it violated the dignity of those involved—a value outlined within the Canadian Nurses Association's (2008) *Code of Ethics for Registered Nurses*. Subsequently, although the hospital policy did not change, as a collective, the nurses created their own working policy on the unit to address the issue of co-ed rooms. When a patient was admitted, the nurses took factors such as age, physical mobility, cognitive awareness, and so forth into consideration in determining in which room/bed to place them.

LEADERSHIP TO CREATE HEALTHY WORK ENVIRONMENTS

To consider leadership at the point of practice, we have decided to focus on what is perhaps one of the most challenging aspects of nursing leadership—that of creating healthy work environments. Leadership has a direct and reciprocal relationship to work environments. Negative work environments lead to a range of undesirable consequences for nurses such as decreased job satisfaction, bullying, moral distress, and turnover (Boev, 2012; Laschinger, Wong, & Grau, 2013; Neff, Cimiotti, Heusinger, & Aiken, 2011; Pauly, Varcoe, Storch, & Newton, 2009; Silen, Svantesson, Kjellstrom, Sidenvall, & Christensson, 2011; Varcoe, Pauly, Storch, Newton, & Makaroff, 2012; Wong & Laschinger, 2013). In a study of 10 countries in Europe, the quality of leadership was the second highest reason (after nurse–physician relationships) for nurses' intentions to leave the profession (Heinen et al., 2013).

On the other hand, research has consistently shown that positive nursing leadership is related to healthy work environments, higher job satisfaction and job engagement, and lower levels of bullying, burnout, moral distress, and job turnover (Bamford, Wong, & Laschinger, 2013; Bell & Breslin, 2008; Kelly, McHugh, & Aiken, 2012; Laschinger, Fineman, Shamian, & Casier, 2000; Laschinger et al., 2012). Positive work environments both support and are created through formal and informal leadership. Positive work environments are characterized by fair and supportive leadership and low levels of role ambiguity and role conflict (Hauge et al., 2011). Research consistently shows both that effective leadership fosters positive work environments for nurses (Bamford et al., 2013; Wong & Laschinger, 2013) and that positive work environments are linked to patient satisfaction with care (Boev, 2012).

To help you actively explore how you might develop and exercise your leadership skills and capacity, below we consider three of the most pervasive workplace challenges that nurses experience—bullying, moral distress, and burnout (Bell & Breslin, 2008; Hutchinson, Wilkes, Jackson, & Vickers, 2010; Laschinger et al., 2012; Pauly et al., 2009; Taylor & Barling, 2004). These challenges have a direct impact on the quality of nursing care and, subsequently, the quality of the experiences of those receiving care. This is particularly important to new graduates who experience high levels of bullying, burnout, and job turnover. For example, studies in the United States and Canada (Laschinger, Grau, Finegan, & Wilk, 2010; Simons, 2008) found that over 30% of new nurses reported being bullied.

We begin by summarizing some of the current research around each of these challenges and then in Try It Out 11.4 invite you to enlist the core leadership practices and the relational inquiry toolbox to imagine possibilities for action to affect these challenges.

Minimizing Workplace Bullying

Hutchinson and Hurley (2013) explain that *workplace bullying* is the term now used for what was previously described in nursing as horizontal or lateral violence. They describe bullying as including "behaviours such as verbal abuse or threat of harm, continual criticism, demeaning remarks, intimidation and undermining, as well as more subtle behaviours such as refusing to cooperate, being unavailable to give assistance, hampering another's performance, and making their work difficult" (p. 554). Bullying has negative consequences for targets including anxiety depression, posttraumatic stress disorder, lower job satisfaction, higher turnover intention, and absenteeism (Hauge, Skogstad, & Einarsen, 2010; Matthiesen & Einarsen, 2004; Nielsen, Hetland, Matthiesen, & Einarsen, 2012).

Although early efforts to understand workplace bullying focused primarily on individual perpetrators and victims, bullying is increasingly being understood relationally. Bullying is now understood to arise from the characteristics of workplaces (Hauge et al., 2011; Hauge et al., 2010; Hutchinson, Jackson, Wilkes, & Vickers, 2008; Hutchinson et al., 2010). Hutchinson and colleagues (2009) studied nurses who had experienced workplace bullying and conceptualized bullying as organizational corruption. This challenges the idea that bullying is an isolated event that arises from interpersonal conflict, organizational pressures, or poor work design. Rather, bullying is a pattern that arises from the interplay among contexts and people. Matthiesen and Einarsen (2007) hypothesize that "workplace bullying may be generated in stressful workplace situations, intolerant organizational climates, or where leadership is characterized as tyrannical or avoidant" (Hutchinson & Hurley, 2013, p. 554). Minimizing bullying begins with understanding it as an organizational problem.

Hutchinson and Hurley (2013) describe that organizations that are rule- and outcome-oriented are more likely to blame workplace problems on individuals. Thus, bullying is seen as "a personality conflict rather than a reflection of organizational practices." When bullying is seen as merely the problem of specific individuals, it "may be seen as a normal part of how the workplace functions, and raising a grievance about bullying may result in further victimization" (p. 557). Moreover, they cite evidence suggesting that transactional leaders may strategically employ bullying as a tactic to achieve goals and improve productivity. Tyrannical leaders rely on splitting strategies that play individuals and groups off each other. Indeed, there is evidence that bullying behaviors can be masked as legitimate organizational processes (Hutchinson, Vickers, Jackson, & Wilkes, 2005).

Positive leadership is important for reducing bullying (McKenna, Smith, Poole, & Coverdale, 2003; Read & Laschinger, 2013) and is linked to lower levels of bullying (Hauge et al., 2011; Laschinger et al., 2012). Creating workplace environments that minimize bullying requires leadership characterized by emotional intelligence and attention to the moral climate so that the values and obligations of nursing can be enacted. In their research on bullying, Hauge and colleagues (2010) deemed leadership adequate or inadequate depending on the extent to which it was judged fair and supportive. Others examining leader's approaches to conflict related to bullying found that forcing solutions and avoiding conflict were associated with more bullying, and problem-solving approaches were associated with less (Baillien, Notelaers, De Witte, & Matthiesen, 2011).

TO ILLUSTRATE
Eating Their Young

Unfortunately, the fact that many new nurses are bullied in nursing has given rise to a pernicious saying that "nurses eat their young." Think about how this saying positions nurses as responsible without pointing to the conditions of work that may foster bullying. Think about how the problem of more experienced nurses bullying newer nurses contrasts with espoused nursing values such as compassion, caring, and fairness. Now, think about what you have just read about bullying. How might you reconceptualize the phenomenon underlying the saying, and how might you respond next time you hear it? I (Colleen) respond to this saying by drawing attention to organizations, saying something such as, "We have to create better organizations that help nurses constructively use their power and that don't tolerate or promote bullying." I (Gweneth) often focus attention at the intrapersonal and interpersonal levels, inviting myself and those I am speaking with to think about that saying in a literal way—what images and sensations come to mind when you think about "eating our young?" The response is most often a visceral one—it becomes clear that it is not an experience nurses want to have or condone. So then the question becomes, how do I/we need to be and relate intrapersonally and interpersonally to produce situations (and health care contexts) of a desired kind?

Preventing Moral Distress

Because leadership to minimize bullying focuses on values and supporting nursing values, it can also minimize moral distress. *Moral distress* refers to the experience of being seriously compromised in being able to practice in accordance with accepted professional values and standards. It is a relational experience shaped by multiple contexts, including the sociopolitical and cultural contexts of the workplace environment (Varcoe, Pauly, Webster, & Storch, 2012). Nurses experience distress when they are unable to meet professional values and standards (McCarthy & Deady, 2008; Rice, Rady, Hamrick, Verheijde, & Pendergast, 2008). Although moral distress has sometimes been conceptualized as a problem of individuals or as arising from errors in personal judgment, it is increasingly seen as arising from the interplay between individuals and their work environments. As Wendy Austin (2012) highlights, it is the canary in the coal mine that alerts us to broader contextual factors that impact the abilities of nurses and other health care providers to enact ethical practice in the best interests of those for whom they care. For example, recall the story in Chapter 1 in which a nurse was caring for a man dying following transfer from emergency. That nurse was distressed because her professional values (for a death with dignity, support for grieving family members) were compromised. The compromises arose not from her competence but from organizational arrangements and norms.

Moral distress arises from constraints within the immediate workplace and from wider social contexts. It can also arise from differences in values and practices between colleagues and when working between competing obligations. Research by our team and others has shown that nurses experience moral distress when they are unable to provide equitable care (Austin, Bergum, & Goldberg, 2003; Hartrick Doane et al., 2009; Storch et al., 2009). Neoliberal sociopolitical contexts are increasing inequities in health and health care access and treatment. These inequities are stratified by poverty, stigma related to ability, mental illness and substance use, and racism and other forms of discrimination, and they shape nurses' abilities to provide care. For example, people who have mobility disabilities are likely to be impoverished due to limited employment opportunities. Poverty and such disabilities work together to create barriers to access to health care, such as through transportation and affordability, and they create barriers to health-promoting nursing practice. In turn, when nurses are unable to provide good care (e.g., picture a woman in a wheelchair with a life-threatening illness living in a rooming house in poor condition and unable to get to her appointments), they often experience distress.

Moral distress cannot be prevented or resolved by individuals trying to "suck it up" or acting alone. Minimizing moral distress requires action at all levels because it arises from constraints within the immediate workplace and wider social contexts, from differences in values and practices between colleagues, and from competing obligations. Some health care places have dealt with moral distress among staff by simply encouraging them with ideas such as "learning to do more with less" or "lowering expectations." Other health care workplaces have instituted strategies to reduce moral distress that are aimed at individuals or follow particular incidents. An example of this is critical incident stress debriefing. This refers to an opportunity for people involved in a particularly distressing experience to discuss the situation, usually with a trained facilitator or counselor. In the situation that I (Colleen) mentioned in Chapter 4 in which two preschool children died after being beaten by their father, all the staff members were offered debriefing to help them cope with their feelings. While this may be useful in particularly intense circumstances, it does not necessarily help address the everyday challenges of providing good care to all. Indeed, in that situation, because the workplace was fraught with bullying behaviors, the critical incident stress debriefing worsened the situation for at least two of the nurses who felt further demeaned by their colleagues after they shared their grief in the group setting.

Rather than seeing moral distress through an individualist lens and placing responsibility only on individuals or focusing on single challenging incidents, bringing a relational understanding to moral distress emphasizes that action is required at all levels to affect the daily circumstances of work and thus prevent moral distress. That is, all players must contribute to the creation of social contexts in which health and health care are viewed as a right for all, and it is widely understood that social position and the conditions in which people live shape health and access to health care resources (Varcoe et al., 2012). When nurses are put in the position of having to ration care, and when they must do so on the basis of unfair criteria or stereotypes, they experience distress. When they work together toward fairness, even in the context of scarce resources, their distress is lessened.

Preventing and reducing moral distress requires the creation of ethical moral climates (Pauly et al., 2009; Schluter, Winch, Holzhauser, & Henderson, 2008;

Silen et al., 2011) through people's actions intrapersonally and interpersonally, including how they enact leadership informally and formally to promote such climates (Bell & Breslin, 2008). This means that creating a climate in which values are made explicit and upholding those values is a collective effort. Promoting a climate in which nursing values can be enacted requires a leadership style that supports those values and that promotes equity and social justice. As you think about the core leadership practices we have identified, how might you act to affect moral distress? For example, if moral distress arises through a combination of intrapersonal, interpersonal, and contextual elements, what is one specific action you might take or one strategy you might enlist at each of those levels?

Reducing Burnout

Burnout is a psychological response to chronic job stressors (Laschinger et al., 2013; Leiter & Maslach, 2009). Such job stressors can include bullying and moral distress. Given the evidence that some nurses experience significantly higher stress and moral distress, for example, African American nurses in the United States compared to others in their workplaces (Corley, Minick, Elswick, & Jacobs, 2005; Kovner, Brewer, Wu, Cheng, & Suzuki, 2006; Ulrich et al., 2007), chronic job stressors often may include racism. Burnout has also been associated with vicarious traumatization, the negative changes experienced by those working with the survivors of violence and trauma due to the repetitive invasion of other's trauma experiences (Tabor, 2011) and compassion fatigue, the final cumulative result of prolonged exposure to workplace stress (Neville & Cole, 2013; Smart et al., 2013). Neville and Cole (2013) describe that compassion fatigue is a newer concept that some claim encompasses both burnout and secondary stress from thinking about the suffering of those to whom care has been provided. They also note that others claim that compassion fatigue should replace burnout as a more accurate depiction of the experience.

Leiter and Maslach (2009) explain that burnout consists of three dimensions: (1) overwhelming exhaustion, (2) cynicism and detachment from the job, and (3) a sense of ineffectiveness and lack of accomplishment. They further explain that a nurse's work experiences can be described in relation to the continuum from burnout to the other end at which nurses feel energized, involved, and effective. Burnout occurs at high levels in nursing (Aiken, Clarke, & Sloane, 2002; Maslach & Leiter, 2008; Neff et al., 2011; Sherman, Edwards, Simonton, & Mehta, 2006), particularly among new graduates (Laschinger et al., 2013; Leiter & Maslach, 2009). Although one study of students did not find significant differences between different levels of students as they progressed through their education and actually found higher levels of feelings of accomplishment among fourth-year students, students were concerned that burnout would be inevitable at some point during their professional careers (Michalec, Diefenbeck, & Mahoney, 2013).

Burnout has been shown to be associated with the intention to leave the profession and is predictive of leaving (Laschinger et al., 2012; Leiter & Maslach, 2009; Neff et al., 2011). For example, in a study of 10 European countries, burnout was one of the seven factors associated with nurses' intentions to leave the profession (Heinen et al., 2013). Again, because burnout is related to organizational stressors, the prevention of burnout and its detrimental consequences requires positive organizational climates and positive leadership.

How we frame situations can strongly influence how nurses respond and the subsequent burnout they experience. Extending your view to see the landscape and the texture of your nursing experiences is a way of seeing burnout as not merely an individual experience but a collective one. Doing so positions you to engage with others, including colleagues and formal leaders, in ways that will enhance your work environment, the care you are able to provide, and your job satisfaction.

TO ILLUSTRATE
Extinguishing the Flames of Burnout

I (Gweneth) have had the privilege of teaching registered nurses who return to university to complete their baccalaureate degrees after practicing for several years. One of the most common things those nurses experience is a reinvestment in nursing. Many describe how they are feeling burned out and have been contemplating leaving the profession. Returning to school is one way of making the decision about whether they will be able to stay in nursing by extending their career possibilities. Interestingly, when they have the opportunity to really examine their practice, reconnect with what really matters to them as nurses (why they entered nursing in the first place), and meet other nurses who share their nursing values and who echo their own deeply held concerns, they find their sense of burnout lessening. This burnout is further reduced as they develop knowledge of research that provides an evidence base for their nursing concerns (they come to see that it is not just about them) and learn strategies to more effectively navigate the complexities of contemporary work environments. Many end up staying in their current roles and clinical settings because by fanning the flames of nursing and connecting their own concerns with those of others, they've tempered the flames of burnout.

TRY IT OUT 11.4
Address a Challenge

Choose one of the three challenges above (bullying, moral distress, or burnout) as a site to consider ways that you as a nurse might be a leader in cultivating a healthy work environment. Revisit the relational inquiry strategies throughout the different chapters to see how they might inform and guide your actions. For example, how might the HP and critical lenses and the three levels of inquiry help focus your attention and enable you to identify the complexities? How might they support your emotional intelligence? How might you enlist the five Cs, five Ws, or the checkpoints outlined in Chapter 9? How might the interprofessional strategies outlined in Chapter 10 be helpful?

continued on page 443

> **TRY IT OUT** *continued*
> ## Address a Challenge
>
> Once you have considered the specific challenge, consider how action to affect that might also impact the other two challenges. For example, how might one action that you target toward addressing bullying simultaneously address moral distress and/or burnout? If you have colleagues or classmates undertaking the same exercise, compare notes on addressing these challenges.

Developing a Leadership Plan for Your Career

Pate (2013) points out that leaders are not born, they are developed, and that like clinical skills, leadership skills develop over time. However, she claims that nurses need to take on the identity of leader before they will be seen by others as leaders.

> *Nurses interested in refining their leadership skills must take time to engage in personal self-assessment and reflection. If the nurse believes that people are born leaders instead of learning to become leaders, then he or she may not take time to consider short- and long-term leadership goals. Working in an unfocused manner concerning one's career trajectory may leave the individual unprepared for new challenges and potentially dissatisfied with work and the profession. Self-awareness of personal strengths and opportunities for professional development allow nurses to focus their efforts on learning specific skills that will help meet career goals. Equipped with the knowledge of what goals to attain, nurses can be poised to make the experiences happen by making sure that they are in the right place at the right time doing the right thing. For instance, a nurse wanting to increase skill in meeting facilitation might start by leading a unit committee. The nurse will gain experience, but others will be given the chance to see the individual in an expanded role. (Pate, 2013, p. 187)*

As a nurse, you are a leader. Initially, you may be leading a small initiative to solve a clinical issue, or you may be serving as a team leader. As you mentor new staff and students, you are leading. Whether or not you choose to take on a formal leadership role, you can take stock of your strengths, identify your goals, and identify opportunities to enhance your leadership skills.

> # TRY IT OUT 11.5
> ## Outline a Plan
>
> Begin by listing the skills that you have gleaned from your reading in this chapter as being important to good leadership. Then, assess yourself on each of these skills. What are your strengths and challenges in relation to each skill you have identified? For example, you might have listed skills related to articulating and communicating a vision. How able are you to frame

continued on page 444

TRY IT OUT *continued*

Outline a Plan

your vision of good care for a particular patient to others? Does this vary depending on the power position of people with whom you are communicating? You might have listed some of the skills of emotional intelligence, such as the ability to perceive emotions in oneself and others accurately. How able are you to discern how others are feeling and verify those with people? I (Colleen) am reasonably good at accurately identifying and checking out how people are feeling, but Gweneth is much more skilled than I at using emotions to facilitate thinking. Gweneth will say to nurses, "Now, let's think about that—how you are feeling, what are you feeling; let's explore and track those feelings to see how they might be connected to particular thoughts or assumptions and/or to what is happening in the situation." When she does this, nurses quickly turn their feelings into a deeper understanding.

Next, having taken stock of your current level of skill, set some goals. For example, one of my goals is to take more time to invite people to analyze their feelings fully, such as when they are angry or frustrated. The table below provides a possible format for you to use. I (Colleen) have filled in one example for myself with a short-term goal. Your plan should have short-term (right now), mid-range (1 to 2 years), and long-term goals (5 to 10 years).

Skill	Strength	Challenge	Goal	Opportunity
Problem-solving	I can see the big picture easily; I am a good listener.	I tend to jump to conclusions about solutions without fully analyzing a situation. Sometimes, this overlooks others' input.	Short-term: More thorough attention to understanding problems from various angles before moving to solutions.	On a current team, I could ask a trusted colleague to help me spend more time gathering information, listening, and analyzing.

THIS WEEK IN PRACTICE
Practicing Leadership

This week in your practice setting, take one goal from your leadership development plan. Find an opportunity to start working toward that goal. Volunteer for something, or try a different approach to someone or an issue. Draw power dynamics, values, or contextual features to attention. Listen more carefully. Try to shift understanding. Try to help others be better nurses as you become better yourself.

YOUR RELATIONAL INQUIRY TOOLBOX

Add these tools to your relational inquiry toolbox.

■ See leadership as a relational process of engaging others toward well-being.

■ Understand the different ways that formal and informal leaders are positioned within organizations.

■ Analyze both formal and informal leaders in action.

■ Identify your own leadership strengths and areas for development.

■ Link your nursing goals to your leadership actions.

■ Lead by influencing formal leaders.

■ Experiment with core leadership practices.

■ Work to minimize workplace bullying by contributing to positive workplace climates.

■ Prevent moral distress by acting at all levels to enhance daily circumstances of work and the upholding of nursing values.

■ Reduce burnout by engaging collaboratively with colleagues and leaders to enhance work environments.

■ Plan leadership across your career.

REFERENCES

Aiken, L. H., Clarke, S. P., & Sloane, D. M. (2002). Hospital staffing, organization, and quality of care: Cross-national findings. *International Journal for Quality in Health Care, 14*(1), 5–13.

Austin, W. (2012). Moral distress and the contemporary plight of health professionals. *HEC Forum: An Interdisciplinary Journal on Hospitals' Ethical And Legal Issues, 24*(1), 27–38.

Austin, W., Bergum, V., & Goldberg, L. (2003). Unable to answer the call of our patients: Mental health nurses' experience of moral distress. *Nursing Inquiry, 10*, 177–183.

Avolio, B. J., Walumbwa, F. O., & Weber, T. J. (2009). Leadership: Current theories, research, and future directions. *Annual Review of Psychology, 60*(1), 421–449.

Baillien, E., Notelaers, G., De Witte, H., & Matthiesen, S. B. (2011). The relationship between the work unit's conflict management styles and bullying at work: Moderation by conflict frequency. *Economic and Industrial Democracy, 32*(3), 401–419.

Bamford, M., Wong, C. A., & Laschinger, H. (2013). The influence of authentic leadership and areas of worklife on work engagement of registered nurses. *Journal of Nursing Management, 21*(3), 529–540.

Bass, M. B., & Riggio, E. G. (2006). *Transformational leadership* (2nd ed.). Mahwah, NJ: Lawrence Erlbaum Associates.

Bell, J., & Breslin, J. M. (2008). Health care provider moral distress as a leadership challenge. *JONA's Health care Law, Ethics and Regulation, 10*(4), 94–97.

Boev, C. (2012). The relationship between nurses' perception of work environment and patient satisfaction in adult critical care. *Journal of Nursing Scholarship, 44*(4), 368–375.

Canadian Nurses Association. (2008). *Code of ethics for registered nurses*. Retrieved August 19, 2013, from http://www.cna-aiic.ca/cna/documents/pdf/publications/Code_of_Ethics_2008_e.pdf

Corley, M. C., Minick, P., Elswick, R. K., & Jacobs, M. (2005). Nurse moral distress and ethical work environment. *Nursing Ethics, 12*(4), 381–390.

Fontenot, T. (2012). Leading ladies: Women in health care leadership. *Frontiers of Health Services Management, 28*(4), 11–12.

Ghomeshi, J. (2013, June 14). Ireland's first female President Mary Robinson. Q with Jian Ghomeshi (Interviewer). [Radio broadcast]. CBC Radio. Retrieved August 19, 2013, from http://www.cbc.ca/q/blog/2013/06/14/irelands-first-female-president-mary-robinson/

Hartrick Doane, G. A., Storch, J., & Pauly, B. (2009). Ethical nursing practice: Inquiry-in-action. *Nursing Inquiry, 16*(3), 232–240.

Hartung, S. Q., & Miller, M. (2013). Communication and the healthy work environment: nurse managers' perceptions. *The Journal of Nursing Administration, 43*(5), 266–273.

Hauge, L. J., Einarsen, S., Knardahl, S., Lau, B., Notelaers, G., & Skogstad, A. (2011). Leadership and role stressors as departmental level predictors of workplace bullying. *International Journal of Stress Management, 18*(4), 305–323.

Hauge, L. J., Skogstad, A., & Einarsen, S. (2010). The relative impact of workplace bullying as a social stressor at work. *Scandinavian Journal of Psychology, 51*(5), 426–433.

Heifetz, R. A., Grashow, A., & Linsky, M. (2009). *The practice of adaptive leadership*. Boston: Cambridge Leadership Associates.

Heifetz, R. A., & Linsky, M. (2002). *Leadership on the line. Staying alive through the dangers of leading.* Boston: Harvard Business Review.

Heinen, M. M., van Achterberg, T., Schwendimann, R., Zander, B., Matthews, A., Kózka, M., et al. (2013). Nurses' intention to leave their profession: A cross sectional observational study in 10 European countries. *International Journal of Nursing Studies, 50*(2), 174–184.

Hutchinson, M., & Hurley, J. (2013). Exploring leadership capability and emotional intelligence as moderators of workplace bullying. *Journal of Nursing Management, 21*(3), 553–562.

Hutchinson, M., & Jackson, D. (2013). Transformational leadership in nursing: Towards a more critical interpretation. *Nursing Inquiry, 20*(1), 11–22.

Hutchinson, M., Jackson, D., Wilkes, L., & Vickers, M. H. (2008). A new model of bullying in the nursing workplace: Organizational characteristics as critical antecedents. *Advances in Nursing Science, 31*(2), E60–E71.

Hutchinson, M., Vickers, M. H., Jackson, D., & Wilkes, L. (2005). "I'm gonna do what i wanna do." Organizational change as a legitimized vehicle for bullies. *Health Care Management Review, 30*(4), 331–336.

Hutchinson, M., Vickers, M., Jackson, D., & Wilkes, L. (2009). The worse you behave, the more you seem to be rewarded: Bullying in nursing as organizational corruption. *Journal of Employee Responsibilities and Rights, 21*, 213–229.

Hutchinson, M., Wilkes, L., Jackson, D., & Vickers, M. H. (2010). Integrating individual, work group and organizational factors: Testing a multidimensional model of bullying in the nursing workplace. *Journal of Nursing Management, 18*(2), 173–181.

Institute of Medicine. (2011). *The future of nursing: Leading change, advancing health*. Washington, DC: The National Academies Press.

Kelly, L. A., McHugh, M. D., & Aiken, L. H. (2012). Nurse outcomes in magnet and non-magnet hospitals. *Journal of Nursing Administration, 42*(10), S44–S49.

Kovner, C., Brewer, C., Wu, Y.-W., Cheng, Y., & Suzuki, M. (2006). Factors associated with work satisfaction of registered nurses. *Journal of Nursing Scholarship, 38*(1), 71–79.

Laschinger, H. K. S., Fineman, J., Shamian, J., & Casier, S. (2000). Organizational trust and empowerment in restructured health care settings: Effects on staff nurse commitment. *Journal of Nursing Administration, 30*(9), 413–425.

Laschinger, H. K. S., Grau, A. L., Finegan, J., & Wilk, P. (2010). New graduate nurses' experiences of bullying and burnout in hospitals settings. *Journal of Advanced Nursing, 66*(12), 2732–2742.

Laschinger, H. K. S., & Smith, L. M. (2013). The influence of authentic leadership and empowerment on new-graduate nurses' perceptions of interprofessional collaboration. *Journal of Nursing Administration, 43*(1), 24–29.

Laschinger, H. K. S., Wong, C. A., & Grau, A. L. (2012). The influence of authentic leadership on newly graduated nurses' experiences of workplace bullying, burnout and retention outcomes: A cross-sectional study. *International Journal of Nursing Studies, 49*(10), 1266–1276.

Laschinger, H. K. S., Wong, C. A., & Grau, A. L. (2013). Authentic leadership, empowerment and burnout: A comparison in new graduates and experienced nurses. *Journal of Nursing Management, 21*(3), 541–552.

Leiter, M. P., & Maslach, C. (2009). Nurse turnover: The mediating role of burnout. *Journal of Nursing Management, 17*(3), 331–339.

Maslach, C., & Leiter, M. P. (2008). Early predictors of job burnout and engagement. *The Journal of Applied Psychology, 93*(3), 498–512.

Matthiesen, S. B., & Einarsen, S. (2004). Psychiatric distress and symptoms of PTSD among victims of bullying at work. *British Journal of Guidance & Counselling, 32*(3), 335–356.

Matthiesen, S. B., & Einarsen, S. (2007). Perpetrators and targets of bullying at work: Role stress and individual differences. *Violence and Victims, 22*(6), 735–753.

McCarthy, J., & Deady, R. (2008). Moral distress reconsidered. *Nursing Ethics, 15*(2), 254–262.

McKenna, B. G., Smith, N. A., Poole, S. J., & Coverdale, J. H. (2003). Horizontal violence: Experiences of registered nurses in their first year of practice. *Journal of Advanced Nursing, 42*(1), 90–96.

Michalec, B., Diefenbeck, C., & Mahoney, M. (2013). The calm before the storm? Burnout and compassion fatigue among undergraduate nursing students. *Nurse Education Today, 33*(4), 314–320.

Neff, D. F., Cimiotti, J. P., Heusinger, A. S., & Aiken, L. H. (2011). Nurse reports from the frontlines: Analysis of a statewide nurse survey. *Nursing Forum, 46*(1), 4–10.

Neville, K., & Cole, D. A. (2013). The relationships among health promotion behaviors, compassion fatigue, burnout, and compassion satisfaction in nurses practicing in a community medical center. *The Journal of Nursing Administration, 43*(6), 348–354.

Nielsen, M. B., Hetland, J., Matthiesen, S. B., & Einarsen, S. (2012). Longitudinal relationships between workplace bullying and psychological distress. *Scandinavian Journal of Work, Environment & Health, 38*(1), 38–46.

Parks, S. D. (2005). *Leadership can be taught.* Boston: Harvard Business School Press.

Pate, M. F. D. (2013). Nursing leadership from the bedside to the boardroom. *AACN Advanced Critical Care, 24*(2), 186–193.

Pauly, B., Varcoe, C., Storch, J., & Newton, L. (2009). Registered nurses' perceptions of moral distress and ethical climate. *Nursing Ethics, 16*(5), 561–573.

Read, E., & Laschinger, H. K. (2013). Correlates of new graduate nurses' experiences of workplace mistreatment. *Journal of Nursing Administration, 43*(4), 221–228.

Rice, E. M., Rady, M. Y., Hamrick, A., Verheijde, J. L., & Pendergast, D. K. (2008). Determinants of moral distress in medical and surgical nurses at an adult acute tertiary care hospital. *Journal of Nursing Management, 16*, 360–373.

Scharmer, C. O. (2008). Uncovering the blind spots of leadership. *Leader to Leader, 47*, 52–59.

Schluter, J., Winch, S., Holzhauser, K., & Henderson, A. (2008). Nurses' moral sensitivity and hospital ethical climate: A literature review. *Nursing Ethics, 15*, 304–321.

Sherman, A. C., Edwards, D., Simonton, S., & Mehta, P. (2006). Caregiver stress and burnout in an oncology unit. *Palliative & Supportive Care, 4*(1), 65–80.

Silen, M., Svantesson, M., Kjellstrom, S., Sidenvall, B., & Christensson, L. (2011). Moral distress and ethical climate in a Swedish nursing context: Perceptions and instrument usability. *Journal of Clinical Nursing, 20*(23–24), 3483–3493.

Simons, S. (2008). Workplace bullying experienced by Massachusetts registered nurses and the relationship to intention to leave the organization. *Advances in Nursing Science, 31*(2), E48–E59.

Smart, D., English, A., James, J., Wilson, M., Daratha, K. B., Childers, B., et al. (2013). Compassion fatigue and satisfaction: A cross-sectional survey among U.S. health care workers. *Nursing & Health Sciences.* Advance online publication.

Stanley, D. (2008). Congruent leadership: Values in action. *Journal of Nursing Management, 16*(5), 519–524.

Stanley, D., & Sherratt, A. (2010). Lamp light on leadership: Clinical leadership and Florence Nightingale.

Journal of Nursing Management, 18(2), 115–121.

Stewart, L., Holmes, C., & Usher, K. (2012). Reclaiming caring in nursing leadership: A deconstruction of leadership using a Habermasian lens. *Collegian, 19*(4), 223–229.

Storch, J., Rodney, P., Pauly, B., Fulton, T. R., Stevenson, L., Newton, L., et al. (2009). Enhancing ethical climates in nursing work environments. *Canadian Nurse, 105*(3), 20–25.

Storch, J., Schick Makaroff, K., Pauly, B., & Newton, L. (2013). Take me to my leader: The importance of ethical leadership among formal nurse leaders. *Nursing Ethics, 20*(2), 150–157.

Tabor, P. D. (2011). Vicarious traumatization: Concept analysis. *Journal of Forensic Nursing, 7*(4), 203–208.

Taylor, B., & Barling, J. (2004). Identifying sources and effects of carer fatigue and burnout for mental health nurses: A qualitative approach. *International Journal of Mental Health Nursing, 13*(2), 117–125.

Ulrich, C., O'Donnell, P., Taylor, C., Farrar, A., Danis, M., & Grady, C. (2007). Ethical climate, ethics stress, and the job satisfaction of nurses and social workers in the United States. *Social Science & Medicine, 65*(8), 1708–1719.

Varcoe, C., Pauly, B., Storch, J., Newton, L., & Makaroff, K. (2012). Nurses' perceptions of and responses to morally distressing situations. *Nursing Ethics, 19*(4), 488–500.

Varcoe, C., Pauly, B., Webster, G., & Storch, J. (2012). Moral distress: Tensions as springboards for action. *HEC Forum: An Interdisciplinary Journal On Hospitals' Ethical and Legal Issues, 24*(1), 51–62.

Wong, C. A., & Laschinger, H. K. S. (2013). Authentic leadership, performance, and job satisfaction: The mediating role of empowerment. *Journal of Advanced Nursing, 69*(4), 947–959.

Zander, R., & Zander, B. (2000). *The art of possibility*. New York: Penguin Books.

Index